T0348506

2011
YEAR BOOK OF
VASCULAR SURGERY®

The 2011 Year Book Series

Year Book of Anesthesiology and Pain Management™: Drs Chestnut, Abram, Black, Gravlee, Lien, Mathru, and Roizen

Year Book of Cardiology®: Drs Gersh, Cheitlin, Elliott, Gold, Graham, and Thourani

Year Book of Critical Care Medicine®: Drs Dellinger, Parrillo, Balk, Dorman, Dries, and Zanotti-Cavazzoni

Year Book of Dermatology and Dermatologic Surgery™: Dr Del Rosso

Year Book of Diagnostic Radiology®: Drs Osborn, Abbara, Elster, Manaster, Oestreich, Offiah, Rosado de Christenson, Stephens, and Walker

Year Book of Emergency Medicine®: Drs Hamilton, Bruno, Handly, Mullin, Quintana, and Ramoska

Year Book of Endocrinology®: Drs Schott, Apovian, Clarke, Eugster, Ludlam, Meikle, Schinner, Schteingart, and Toth

Year Book of Gastroenterology™: Drs Talley, DeVault, Harnois, Murray, Pearson, Philcox, Picco, and Smith

Year Book of Hand and Upper Limb Surgery®: Drs Yao and Steinmann

Year Book of Medicine®: Drs Barker, Garrick, Gersh, Khardori, LeRoith, Seo, Talley, and Thigpen

Year Book of Neonatal and Perinatal Medicine®: Drs Fanaroff, Benitz, Donn, Neu, Papile, Polin, and van Marter

Year Book of Neurology and Neurosurgery®: Drs Klimo and Rabinstein

Year Book of Obstetrics, Gynecology, and Women's Health®: Drs Dungan and Shulman

Year Book of Oncology®: Drs Arceci, Bauer, Chiorean, Gordon, Lawton, Murphy, Thigpen, and Tsao

Year Book of Ophthalmology®: Drs Rapuano, Cohen, Flanders, Fudemberg, Hammersmith, Milman, Myers, Nagra, Nelson, Penne, Pyfer, Sergott, Shields, Talekar, and Vander

Year Book of Orthopedics®: Drs Morrey, Beauchamp, Huddleston, Swiontkowski, and Trigg

Year Book of Otolaryngology-Head and Neck Surgery®: Drs Sindwani, Balough, Franco, Gapany, and Mitchell

Year Book of Pathology and Laboratory Medicine®: Drs Raab, Parwani, Bejarano, and Bissell

Year Book of Pediatrics®: Dr Stockman

Year Book of Plastic and Aesthetic Surgery™: Drs Miller, Gosain, Gurtner, Gutowski, Ruberg, Salisbury, and Smith

Year Book of Psychiatry and Applied Mental Health®: Drs Talbott, Ballenger, Buckley, Frances, Krupnick, and Mack

Year Book of Pulmonary Disease®: Drs Barker, Jones, Maurer, Raza, Tanoue, and Willsie

Year Book of Sports Medicine®: Drs Shephard, Cantu, Feldman, Jankowski, Khan, Lebrun, Nieman, Pierrynowski, and Rowland

Year Book of Surgery®: Drs Copeland, Behrns, Daly, Eberlein, Fahey, Huber, Klodell, Mozingo, and Pruett

Year Book of Urology®: Drs Andriole and Coplen

Year Book of Vascular Surgery®: Drs Moneta, Gillespie, Starnes, and Watkins

2011

The Year Book of
VASCULAR
SURGERY®

Editor-in-Chief
Gregory L. Moneta, MD
Professor and Chief of Vascular Surgery, Oregon Health and Science University; and Chief of Vascular Surgery, Oregon Health and Science University Hospital, Portland, Oregon

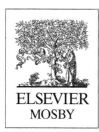

ELSEVIER
MOSBY

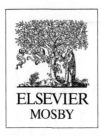

ELSEVIER
MOSBY

Vice President, Continuity: Kimberly Murphy
Editor: Teia Stone
Production Supervisor, Electronic Year Books: Donna M. Skelton
Electronic Article Manager: Emily Ogle
Illustrations and Permissions Coordinator: Dawn Vohsen

Composition by TNQ Books and Journals Pvt Ltd, India

Editorial Office:
Elsevier
Suite 1800
1600 John F. Kennedy Blvd.
Philadelphia, PA 19103-2899

International Standard Serial Number: 0749-4041
International Standard Book Number: 978-0-323-08429-1

Printed and bound by CPI Group (UK) Ltd, Croydon, CR0 4YY
Transferred to Digital Print 2011

Associate Editors

David L. Gillespie, MD, RVT, FACS
Professor of Surgery, Division of Vascular Surgery; University of Rochester School of Medicine and Dentistry, Rochester, New York

Benjamin W. Starnes, MD
Professor of Surgery and Chief, Division of Vascular Surgery; University of Washington, Seattle, Washington

Michael T. Watkins, MD
Associate Professor of Surgery, Harvard Medical School; and Director, Vascular Surgery Research Laboratory, Massachusetts General Hospital, Boston, Massachusetts

Contributors

Zachary M. Arthurs, MD
Assistant Professor, Department of Vascular Surgery, Uniformed Services University of Health Sciences, San Antonio Military Medical Center, San Antonio, Texas

Robert S. Crawford, MD
Assistant Professor, Division of Vascular Surgery, University of Maryland Medical Center, Baltimore, Maryland

Marc A. Passman, MD
Professor of Surgery, Section of Vascular Surgery and Endovascular Therapy, University of Alabama at Birmingham, Birmingham, Alabama

Joseph D. Raffetto, MD, FACS, FSVM
Assistant Professor of Surgery, Harvard Medical School, Brigham and Women's Hospital; Chief, Vascular Surgery Division, VA Boston Healthcare System, West Roxbury, Massachusetts

LTC Niten Singh, MD
Chief, Endovascular Surgery, Madigan Army Medical Center; and Assistant Professor of Surgery, Uniformed Services University of Health Sciences, Tacoma, Washington

Table of Contents

Journals Represented

Plastic and Reconstructive Surgery
Science
Stroke
Surgery
Thrombosis Research

STANDARD ABBREVIATIONS

The following terms are abbreviated in this edition: acquired immunodeficiency syndrome (AIDS), cardiopulmonary resuscitation (CPR), central nervous system (CNS), cerebrospinal fluid (CSF), computed tomography (CT), deoxyribonucleic acid (DNA), electrocardiography (ECG), health maintenance organization (HMO), human immunodeficiency virus (HIV), intensive care unit (ICU), intramuscular (IM), intravenous (IV), magnetic resonance (MR) imaging (MRI), ribonucleic acid (RNA), and ultrasound (US).

NOTE

The YEAR BOOK OF VASCULAR SURGERY® is a literature survey service providing abstracts of articles published in the professional literature. Every effort is made to assure the accuracy of the information presented in these pages. Neither the editors nor the publisher of the YEAR BOOK OF VASCULAR SURGERY® can be responsible for errors in the original materials. The editors' comments are their own opinions. Mention of specific products within this publication does not constitute endorsement.

To facilitate the use of the YEAR BOOK OF VASCULAR SURGERY® as a reference tool, all illustrations and tables included in this publication are now identified as they appear in the original article. This change is meant to help the reader recognize that any illustration or table appearing in the YEAR BOOK OF VASCULAR SURGERY® may be only one of many in the original article. For this reason, figure and table numbers will often appear to be out of sequence within the YEAR BOOK OF VASCULAR SURGERY®.

1 Basic Considerations

The Phosphodiesterase Inhibitor Cilostazol Induces Regression of Carotid Atherosclerosis in Subjects With Type 2 Diabetes Mellitus: Principal Results of the Diabetic Atherosclerosis Prevention by Cilostazol (DAPC) Study: A Randomized Trial

Katakami N, Kim Y-S, Kawamori R, et al (Osaka Univ Graduate School of Medicine, Japan; Kyung Hee Univ College of Medicine, Seoul, Korea; Juntendo Univ School of Medicine, Tokyo, Japan)

Circulation 121:2584-2591, 2010

Background.—Antiplatelet drugs are effective in preventing recurrence of atherosclerosis in type 2 diabetic patients. However, the efficacy and usefulness of 2 different antiplatelet drugs, aspirin and cilostazol, in the progression of carotid intima-media thickening are unknown.

Methods and Results.—To compare prevention by cilostazol and aspirin of progression of atherosclerosis, we conducted a prospective, randomized, open, blinded end point study in 4 East Asian countries. A total of 329 type 2 diabetic patients suspected of peripheral artery disease were allocated to either an aspirin-treated (81 to 100 mg/d) group or a cilostazol-treated (100 to 200 mg/d) group. The changes in intima-media thickness of the common carotid artery during a 2-year observation period were examined as the primary end point. The regression in maximum left, maximum right, mean left, and mean right common carotid artery intima-media thickness was significantly greater with cilostazol compared with aspirin (-0.088 ± 0.260 versus 0.059 ± 0.275 mm, $P<0.001$; -0.042 ± 0.274 versus 0.045 ± 0.216 mm, $P=0.003$; -0.043 ± 0.182 versus 0.028 ± 0.202 mm, $P=0.004$; and -0.024 ± 0.182 versus 0.048 ± 0.169 mm, $P<0.001$). In a regression analysis adjusted for possible confounding factors such as lipid levels and hemoglobin A_{1c}, the improvements in common carotid artery intima-media thickness with cilostazol treatment over aspirin treatment remained significant.

Conclusions.—Compared with aspirin, cilostazol potently inhibited progression of carotid intima-media thickness, an established surrogate marker of cardiovascular events, in patients with type 2 diabetes mellitus.

Clinical Trial Registration.—URL: http://www.clinicaltrials.gov. Unique identifier: C000000215.

▶ It appears patients with diabetes without previous myocardial infarction have as high a risk of myocardial infarction as patients without diabetes and previous myocardial infarction.[1] Based on this, it is advocated by some that primary

1

prevention in patients with diabetes may be indicated. Guidelines suggest that individuals with risk factors for coronary heart disease, such as diabetes mellitus, should take aspirin for primary and secondary prevention, although the ability of aspirin to effectively serve as a primary preventive agent is controversial.[2] There has been some suggestion that cilostazol may be effective in preventing cardiovascular events in patients with type 2 diabetes mellitus.[3] This study therefore compared the ability of two antiplatelet agents, aspirin and cilostazol, to prevent progression of carotid intima-media thickness. Cilostazol is a phosphodiesterase-3 inhibitor and has antiplatelet, antithrombotic, and vaso-dilatory effects. It is approved for treatment of claudication in the United States and for secondary prevention of cerebral infarction in Asia. The ability of antiplatelet agents to serve as effective primary prevention in patients with diabetes is controversial. This study suggests that perhaps the wrong antiplatelet agent is being evaluated in diabetic patients. Progression of intima-media thickness serves only as a surrogate marker for progression of atherosclerosis and has not been shown to predict clinical events in patients with type 2 diabetes. The results here are interesting and suggest a large-scale prospective study of cilostazol for primary prevention in type 2 diabetic patients should be considered.

G. L. Moneta, MD

References

1. Haffner SM, Lehto S, Rönnemaa T, Pyörälä K, Laakso M. Mortality from coronary heart disease in subjects with type 2 diabetes and in nondiabetic subjects with and without prior myocardial infarction. *N Engl J Med.* 1998;339:229-234.
2. American Diabetes Association. Standards of medical care in diabetes—2007. *Diabetes Care.* 2007;30:s4-s41.
3. Shinohara Y, Gotoh F, Tohgi H, et al. Antiplatelet cilostazol is beneficial in diabetic and/or hypertensive ischemic stroke patients. Subgroup analysis of the cilostazol stroke prevention study. *Cerebrovasc Dis.* 2008;26:63-70.

Angiotensin II Type 2 Receptor Signaling Attenuates Aortic Aneurysm in Mice Through ERK Antagonism

Habashi JP, Doyle JJ, Holm TM, et al (Johns Hopkins Univ School of Medicine, Baltimore, MD)
Science 332:361-365, 2011

Angiotensin II (AngII) mediates progression of aortic aneurysm, but the relative contribution of its type 1 (AT1) and type 2 (AT2) receptors remains unknown. We show that loss of AT2 expression accelerates the aberrant growth and rupture of the aorta in a mouse model of Marfan syndrome (MFS). The selective AT1 receptor blocker (ARB) losartan abrogated aneurysm progression in the mice; full protection required intact AT2 signaling. The angiotensin-converting enzyme inhibitor (ACEi) enalapril, which limits signaling through both receptors, was less effective. Both drugs attenuated canonical transforming growth factor−β (TGFβ) signaling in the aorta, but losartan uniquely inhibited TGFβ-mediated activation of extracellular signal—regulated kinase (ERK), by allowing continued signaling through AT2. These data highlight the protective nature of AT2 signaling and potentially inform the choice of therapies in MFS and related disorders.

▶ Marfan syndrome is an autosomal dominant disorder caused by deficiency of microfibrillar constituent protein fibrillin-1. The most common class of mutation in people with Marfan syndrome involves a cysteine substitution in the epidermal growth factor—like domain of fibrillin-1. In a mouse model of fibrillin-1—deficient mice, the effects of the fibrillin-1 mutation were attenuated by administration of polyclonal transforming growth factor-β—neutralizing antibodies. Similar protection can also be obtained by treating fribillin-1—mutated mice with the angiotensin II type I (AT1) receptor blocker losartan. In this article, the authors demonstrate that loss of angiotensin II expression accelerates the aneurysm process in the mouse model of Marfan syndrome. Full protection of aneurysm degeneration in the mouse model of Marfan syndrome required intact angiotensin II receptor signaling. These authors have previously demonstrated remarkable effects of losartan in decreasing aneurysmal degeneration in a mouse model of Marfan syndrome. This study further extends their previous work and indicates that in the presence of AT1 receptor blocking, ongoing AT2 receptor signaling is required for attenuation of extracellular signal—regulated kinase (ERK) phosphorylation. This appears to be required for losartan's favorable effect in attenuating aneurysmal degeneration in the mouse model of Marfan disease. Modification of the ERK 1/2 signaling cascade is potentially a therapeutic target for the treatment of aneurysmal degeneration in patients with the cysteine substitution of mutation of the fibrillin-1 gene, the most common underlying mutation in human Marfan syndrome.

G. L. Moneta, MD

Apolipoprotein(a) Isoforms and the Risk of Vascular Disease Systematic Review of 40 Studies Involving 58,000 Participants

Erqou S, Thompson A, Di Angelantonio E, et al (Univ of Cambridge, UK; et al)
J Am Coll Cardiol 55:2160-2167, 2010

Objectives.—The purpose of this study was to assess the association of apolipoprotein(a) (apo[a]) isoforms with cardiovascular disease risk.

Background.—Although circulating lipoprotein(a) (Lp[a]) is likely to be a causal risk factor in coronary heart disease (CHD), the magnitude of this association is modest. Lipoprotein(a) particles with smaller, rather than larger, apo(a) isoforms may be stronger risk factors.

Methods.—Information was collated from 40 studies published between January 1970 and June 2009 that reported on associations between apo(a) isoforms and risk of CHD or ischemic stroke (involving a total of 11,396 patients and 46,938 controls).

Results.—Thirty-six studies used broadly comparable phenotyping and analytic methods to assess apo(a) isoform size. These studies yielded a combined relative risk for CHD of 2.08 (95% confidence intervals [CI]: 1.67 to 2.58) for individuals with smaller versus larger apo(a) isoforms (corresponding approximately to 22 or fewer kringle IV type 2 repeats vs. >22 repeats or analogously an apo[a] molecular weight of <640 kDa vs. _640 kDa). There was substantial heterogeneity among these studies ($I^2 = 85\%$, 80% to 89%), which was mainly explained by differences in the laboratory methods and analytic approaches used. In the 6 studies of ischemic stroke that used comparable phenotypic methods, the combined relative risk was 2.14 (1.85 to 2.97). Overall, however, only 3 studies made allowances for Lp(a) concentration.

Conclusions.—People with smaller apo(a) isoforms have an approximately 2-fold higher risk of CHD or ischemic stroke than those with larger proteins. Further studies are needed to determine whether the impact of smaller apo(a) isoforms is independent from Lp(a) concentration and other risk factors.

▶ Lipoprotein (a) (Lp[a]) is composed of a glycoprotein molecule, apolipoprotein (a) (apo[a]), and a low-density lipoprotein (LDL) particle. Apo(a) is responsible for the properties of Lp(a).[1,2] Circulating Lp(a) concentration is associated with increased risk of coronary heart disease and stroke. This risk is independent of other conventional risk factors for vascular disease, including total cholesterol levels. There are significant associations and variations of Lp(a) risk related to genetic variations of Lp(a). Apo(a) size heterogeneity is a function of copy number variation of one of its protein domains, kringle IV type 2. This gene exists in 5 to 50 identically repeated copies. Copy number variation of the gene confers marked heterogeneity in the molecular mass of the apo(a) isoform.[3] The use of apo(a) subtyping has been clinically limited by the fact that it overall adds relatively modest incremental risk compared with other biomarkers for cardiovascular disease. This study, however, indicates that there are subtypes of apo(a) that may be worth looking for. It remains to be seen whether smaller apo(a) isoforms have sufficient relevance to the determination of vascular risk and disease independent from Lp(a) concentration and other more conventional risk factors for atherosclerosis that indicate whether the additional trouble of determining apo(a) isoforms is clinically important.

G. L. Moneta, MD

References

1. Marcovina SM, Koschinsky ML. Lipoprotein(a) as a risk factor for coronary artery disease. *Am J Cardiol.* 1998;82:57U-66U.
2. McLean JW, Tomlinson JE, Kuang WJ, et al. cDNA sequence of human apolipoprotein(a) is homologous to plasminogen. *Nature.* 1987;330:132-137.
3. Boffa MB, Marcovina SM, Koschinsky ML. Lipoprotein(a) as a risk factor for atherosclerosis and thrombosis: mechanistic insights from animal models. *Clin Biochem.* 2004;37:333-343.

Association of Colony-Forming Units With Coronary Artery and Abdominal Aortic Calcification

Cheng S, Cohen KS, Shaw SY, et al (Framingham Heart Study, MA; Massachusetts General Hosp, Boston; et al)
Circulation 122:1176-1182, 2010

Background.—Certain bone marrow—derived cell populations, called endothelial progenitor cells, have been reported to possess angiogenic activity. Experimental data suggest that depletion of these angiogenic cell populations may promote atherogenesis, but limited data are available on their relation to subclinical atherosclerotic cardiovascular disease in humans.

Methods and Results.—We studied 889 participants of the Framingham Heart Study who were free of clinically apparent cardiovascular disease (mean age, 65 years; 55% women). Participants underwent endothelial progenitor cell phenotyping with an early-outgrowth colony-forming unit assay and cell surface markers. Participants also underwent noncontrast multidetector computed tomography to assess the presence of subclinical atherosclerosis, as reflected by the burden of coronary artery calcification and abdominal aortic calcification. Across decreasing tertiles of colony-forming units, there was a progressive increase in median coronary artery calcification and abdominal aortic calcification scores. In multivariable analyses adjusting for traditional cardiovascular risk factors, each 1-SD increase in colony-forming units was associated with a ≈16% decrease in coronary artery calcification ($P=0.02$) and 17% decrease in abdominal aortic calcification ($P=0.03$). In contrast, neither CD34$^+$/KDR$^+$ nor CD34$^+$ variation was associated with significant differences in coronary or aortic calcification.

Conclusions.—In this large, community-based sample of men and women, lower colony-forming unit number was associated with a higher burden of subclinical atherosclerosis in the coronary arteries and aorta. Decreased angiogenic potential could contribute to the development of atherosclerosis in humans.

▶ Calcified plaques of the aorta and coronary arteries are considered markers of atherosclerosis and predictive of future cardiovascular events.[1] Some peripherally circulating cell populations appear to have endothelial angiogenic and reparative properties. These have been termed as endothelial progenitor cells (EPCs). There are data to suggest that decreased EPC number results in increased risk of adverse cardiovascular outcomes.[2] The authors sought to clarify the link between EPC number and atherosclerosis by correlating EPC numbers with arterial calcification. They reason that an association of EPCs with arterial calcification would support the hypothesis that depletion of EPCs contributes to progression from subclinical endothelial dysfunction to cardiovascular disease in humans. The results are consistent with the theory that EPC colony-forming units and CD34$^+$-related cells represent different functional types of EPCs. Each may have distinct roles in mediating the vascular response to atherogenic exposures. A decreased angiogenic potential reflected in decreased colony-forming units of EPC cells could contribute, in some way, to development of human atherosclerosis. Stimulation of EPC production may someday serve as potential therapy in patients with atherogenic risk factors.

G. L. Moneta, MD

References

1. Detrano R, Guerci AD, Carr JJ, et al. Coronary calcium as a predictor of coronary events in four racial or ethnic groups. N Engl J Med. 2008;358:1336-1345.
2. Schmidt-Lucke C, Rössig L, Fichtlscherer S, et al. Reduced number of circulating endothelial progenitor cells predicts future cardiovascular events: proof of concept for the clinical importance of endogenous vascular repair. Circulation. 2005;111:2981-2987.

Cholesterol Efflux Capacity, High-Density Lipoprotein Function, and Atherosclerosis

Khera AV, Cuchel M, de la Llera-Moya M, et al (Univ of Pennsylvania, Philadelphia; et al)
N Engl J Med 364:127-135, 2011

Background.—High-density lipoprotein (HDL) may provide cardiovascular protection by promoting reverse cholesterol transport from macrophages. We hypothesized that the capacity of HDL to accept cholesterol from macrophages would serve as a predictor of atherosclerotic burden.

Methods.—We measured cholesterol efflux capacity in 203 healthy volunteers who underwent assessment of carotid artery intima–media thickness, 442 patients with angiographically confirmed coronary artery disease, and 351 patients without such angiographically confirmed disease. We quantified efflux capacity by using a validated ex vivo system that involved incubation of macrophages with apolipoprotein B–depleted serum from the study participants.

Results.—The levels of HDL cholesterol and apolipoprotein A-I were significant determinants of cholesterol efflux capacity but accounted for less than 40% of the observed variation. An inverse relationship was noted between efflux capacity and carotid intima–media thickness both before and after adjustment for the HDL cholesterol level. Furthermore, efflux capacity was a strong inverse predictor of coronary disease status (adjusted odds ratio for coronary disease per 1-SD increase in efflux capacity, 0.70; 95% confidence interval [CI], 0.59 to 0.83; P<0.001). This relationship was attenuated, but remained significant, after additional adjustment for the HDL cholesterol level (odds ratio per 1-SD increase, 0.75; 95% CI, 0.63 to 0.90; P=0.002) or apolipoprotein A-I level (odds ratio per 1-SD increase, 0.74; 95% CI, 0.61 to 0.89; P=0.002). Additional studies showed enhanced efflux capacity in patients with the metabolic syndrome and low HDL cholesterol levels who were treated with

TABLE 2.—Beta Coefficients for the Association between Cholesterol Efflux Capacity and Carotid Intima—Media Thickness

Linear-Regression Covariates*	Beta Coefficient per 1-SD Increase in Efflux Capacity (95% CI)	P Value
Age and sex	−0.02 (−0.04 to −0.003)	0.02
Age, sex, and cardiovascular risk factors	−0.02 (−0.04 to −0.004)	0.02
Age, sex, cardiovascular risk factors, and high-density lipoprotein cholesterol	−0.03 (−0.06 to −0.01)	0.003
Age, sex, cardiovascular risk factors, and apolipoprotein A-I	−0.04 (−0.06 to −0.01)	0.005

*Cardiovascular risk factors were systolic blood pressure, glycated hemoglobin, and low-density lipoprotein cholesterol.

TABLE 3.—Coronary Artery Disease Status According to Quartile of Efflux Capacity

Variable	No. of Patients	Odds Ratio for Coronary Artery Disease (95% CI)*		
		Adjusted for Cardiovascular Risk Factors	Adjusted for Cardiovascular Risk Factors and HDL Cholesterol	Adjusted for Cardiovascular Risk Factors and Apolipoprotein A-I
Quartile 1	198	1.00	1.00	1.00
Quartile 2	198	0.75 (0.48−1.16)	0.79 (0.51−1.24)	0.77 (0.49−1.21)
Quartile 3	198	0.58 (0.37−0.89)	0.64 (0.41−1.00)	0.63 (0.40−0.99)
Quartile 4	199	0.40 (0.25−0.63)	0.48 (0.30−0.78)	0.46 (0.28−0.75)
P value for trend		<0.001	0.002	0.002

*Cardiovascular risk factors included in the logistic-regression model were age, sex, smoking status, presence or absence of diabetes, presence or absence of hypertension, and low-density lipoprotein cholesterol. HDL denotes highdensity lipoprotein.

pioglitazone, but not in patients with hypercholesterolemia who were treated with statins.

Conclusions.—Cholesterol efflux capacity from macrophages, a metric of HDL function, has a strong inverse association with both carotid intima—media thickness and the likelihood of angiographic coronary artery disease, independently of the HDL cholesterol level. (Funded by the National Heart, Lung, and Blood Institute and others.) (Tables 2 and 3).

▶ There is a strong inverse association between levels of high-density lipoprotein (HDL) cholesterol and cardiovascular disease risk. This inverse association has fostered investigation into whether pharmacologic increases in HDL cholesterol might provide benefit in reducing cardiovascular risk. However, an inhibitor of cholesterol ester transfer protein was found to result in a 72% increase in HDL cholesterol levels, but was actually associated with an increase in the number of cardiovascular events.[1] This may in part be explained by the fact that HDL appears to have marked heterogeneity in particle composition. This heterogeneity affects biologic properties. Emphasis has therefore shifted on not only measurement of HDL cholesterol levels but on the development of a validated measure of HDL function.[2] There may be many components of HDL-mediated atheroprotection, and it appears that the ability of HDL to promote reverse cholesterol transport by accepting cholesterol from lipid-laden macrophages may be important. This is termed "cholesterol efflux capacity."[3] The study has addressed an important issue as to why static measurements of HDL cholesterol have inherent limitations predicting functional affects of HDL (Tables 2 and 3). Clearly, simple assessment of HDL levels and modulation of only HDL levels is not likely, based on these data, to result in predictable modification of cardiovascular risk factors. Drug therapy targeting cholesterol efflux capacity may be a more fruitful target for modulation of the antiatherogenic effects of HDL cholesterol.

G. L. Moneta, MD

References

1. Barter PJ, Caulfield M, Eriksson M, et al. Effects of torcetrapib in patients at high risk for coronary events. *N Engl J Med.* 2007;357:2109-2122.
2. Vaisar T, Pennathur S, Green PS, et al. Shotgun proteomics implicates protease inhibition and complement activation in the antiinflammatory properties of HDL. *J Clin Invest.* 2007;117:746-756.
3. Tall AR. Cholesterol efflux pathways and other potential mechanisms involved in the athero-protective effect of high density lipoproteins. *J Intern Med.* 2008;263: 256-273.

---

eNOS and ACE genes influence peripheral arterial disease predisposition in smokers
Sticchi E, Sofi F, Romagnuolo I, et al (Univ of Florence, Italy)
J Vasc Surg 52:97-102, 2010

Objective.—Several biologic mediators and genetic predisposing factors may contribute to the development of peripheral arterial disease (PAD). The *eNOS* gene, encoding for endothelial nitric oxide synthase, has been proposed as a candidate gene in the predisposition to the disease. In this study, we evaluated the role of *eNOS-786T>C, -894G>T* and *4a/4b* polymorphisms as markers of PAD per se and in the presence of the *ACE D* allele in patients previously investigated.

Methods.—We analyzed 281 consecutive patients (220 men, 61 women; median age, 72 years) with PAD and 562 healthy controls, comparable for sex and age.

Results.—eNOS-786C, but not -894T and 4a, allele frequency was significantly higher in PAD patients than in controls (P = .03). An association with the predisposition to PAD was found for the *eNOS-786C* allele (odds ratio [OR], 1.52; 95% confidence interval [CI], 1.11-2.09; P = .009) and the *eNOS-786C/4a* haplotype (OR, 1.41; 95% CI, 1.02-1.94, P = .04) at univariate analysis but not after adjustment for traditional risk factors. When smoking habit was considered, we observed that *eNOS-786C/4a* haplotype, but not the *eNOS-786C* allele, influenced PAD predisposition after adjustment for traditional risk factors in smokers (OR, 2.71; 95% CI, 1.38-5.30; $P = .004$). The *eNOS-786C* and *eNOS-786C/4a* haplotype did not modify the susceptibility to PAD in patients carrying the *ACE D* allele. Nevertheless, the presence of the *eNOS-786C/4a* haplotype increased PAD predisposition in smokers also carrying *ACE D* allele (OR, 2.71 to 3.79; $P > .05$ for interaction).

Conclusions.—This study demonstrated an association between *eNOS* and *ACE* genes in increasing PAD susceptibility in smokers, thus providing evidence for a gene-environment interaction in modulating predisposition to the disease.

▶ Nitric oxide (NO) modulates much of the endothelial dysfunction that serves as a key step in the initiation and progression of atherosclerosis. This likely occurs through NO-mediated changes in platelet inhibition, leukocyte adherence to vascular endothelium, inhibition of smooth muscle cell proliferation and migration, and effects on vascular tone regulation. There are at least 3 isoforms of NO synthase (NOS). Changes in NO availability may be genetically determined through up- or downregulation of NO synthesis. It also appears that polymorphisms in the gene coding for angiotensin converting enzyme (*ACE*) may also be involved in predisposition to peripheral arterial disease (PAD). The data provide evidence that the combined effects of ACE and endothelial NOS, perhaps through combined effects on endothelial dysfunction, play a role in predisposing significant risks of PAD development in those who smoke. Clearly this occurs on a background of environmental factors, and it is most likely a combination of genetic and environmental factors that modulate PAD predisposition. There are certainly a number of variables that may have been unappreciated in the analysis. Perhaps someday those who are unable to cease smoking may be treated with additional strategies such as supplementation of the substrate for NO synthesis (L-arginine) and other donors of NO. Such an approach, of course, would be a bit overly focused in that there is a small chance that it may protect patients who smoke from developing more severe PAD. However, it would be unlikely to mitigate the carcinogenic effects of tobacco abuse.

G. L. Moneta, MD

Infectious Burden and Carotid Plaque Thickness: The Northern Manhattan Study
Elkind MSV, Luna JM, Moon YP, et al (College of Physicians and Surgeons, Columbia Univ, NY; Mailman School of Public Health, Columbia Univ, NY; et al)
Stroke 41:e117-e122, 2010

Background and Purpose.—The overall burden of prior infections may contribute to atherosclerosis and stroke risk. We hypothesized that serological evidence of common infections would be associated with carotid plaque thickness in a multiethnic cohort.

Methods.—Antibody titers to 5 common infectious microorganisms (ie, *Chlamydia pneumoniae, Helicobacter pylori,* cytomegalovirus, and herpesvirus 1 and 2) were measured among stroke-free community participants and a weighted index of infectious burden was calculated based on Cox models previously derived for the association of each infection with stroke risk. High-resolution carotid duplex Doppler studies were used to assess maximum carotid plaque thickness. Weighted least squares regression was used to measure the association between infectious burden and maximum carotid plaque thickness after adjusting for other risk factors.

Results.—Serological results for all 5 infectious organisms were available in 861 participants with maximum carotid plaque thickness measurements available (mean age, 67.2 ± 9.6 years). Each individual infection was associated with stroke risk after adjusting for other risk factors. The infectious burden index (n = 861) had a mean of 1.00 ± 0.35 SD and a median of 1.08. Plaque was present in 52% of participants (mean, 0.90 ± 1.04 mm). Infectious burden was associated with maximum carotid plaque thickness (adjusted increase in maximum carotid plaque thickness 0.09 mm; 95% CI, 0.03 to 0.15 mm per SD increase of infectious burden).

Conclusions.—A quantitative weighted index of infectious burden, derived from the magnitude of association of individual infections with stroke, was associated with carotid plaque thickness in this multiethnic cohort. These results lend support to the notion that past or chronic exposure to common infections, perhaps by exacerbating inflammation, contributes to atherosclerosis. Future studies are needed to confirm this hypothesis and to define optimal measures of infectious burden as a vascular risk factor.

▶ Atherosclerosis is an inflammatory process and begins with endothelial damage and upregulation of adhesion molecules recruiting monocytes and lymphocytes into the subendothelial space. In the subendothelial space, monocytes become macrophages that secrete proinflammatory cytokines and ingest oxidized low-density lipoprotein (LDL).[1] The endothelial injury that precipitates the cascade of events that ultimately leads to atherosclerosis is related to well-known risk factors such as tobacco smoke, shear stress, oxidized LDL, and hypertension, but may also include infections. A number of studies have linked chronic exposure to infectious agents such as *Helicobacter pylori, Chlamydia pneumoniae,* and herpes viruses to coronary artery disease and stroke.[2,3] It has been thought that chronic infections may lead to this inflammatory process through remote signaling of inflammatory mediators that ultimately begin the process of atherosclerosis. This is another of a number of previous articles that suggest past or chronic exposure to common infections contributes to atherosclerosis. The mechanism of such a contribution is unclear, but given the inflammatory nature of atherosclerosis, it is postulated to act by exacerbating inflammation. An implication of the study is that infectious burden may be a modifiable risk of atherosclerosis and that measurement of carotid plaque thickness may provide a way to assess the effects of an anti-infective strategy. A weakness of the study, of course, is that serologic measurements of infection and carotid plaque thickness were determined at only a single point in time. Temporal relationships between carotid plaque thickness and infectious burden cannot be determined from these data. Another problem with the infectious etiology of atherosclerosis theory is that clinical trials of antibiotic therapy for infectious agents thought to be associated with atherosclerosis have not been shown to reduce vascular risk.[4,5] However, such studies may have included patients without serologic evidence of infection and used therapy perhaps late in the course of the disease. Clearly the infection and atherosclerosis concept is not going away.

G. L. Moneta, MD

References

1. Ross R. Atherosclerosis—an inflammatory disease. *N Engl J Med*. 1999;340: 115-126.
2. Wimmer ML, Sandmann-Strupp R, Saikku P, Haberl RL. Association of chlamydial infection with cerebrovascular disease. *Stroke*. 1996;27:2207-2210.
3. Ridker PM, Hennekens CH, Stampfer MJ, Wang F. Prospective study of herpes simplex virus, cytomegalovirus, and the risk of future myocardial infarction and stroke. *Circulation*. 1998;98:2796-2799.
4. O'Connor CM, Dunne MW, Pfeffer MA, et al. Azithromycin for the secondary prevention of coronary heart disease events: the WIZARD study: a randomized controlled trial. *JAMA*. 2003;290:1459-1466.
5. Cannon CP, Braunwald E, McCabe CH, et al. Antibiotic treatment of *Chlamydia pneumoniae* after acute coronary syndrome. *N Engl J Med*. 2005;352:1646-1654.

Inhibitory Effects of Calcitonin Gene-Related Peptides on Experimental Vein Graft Disease

Zhang X, Zhuang J, Wu H, et al (Guangdong General Hosp, Guangzhou, China)
Ann Thorac Surg 90:117-123, 2010

Background.—Vein graft disease is a chronic inflammatory disease and limits the long-term clinical outcome of coronary revascularization. Because calcitonin gene-related peptide (CGRP) inhibits macrophage infiltration and inflammatory mediators, we hypothesized that transfected CGRP gene would inhibit macrophage infiltration and expression of inflammatory mediators in vein graft disease.

Methods.—Autologous rabbit jugular vein grafts were incubated ex vivo in a solution of mosaic adeno-associated virus vectors containing CGRP gene (AAV2/1.CGRP) or *Escherichia coli* B-galactosidase gene (LacZ) or a saline solution and then interposed in the carotid artery. Expression of CGRP gene was identified by reverse transcription—polymerase chain reaction, and *E. coli* LacZ gene expression was identified by X-gal staining. Intima to media ratios were evaluated at postoperative 4 weeks. Macrophages were identified with CD68 antibody by immunocytochemistry. Inflammatory mediators were measured with real-time polymerase chain reaction.

Results.—The CGRP and LacZ gene expression were positive at postoperative 4 weeks. The intima to media ratio was significantly inhibited in the AAV2/1.CGRP group. Macrophage infiltration and expression of inflammatory mediators including monocyte chemoattractant protein-1, tumor necrosis factor-α, inducible nitric oxide synthase, and matrix metalloproteinase-9 were also significantly inhibited in the AAV2/1.CGRP group.

Conclusions.—Transfection of AAV2/1.CGRP inhibited inflammatory mediator expression, macrophage infiltration, and neointimal hyperplasia in experimental vein graft disease.

▶ Mechanisms of intimal hyperplasia are complex and include complex interactions with inflammatory cells, inflammatory mediators, and smooth muscle cells. In particular, macrophages appear necessary for initiation of intimal hyperplasia. Calcitonin gene-related peptide (CGRP) is a biologically active aminopeptide, 37 amino acids in length. Studies have shown that CGRP can inhibit inflammatory cells and expression of inflammatory mediators, such as tumor necrosis factor-α and monocyte chemoattractant protein-1, that appear important in intimal hyperplasia.[1] CGRP can also inhibit hyperplasia of vascular smooth muscle and protect endothelial cell function.[2,3] The authors sought to evaluate the effects of CGRP expressed by an adeno-associated virus vector, gene transfer on macrophage infiltration, and inflammatory mediators of vein graft disease in a rabbit model. The authors' experiment supported their hypothesis. The report is brief and does not delineate specific patterns of gene expression and thus does not allow precise determination of mechanisms. However, the end result is interesting: very effective inhibition of intimal hyperplasia. Vascular and cardiovascular surgeons remember the recent disappointments of the Prevent 3 and Prevent 4 trials, where novel therapy directed at the genetic level failed to suppress intimal hyperplasia. With respect to inhibiting intimal hyperplasia, the chasm between promising basic bench research and clinical relevance in humans remains wide. This is interesting work, but given the history of this field, any optimism should be tempered with caution.

G. L. Moneta, MD

References

1. Li W, Wang T, Ma C, Xiong T, Zhu Y, Wang X. Calcitonin gene-related peptide inhibits interleukin-1beta-induced endogenous monocyte chemoattractant protein-1 secretion in type II alveolar epithelial cells. *Am J Physiol Cell Physiol.* 2006;291:C456-C465.
2. Deng W, St Hilaire RC, Chattergoon NN, Jeter JR Jr, Kadowitz PJ. Inhibition of vascular smooth muscle cell proliferation in vitro by genetically engineered marrow stromal cells secreting calcitonin gene-related peptide. *Life Sci.* 2006; 78:1830-1838.
3. Ye F, Deng PY, Li D, et al. Involvement of endothelial cell-derived CGRP in heat stress-induced protection of endothelial function. *Vascul Pharmacol.* 2007;46: 238-246.

A novel cell permeant peptide inhibitor of MAPKAP kinase II inhibits intimal hyperplasia in a human saphenous vein organ culture model

Lopes LB, Brophy CM, Flynn CR, et al (Arizona State Univ, Tempe; et al)
J Vasc Surg 52:1596-1607, 2010

Objective.—The present study was aimed at developing a new cell-permeant peptide inhibitor (MK2i) of the kinase that phosphorylates and activates heat-shock protein (HSP)27 (MAPKAP kinase II), and evaluating the ability of this peptide to inhibit HSP27 phosphorylation and intimal thickening.

Methods.—The ability of MK2i to reduce HSP27 phosphorylation and cell migration was evaluated in A7R5 cells stimulated with arsenite or lysophosphatidic acid. Stable isotopic labeling using amino acids in cell culture, in combination with liquid chromatography mass spectrometry, was used to characterize the effect of MK2i on global protein expression in fibroblasts. The effect of MK2i on intimal thickening and connective tissue growth factor expression was evaluated in human saphenous vein (HSV) rings maintained with 30% fetal bovine serum for 14 days by light microscopy and immunoblotting.

Results.—Pretreatment of cells with MK2i (10 μM) prior to arsenite or lysophosphatidic acid stimulation decreased phosphorylation of HSP27 (36% ± 9% and 33% ± 10%, respectively) compared with control (not pretreated) cells. MK2i also inhibited A7R5 migration, and downregulated the transforming growth factor-induced expression of collagen and fibronectin in keloid cells, two major matrix proteins involved in the development of intimal hyperplasia. Treatment of HSV segments with MK2i enhanced relaxation, reduced HSP27 phosphorylation (40% ± 17%), connective tissue growth factor expression (17% ± 5%), and intimal thickness (48.2% ± 10.5%) compared with untreated segments. On the other hand, treatment with a recombinant fusion protein containing a cell-permeant peptide attached to the HSP27 sequence increased intimal thickness of HSV segments by 48% ± 14%.

Conclusion.—Our results suggest that HSP27 may play a role in the development of processes leading to intimal hyperplasia in HSV, and reduction of HSP27 phosphorylation by MK2i may be a potential strategy to inhibit the development of intimal hyperplasia in HSV to prevent the autologous vascular graft failure.

▶ In this study, investigators developed a cell-permeant peptide inhibitor (named MK2i) of the kinase that phosphorylates and activates heat-shock protein (HSP) 27 and evaluated its potential as a new strategy to prevent intimal hyperplasia. These experiments are logical extensions of extensive pre-existing work, which defined the role of HSP27 in the development of intimal hyperplasia, smooth muscle proliferation, and migration. To make the preexisting work translationally relevant, it's essential to show that MK2i can be delivered effectively to clinically relevant tissues in doses that are not toxic. They developed MK2i using a protein transduction domain that binds to and inhibits the catalytic site of mitogen-activated protein kinase-activated protein (MAP-KAP) kinase II. Protein transduction domains were used because of their ability to carry other peptides, proteins, and even small particles across cell membranes. This strategy should lead to concentrated delivery of the inhibitor to tissue at risk. The cell-permeant inhibitor significantly reduced stimulated phosphorylation of HSP27 in commercially available embryonic smooth muscle cells obtained from rats. The authors provided an important control by including experiments using an inhibitor upstream of MAPKAP kinase, which also inhibited phosphorylation of HSP27. A crucial component of the experiments in this report included an assessment of how well this cell-permeant inhibitor worked in a model of human intimal hyperplasia. These investigators demonstrated that the inhibitor decreased intimal hyperplasia in an organ culture model of intimal hyperplasia using human saphenous vein. These experiments are well described and logical in their design. The major drawback to the experiments is that they were performed in static conditions with no mechanical stress. Shear stress[1-3] and cyclic stretch[4] are known to modulate HSP27 phosphorylation in vascular endothelial cells. It is not clear whether there will be an effective inhibition of HSP27 phosphorylation in smooth muscle cells exposed to mechanical stress. Nevertheless, these experiments are important in the progression of this treatment concept from the bench to bedside.

M. T. Watkins, MD

References

1. Chang E, Heo KS, Woo CH, et al. MK2 SUMOylation regulates actin filament remodeling and subsequent migration in endothelial cells by inhibiting MK2 kinase and HSP27 phosphorylation. *Blood.* 2011;117:2527-2537.
2. Cai H, Liu D, Garcia JG. CaM Kinase II-dependent pathophysiological signalling in endothelial cells. *Cardiovasc Res.* 2008;77:30-34.
3. Li S, Piotrowicz RS, Levin EG, Shyy YJ, Chien S. Fluid shear stress induces the phosphorylation of small heat shock proteins in vascular endothelial cells. *Am J Physiol.* 1996;271:C994-1000.
4. Birukova AA, Rios A, Birukov KG. Long-term cyclic stretch controls pulmonary endothelial permeability at translational and post-translational levels. *Exp Cell Res.* 2008;314:3466-3477.

Adipokine Resistin is a Key Player to Modulate Monocytes, Endothelial Cells, and Smooth Muscle Cells, Leading to Progression of Atherosclerosis in Rabbit Carotid Artery

Cho Y, Lee S-E, Lee H-C, et al (Seoul Natl Univ College of Medicine, Korea; Seoul Natl Univ Hosp, Korea)
J Am Coll Cardiol 57:99-109, 2010

Objectives.—We investigated the effects of human resistin on atherosclerotic progression and clarified its underlying mechanisms.

Background.—Resistin is an adipokine first identified as a mediator of insulin resistance in murine obesity models. But, its role in human pathology is under debate. Although a few recent studies suggested the relationship between resistin and atherosclerosis in humans, the causal relationship and underlying mechanism have not been clarified.

Methods.—We cloned rabbit resistin, which showed 78% identity to human resistin at the complementary deoxyribonucleic acid level, and its expression was examined in 3 different atherosclerotic rabbit models. To evaluate direct role of resistin on atherosclerosis, collared rabbit carotid arteries were used. Histological and cell biologic analyses were performed.

Results.—Rabbit resistin was expressed by macrophages of the plaque in the 3 different atherosclerotic models. Peri-adventitial resistin gene transfer induced macrophage infiltration and expression of various inflammatory cytokines, resulting in the acceleration of plaque growth and destabilization. In vitro experiments elucidated that resistin increased monocyte-endothelial cell adhesion by upregulating very late antigen-4 on monocytes and their counterpart vascular cell adhesion molecule-1 on endothelial cells. Resistin augmented monocyte infiltration in collagen by direct chemoattractive effect as well as by enhancing migration toward monocyte chemotactic protein-1. Administration of connecting segment-1 peptide, which blocks very late antigen-4 × vascular cell adhesion molecule-1 interaction, ameliorated neointimal growth induced by resistin in vivo.

Conclusions.—Our results indicate that resistin aggravates atherosclerosis by stimulating monocytes, endothelial cells, and vascular smooth muscle cells to induce vascular inflammation. These findings provide the first insight on the causal relationship between resistin and atherosclerosis.

▶ The convergence of insulin resistance and inflammation in the pathogenesis of atherosclerotic cardiovascular disease had been recognized over the past decade. Resistin has emerged as a new molecule to stand at the nodal point of signaling pathways to link metabolic disorders and inflammation. These investigators provide a causal link between the expression of resistin and the progression of vascular disease in 3 different models of atherosclerosis in a rabbit model. The rationale for using the rabbit rather than the murine model of atherosclerosis is based on the fact that murine resistin is different from that of human in amino acid sequence, expression patterns, and functions. Rabbit was one of the best candidates for this study because it has established experimental models mimicking human atherosclerosis. These investigators then cloned rabbit resistin and revealed that it has high homology to that of human (78% and 69% identity at complementary deoxyribonucleic acid and amino acid level, respectively). The importance of this study and the ability of the authors to make such a strong causal relationship between resistin expression and arterial inflammation is based on the fact that they were able to specifically block the effects of resistin with a downstream inhibitor of resistin. This obviously has considerable clinical implications and deserves further investigation.

M. T. Watkins, MD

Beyond Thrombosis: The Versatile Platelet in Critical Illness

Katz JN, Kolappa KP, Becker RC (The Univ of North Carolina, Chapel Hill; Duke Univ Med Ctr, Durham, NC)
Chest 139:658-668, 2011

Sepsis, acute lung injury, and ARDS contribute substantially to the expanding burden of critical illness within our ICUs. Each of these processes is characterized by a myriad of injurious events, including apoptosis, microvascular dysfunction, abnormal coagulation, and dysregulated host immunity. Only recently have platelets—long considered merely effectors of thrombosis—been implicated in inflammatory conditions and the pathobiology of these disease processes. A growing body of evidence suggests a prominent role for maladaptive platelet activation and aggregation during sepsis and ARDS and has begun to underscore the pluripotential influence of platelets on outcomes in critical illness. Not only do platelets enhance vascular injury through thrombotic mechanisms but also appear to help orchestrate pathologic immune responses and are pivotal players in facilitating leukocyte recruitment to vulnerable tissue. These events contribute to the organ damage and poor patient outcomes that still plague the care of these high-risk individuals. An understanding of the role of platelets in critical illness also highlights the potential for both the development of risk stratification schema and the use of novel, targeted therapies that might alter the natural history of sepsis, acute lung injury, and ARDS. Future studies of adenosine, platelet polyphosphates, and the platelet transcriptome/proteome also should add considerably to our ability to unravel the mysteries of the versatile platelet.

▶ In this outstanding review, the authors discuss the role for maladaptive platelet activation and aggregation during sepsis and adult respiratory distress syndrome (ARDS). Because sepsis, acute lung injury, and ARDS carry a significant in-hospital mortality of nearly 50% and cost billions of dollars annually in health care expenses, a critical understanding of the functional role of platelets during sepsis and ARDS could provide significant insight in the mechanisms involved and therapeutic targets for treatment. The review provides evidence beyond what platelets are known to do during injury, which is to provide hemostasis. In fact, evidence suggests that platelets enhance vascular injury through thrombotic mechanisms, and during sepsis platelets play a crucial role in coordinating a pathologic immune response that is a key feature in facilitating leukocyte recruitment and attaching leukocytes to vulnerable tissue. These are both evident in the solid organ circulation and in the alveolar-capillary complex. These events contribute to severe inflammation, ultimately leading to organ damage, poor patient outcomes, and high health care costs for critically ill patients. The key features of sepsis, acute lung injury, and ARDS are that all are characterized by abnormally enhanced coagulation, dysregulated host immunity, microvascular dysfunction, and tissue necrosis. The review begins with an overview of the structure and function of platelets and the role of various receptors that lead to platelet activation, how platelets are involved in host immunity by releasing inflammatory mediators and recruitment of leukocytes to platelets and leukocytes to the endothelium by P-selectins, the thrombocytopenia that occurs in up to 50% of patients during critical illness and its implications, and how antiplatelet therapeutic strategies in critical care specifically in sepsis and ARDS may alter outcomes. This is an important review for any clinician who cares for critically ill patients who develop sepsis and ARDS and wants to gain a better understanding of the critical importance of platelets in the pathophysiology of these devastating diseases.

M. T. Watkins, MD

Circulating Levels of Endothelial Progenitor Cell Mobilizing Factors in the Metabolic Syndrome
Jialal I, Fadini GP, Pollock K, et al (Univ of California Davis Med Ctr and the VA Med Ctr, Sacramento; Univ of Padua Med School, Italy)
Am J Cardiol 106:1606-1608, 2010

Endothelial progenitor cells (EPCs) are an emerging biomarker of vascular health. However, there are few data on the biology and mobilizing factors of EPCs in metabolic syndrome (MS). The aim of this study was to assay EPC mobilizing factors, including granulocyte colony-stimulating factor, stem cell factor/c-kit ligand (SCF), vascular endothelial growth factor, and stromal cell–derived factor–1 levels, in patients with MS (n = 36) and age- and gender-matched controls (n = 38). There was a significant reduction of 83% in granulocyte colony-stimulating factor levels in patients with MS. Also, there were decreases in SCF and SCF soluble receptor levels. However, there was no significant difference in stromal cell–derived factor–1 levels, and paradoxically, vascular endothelial growth factor levels were increased, consistent with resistance. In conclusion, in addition to progenitor cell exhaustion as a mechanism for the decrease in EPCs in patients with MS, they also have a mobilization defect, as manifested by decreased levels of granulocyte colony-stimulating factor and SCF, resulting in a decrease in EPCs.

▶ It is well known that patients with atherosclerosis, diabetes, and advanced age have decreased levels of endothelial progenitor cells (EPCs) and CD34+ progenitor cells (PCs). These authors provide the first hard evidence on why there is a reduction in EPCs in patients with metabolic syndrome prior to the onset of diabetes. They describe a reduction of granulocyte colony-stimulating factor (GCSF) and low levels of stem cell factor (SCF)/c-kit ligand. This is an important observation because GCSF and SCF are known to synergize in inducing bone marrow PC mobilization, and plasma levels of SCF have been also taken to represent a measure of PC mobilization. These data indicate that there is an imbalance in the factors responsible for mobilizing EPCs and PCs prior to the onset of frank diabetes. It may be important to evaluate these factors in human patients who progress to full-blown diabetes and those patients who experience problems with wound healing. GCSF is commercially available for treating patients with neutropenia and might be a potential treatment for patients with poor wound healing.

M. T. Watkins, MD

Cyclosporine Up-Regulates Krüppel-Like Factor-4 (KLF4) in Vascular Smooth Muscle Cells and Drives Phenotypic Modulation In Vivo
Garvey SM, Sinden DS, Schoppee Bortz PD, et al (Univ of Virginia, Charlottesville)
J Pharmacol Exp Ther 333:34-42, 2010

Cyclosporine A (CSA, calcineurin inhibitor) has been shown to block both vascular smooth muscle cell (VSMC) proliferation in cell culture and vessel neointimal formation following injury in vivo. The purpose of this study was to determine molecular and pathological effects of CSA on VSMCs. Using real-time reverse transcription-polymerase chain reaction, Western blot analysis, and immunofluorescence microscopy, we show that CSA upregulated the expression of Krüppel-like factor-4 (*KLF4*) in VSMCs. KLF4 plays a key role in regulating VSMC phenotypic modulation. KLF4 antagonizes proliferation, facilitates migration, and down-regulates VSMC differentiation marker gene expression. We show that the VSMC differentiation marker genes smooth muscle α-actin (*ACTA2*), transgelin (*TAGLN*), smoothelin (*SMTN*), and myocardin (*MYOCD*) are all downregulated by CSA in VSMC monoculture, whereas cyclindependent kinase inhibitor-1A (*CDKN1A*) and matrix metalloproteinase-3 (*MMP3*) are up-regulated. CSA did not affect the abundance of the VSMC microRNA (MIR) markers MIR143 and MIR145. Administration of CSA to rat carotid artery in vivo resulted in acute and transient suppression of ACTA2, TAGLN, SMTN, MYOCD, and smooth muscle myosin heavy chain (MYH11) mRNA levels. The tumor suppressor genes *KLF4*, *p53*, and *CDKN1A*, however, were up-regulated, as well as *MMP3*, *MMP9*, and collagen-VIII. CSA-treated arteries showed remarkable remodeling, including breakdown of the internal elastic lamina and reorientation of VSMCs, as well as increased KLF4 immunostaining in VSMCs and endothelial cells. Altogether, these data show that cyclosporin up-regulates KLF4 expression and promotes phenotypic modulation of VSMCs.

▶ This is an important article because it provides seminal information on how cyclosporine may contribute to the development of posttransplant arteriopathy. The authors provide a combination of in vivo and in vitro experiments that implicate cyclosporine-mediated increase in Krüppel-like factor-4 (*KLF4*), which is a pivotal transcription factor involved with vascular smooth muscle cell (VSMC) phenotypic modulation from the contractile phenotype toward proliferative, migratory, and/or inflammatory phenotypes. They show that cyclosporine A (CSA) treatment of rat VSMCs increased both *KLF4* messenger RNA (mRNA) and protein in cell culture. Short interfering RNA oligonucleotides targeting

KLF4 reversed the cyclosporine-mediated change in vascular smooth muscle phenotype. They show that CSA treatment of rat carotid arteries in vivo upregulated *KLF4* and was coincident with the development of intimal hyperplasia. The authors also demonstrate that the ability of cyclosporine to stimulate smooth muscle expression of *KLF4* was more sustained than platelet-derived growth factor-BB, which was thought to be one of the most potent mediators of intimal hyperplasia. The authors exclude the possibility that the effect of cyclosporine on expression of *KLF4* is specific and not related to the fact that CSA decreases mitochondrial membrane permeability and generates reactive oxygen species. These findings alone, however, would not explain the kind of matrix remodeling known to accompany the development of intimal hyperplasia and transplant-associated arteriopathy. The authors did show evidence of increased mRNA for the matrix metalloproteinases 3 and 9 that were associated with changes in smooth muscle cell reorientation and breakdown of the internal elastic lamina. The authors did not show that this increase in mRNA was associated with an increase in metalloproteinase protein or activity. Despite this shortcoming, the article is excellent and may provide insight into therapeutic strategies to modulate transplant-associated arteriopathy.

M. T. Watkins, MD

Does Carotid Intima-Media Thickness Regression Predict Reduction of Cardiovascular Events?: A Meta-Analysis of 41 Randomized Trials

Costanzo P, Perrone-Filardi P, Vassallo E, et al (Federico II Univ, Naples, Italy)
J Am Coll Cardiol 56:2006-2020, 2010

Objectives.—The purpose of this study was to verify whether intima-media thickness (IMT) regression is associated with reduced incidence of cardiovascular events.

Background.—Carotid IMT increase is associated with a raised risk of coronary heart disease (CHD) and cerebrovascular (CBV) events. However, it is undetermined whether favorable changes of IMT reflect prognostic benefits.

Methods.—The MEDLINE database and the Cochrane Database were searched for articles published until August 2009. All randomized trials assessing carotid IMT at baseline, at end of follow-up, and reporting clinical end points were included. A weighted random-effects meta-regression analysis was performed to test the relationship between mean and maximum IMT changes and outcomes. The influence of baseline patients' characteristics, cardiovascular risk profile, IMT at baseline, follow-up, and quality of the trials was also explored. Overall estimates of effect were calculated with a fixed-effects model, random-effects model, or Peto method.

Results.—Forty-one trials enrolling 18,307 participants were included. Despite significant reduction in CHD, CBV events, and all-cause death induced by active treatments (for CHD events, odds ratio [OR]: 0.82, 95% confidence interval [CI]: 0.69 to 0.96, p = 0.02; for CBV events, OR: 0.71, 95% CI: 0.51 to 1.00, p = 0.05; and for all-cause death, OR:

0.71, 95% CI: 0.53 to 0.96, p = 0.03), there was no significant relationship between IMT regression and CHD events (Tau 0.91, p = 0.37), CBV events (Tau −0.32, p = 0.75), and all-cause death (Tau −0.41, p = 0.69). In addition, subjects' baseline characteristics, cardiovascular risk profile, IMT at baseline, follow-up, and quality of the trials did not significantly influence the association between IMT changes and clinical outcomes.

Conclusions.—Regression or slowed progression of carotid IMT, induced by cardiovascular drug therapies, do not reflect reduction in cardiovascular events.

▶ This is a very controversial study that is so important because it is a meta-analysis of 41 trials culled from over 9000 articles on the topic. When all data from the 41 trials were pooled, there was no significant relationship between intima-media thickness changes from baseline to end of follow-up and coronary artery disease, cerebrovascular disease, composite outcome, and all-cause death. Likewise, no relationship was found when only hard cardiovascular events (cardiac death, myocardial infarction, and stroke) were considered. In contrast, meta-regression analysis of lipid-lowering trials demonstrated a significant relationship between low-density lipoprotein lowering and reduction of coronary heart disease events and composite outcome, with a trend for cerebrovascular events. Thus, intima-media changes did not accurately predict the benefits of therapies with proven favorable effects on cardiovascular risk profile. The one potential criticism of this article is that it is not clear that the same level of expertise in measuring carotid intima-media ratio can be assumed.

M. T. Watkins, MD

Endothelial cells are susceptible to rapid siRNA transfection and gene silencing ex vivo
Andersen ND, Chopra A, Monahan TS, et al (Beth Israel Deaconess Med Ctr, Boston, MA; et al)
J Vasc Surg 52:1608-1615, 2010

Background.—Endothelial gene silencing via small interfering RNA (siRNA) transfection represents a promising strategy for the control of vascular disease. Here, we demonstrate endothelial gene silencing in human saphenous vein using three rapid siRNA transfection techniques amenable for use in the operating room.

Methods.—Control siRNA, Cy5 siRNA, or siRNA targeting glyceraldehyde-3-phosphate dehydrogenase (GAPDH) or endothelial specific nitric oxide synthase (eNOS) were applied to surplus human saphenous vein for 10 minutes by (i) soaking, (ii) applying 300 mm Hg hyperbaric pressure, or (iii) 120 mm Hg luminal distending pressure. Transfected vein segments were maintained in organ culture. siRNA delivery and gene silencing were assessed by tissue layer using confocal microscopy and immunohistochemistry.

Results.—Distending pressure transfection yielded the highest levels of endothelial siRNA delivery (22% pixels fluorescing) and gene silencing (60% GAPDH knockdown, 55% eNOS knockdown) as compared with hyperbaric (12% pixels fluorescing, 36% GAPDH knockdown, 30% eNOS knockdown) or non-pressurized transfections (10% pixels fluorescing, 30% GAPDH knockdown, 25% eNOS knockdown). Cumulative endothelial siRNA delivery (16% pixels fluorescing) and gene silencing (46% GAPDH knockdown) exceeded levels achieved in the media/adventitia (8% pixels fluorescing, 24% GAPDH knockdown) across all transfection methods.

Conclusion.—Endothelial gene silencing is possible within the time frame and conditions of surgical application without the use of transfection reagents. The high sensitivity of endothelial cells to siRNA transfection marks the endothelium as a promising target of gene therapy in vascular disease.

▶ A PubMed search using the terms siRNA and clinical trial provided nearly 100 articles published electronically in the last 18 months, indicating the potential clinical importance of the methodology of gene silencing using small interfering RNAs. None of these electronically published articles deal with cardiovascular disease. This article from the LoGerfo laboratory deserves considerable attention primarily because it deals with human tissue and is a logical precursor for use of siRNA technology in a clinical trial for patients undergoing bypass surgery. It is important for surgeons to continue to seek methods to improve the outcome of vein bypass surgery because catheter-based techniques are used as primary strategies for coronary and peripheral revascularizations, the patients who do come to bypass are usually sicker with more extensive disease. This article is important because it studies gene silencing in a scenario that is surgically relevant from a logistical and temporal standpoint. A focused study of gene silencing in vein grafts was needed because the rate of graft failure in veins pressure treated with placebo in the PRoject of Ex-vivo Vein graft ENgineering via Transfection IV trial[1] was found to be higher than in other studies, and the transfection technique was questioned to have heightened the rate of vein graft failure.[2]

M. T. Watkins, MD

References

1. Mann MJ, Whittemore AD, Donaldson MC, et al. Ex-vivo gene therapy of human vascular bypass grafts with E2F decoy: the PREVENT single-centre, randomised, controlled trial. *Lancet.* 1999;354:1493-1498.
2. Desai ND, Fremes SE. Efficacy and safety of edifoligide. *JAMA.* 2006;295:1514. author reply 1514—5.

Exercise Reverses Metabolic Syndrome in High-Fat Diet–Induced Obese Rats

Touati S, Meziri F, Devaux S, et al (UFR Sciences, Avignon, France; Univ of Franche-Comté, Besancon, France; et al)
Med Sci Sports Exerc 43:398-407, 2011

Purpose.—Chronic consumption of a high-fat diet induces obesity. We investigated whether exercise would reverse the cardiometabolic disorders associated with obesity without it being necessary to change from a high- to normal-fat diet.

Methods.—Sprague–Dawley rats were placed on a high-fat (HFD) or control diet (CD) for 12 wk. HFD rats were then divided into four groups: sedentary HFD (HFD-S), exercise trained (motor treadmill for 12 wk) HFD (HFD-Ex), modified diet (HFD to CD; HF/CD-S), and exercise trained with modified diet (HF/CD-Ex). Cardiovascular risk parameters associated with metabolic syndrome were measured, and contents of aortic Akt, phospho-Akt at Ser (473), total endothelial nitric oxide synthase (eNOS), and phospho-eNOS at Ser (1177) were determined by Western blotting.

Results.—Chronic consumption of HFD induced a metabolic syndrome. Exercise and dietary modifications reduced adiposity, improved glucose and insulin levels and plasma lipid profile, and exerted an antihypertensive effect. Exercise was more effective than dietary modification in improving plasma levels of thiobarbituric acid-reacting substance and in correcting the endothelium-dependent relaxation to acetylcholine and insulin. Furthermore, independent of the diet used, exercise increased Akt and eNOS phosphorylation.

Conclusions.—Metabolic syndrome induced by HFD is reversed by exercise and diet modification. It is demonstrated that exercise training induces these beneficial effects without the requirement for dietary modification, and these beneficial effects may be mediated by shear stress-induced Akt/eNOS pathway activation. Thus, exercise may be an effective strategy to reverse almost all the atherosclerotic risk factors linked to obesity, particularly in the vasculature.

▶ Obesity is a major health risk for cardiovascular events. Obesity is on the rise in the United States and leads to the metabolic syndrome (hypertension, dyslipidemia, and insulin resistance). Understanding how diet and exercise can correct the metabolic syndrome is paramount, especially given the increased incidence of obesity, diabetes, and cardiovascular disorders that are observed and affect our everyday clinical practice. In this well-designed study, the main outcomes in rats fed a high-fat diet, in which rats were trained to exercise (on a motorized treadmill) versus remaining sedentary, and in rats fed initially a high-fat diet and then given a modified diet again in rats who were sedentary or exercised, demonstrated that exercise (and not diet) was the key parameter in normalizing endothelial function, as measured by increasing aortic Akt, phospho-Akt at Ser (473), total endothelial nitric oxide synthase (eNOS), and phospho-eNOS at Ser (1177) as determined by Western blotting. In addition, total body weight, blood pressure, and insulin resistance were all reduced, while the skeletal muscle oxidative enzyme activity (a measure of effective skeletal muscle exercise training) was significantly elevated in the exercising rats, and the cholesterol parameters all improved (similar to control diet rats) in the exercised rats compared with sedentary high-fat diet rats. The oxidative stress was significantly reduced in exercising rats. A part of this study that was very interesting was that the authors studied the aortic vasorelaxant effect to acetylcholine in isometric tissue chambers. Rats on either a high-fat diet or converted to a modified diet who exercised had the best functional relaxing response to acetylcholine, indicating excellent endothelial function, compared with the high-fat diet sedentary rats that had reduced endothelial dependent relaxation. Understanding all of the beneficial effects of exercise gives us a good reason to lead healthy lives by exercising regularly and eating modestly. What needs to be determined is how much exercise, type of exercise, and physiologic responses needed (heart rate, blood pressure) to attain the appropriate threshold required to gain the benefit of exercise. Is running 30 minutes the same as walking for 60 minutes?

M. T. Watkins, MD

Nicotine and cotinine affect the release of vasoactive factors by trophoblast cells and human umbilical vein endothelial cells

Romani F, Lanzone A, Tropea A, et al (Università Cattolica del Sacro Cuore (UCSC), Roma, Italy; Istituto di Ricerca "Associazione OASI Maria SS ONLUS", Troina (EN), Italy; et al)
Placenta 32:153-160, 2011

Objective.—To examine nicotine (N) and cotinine (C) effects on trophoblast cells (TCs) and human umbilical vein endothelial cells (HUVEC) secretion of soluble fms-like tyrosine kinase (sFlt-1), soluble endoglin (sENG), placental growth factor (PlGF), transforming growth factor-beta (TGF-beta) and vascular endothelial growth factor (VEGF).

Study Design.—Human placentas and umbilical cords were collected from uncomplicated pregnancies at term from a total of 24 non-smoking women with a history of normal blood pressure. TCs and HUVEC were cultured for 24 h with C or N (from 10^{-12} to 10^{-7} M).

Main Outcome Measures.—sFlt-1, sENG, PlGF, TGF-beta and VEGF release and messenger RNA (mRNA) expression were evaluated by ELISA and real-time polymerase chain reaction (PCR), respectively.

Results.—N and C reduced sFlt-1, sENG and PlGF release by TCs and TGF-beta release by HUVEC. Conversely, N and C increased PlGF secretion, while N alone increased sFlt-1 release by HUVEC. N and C were able to modulate VEGF mRNA expression in HUVEC.

Conclusions.—Our results suggest that N and C affect the balance of some important vasoactive factors released by TCs and HUVEC. This might be one of the possible mechanism through which smoke reduces the risk of hypertensive disorders during pregnancy as well as contributes to the well known detrimental effects of smoking on fetal development.

▶ In a field of vascular disease, smoking has been attributed to many disorders of atherosclerosis and vessels dysfunction. Interestingly, women who smoke during pregnancy have been reported to have a reduced risk of gestational hypertensive disorders and preeclampsia but at the cost of increased premature abortions and a higher incidence of intrauterine growth retardation, as well as increased fetal death in smokers versus nonsmoking pregnant women. This paradoxical effect has not been well studied. In this study, the authors evaluate the effects of nicotine and its active metabolite cotinine on placental tropho-blast cells (TCs) and human umbilical vein endothelial cells (HUVEC) secretion by measuring important growth factors and vasoactive substances (soluble fms-like tyrosine kinase [sFlt-1], soluble endoglin [sENG], placental growth factor [PlGF], transforming growth factor β [TGF-β] and vascular endothelial growth factor [VEGF]). The main tools to assess for expression were by enzyme-linked immunosorbent assay and real-time polymerase chain reaction. The main findings were that nicotine and cotinine reduced sFlt-1, sENG and PlGF release by TCs and TGF-β release by HUVEC. However, nicotine and coti-nine increased PlGF secretion, while nicotine alone increased sFlt-1 release by HUVEC. In preeclamptic women, it has been reported that an excess of soluble VEGF receptor-1 (known as soluble fms-like tyrosine kinase receptor-1 or sFlt-1) and sENG are elevated. This study demonstrated that both nicotine and coti-nine decreased both sFlt-1 and sENG in placental TC, reducing the binding of PLGF and VEGF that are required for proper maternal vascular function and have been found to be increased in the serum of pregnant women who smoke compared with nonsmokers. Both PLGF and VEGF are responsible for the correct placental development and the remodeling of maternal vasculature during pregnancy. By extrapolating from their data, the authors speculate that reducing placental sENG and sFlt-1 release by nicotine and cotinine could possibly explain why pregnant women who smoke have less hypertensive events. Alternatively, nicotine and cotinine were able to influence the balance of vasoactive factors in HUVEC, which may represent one of the possible mech-anisms involved in intrauterine growth retardation by diminishing the avail-ability of oxygen and nutrients. Future study will be required to understand the full mechanisms of these important mediators during pregnancy and the potential for preeclampsia and hypertensive crisis.

M. T. Watkins, MD

Nitric oxide production and blood corpuscle dynamics in response to the endocrine status of female rats
Uematsu K, Katayama T, Katayama H, et al (Fhime Univ Graduate School of Medicine, Japan; et al)
Thromb Res 126:504-510, 2010

Introduction.—Menopause is associated with marked changes in the endocrine profile, and increases the risk of vascular disease. However, the effect of hormones on the vascular system is still unclear. Therefore, the aim of this study was to examine the effects of endocrine status in female rats on nitric oxide (NO) production, inflammatory reactions and thrombus organization potency in the mesenteric microcirculation.

Materials and Methods.—Female Wistar rats were divided into four groups: proestrus, metestrus, ovariectomized (OVX) and OVX plus estradiol treatment (OVX + E_2). NO was imaged using an NO-sensitive dye. The leukocyte and platelet velocities relative to the erythrocyte velocity (V_W/V_{RC} and V_P/V_{RE}, respectively) and thrombi sizes created by laser radiation were measured as thrombogenesis indices.

Results.—Changes in endocrine status did not affect vascular function in the arterioles. However, in venules, NO production, V_W/V_{RC} and V_P/V_{RE} were decreased in the OVX group compared with the proestrus and metestrus states. Thrombus size was significantly greater in the OVX group than in the proestrus and metestrus states. Administration of E_2 for 2 weeks restored NO production, V_W/V_{RC} and V_P/V_{RE} to control levels.

Conclusions.—Changes in endocrine status did not affect arterioles. In contrast, in venules, reduced estrogen levels led to a decrease in NO production, thereby increasing thrombogenesis. Estrogen replacement restored NO production and leukocyte and platelet velocities, reducing thrombus formation relative to OVX. Although it is unclear how E_2 reduces thrombus formation, our results indicate that leukocyte and platelet adhesion to the endothelium is a target for E_2 via NO.

▶ This article sought to shed light on the influence of estrogen on vascular reactivity and nitric oxide (NO) synthesis in arteries and veins of female rats. The underlying important clinical question is why postmenopausal women are more susceptible to cardiovascular disease and whether hormone replacement can modulate cardiovascular risks. To this end, the authors studied mesenteric vascular reactivity and thrombosis in female rats in different menstrual states, along with a group of ovariectomized animals. Most surprisingly, changes in endocrine status altered venous but not mesenteric arteriolar NO synthesis or thrombosis. These studies were well done and used techniques readily available in these investigators' laboratory. The results however are in conflict with what we observe clinically. Specifically, heart attack and stroke are clearly increased in postmenopausal women. Venous thrombosis appears to be exacerbated in women, particularly young women, receiving exogenous estrogens. These studies show the opposite of what is observed in clinical practice. The reason for these disparate results may be related to the fact that these authors evaluated mesenteric, rather than peripheral, arterial tissue (aorta, vena cava, carotid arteries). The mesenteric arterial tissue may not be representative of the arterial beds where clinically relevant cardiovascular or peripheral arteriopathy is identified. These studies need to be repeated in a more clinically relevant arterial bed.

M. T. Watkins, MD

Persistence of Antibodies to the Topical Hemostat Bovine Thrombin
Randleman CD Jr, Singla NK, Renkens KL, et al (Varicosity Vein Ctr, Birmingham, AL; Huntington Memorial Hosp, Pasadena, CA; Indiana Spine Group, Indianapolis; et al)
J Am Coll Surg 211:798-803, 2010

Background.—Immunoassays that detect antibovine thrombin product antibodies are not widely available. However, knowing whether these antibodies are present preoperatively would be useful because re-exposure to bovine thrombin-containing products is contraindicated in patients with pre-existing antiproduct antibodies due to the risk of developing immune-mediated coagulopathies. In these exploratory analyses, we characterized one aspect of immune sensitization, the persistence of circulating antibodies after exposure to bovine thrombin product.

Study Design.—Elapsed time since a historical surgical procedure with documented or highly likely use of bovine thrombin product was determined for 204 patients enrolled in a recently completed trial. After study completion, baseline samples were assayed for antibovine thrombin product antibodies using validated immunoassays. Antibody data were sorted by time elapsed since the historical procedure. The proportion of patients with antibovine thrombin product antibodies and 95% confidence interval (CI) were determined for each 1-year period, providing an estimate for antibody persistence.

Results.—Antibovine thrombin product antibodies were detected in 20.7% of patients (23 of 111; 95% CI 14.2%, 29.2%) with ≤1 year since the historical surgical procedure; 6.8% of patients (3 of 44; 95% CI 1.68%, 18.9%) with 1 to <2 years; 16.1% of patients (5 of 31; 95% CI 6.62%, 33.1%) with 2 to <3 years; and 5.6% of patients (1 of 18; 95% CI 0.00%, 27.6%) with ≥3 years since the historical procedure.

Conclusions.—The proportion of patients with antibovine thrombin product antibodies ranged from 5.6% to 20.7% across the multiyear postoperative window. Clinicians should be aware that antibodies to bovine thrombin products may persist for years after exposure.

▶ While the results of this investigation largely confirm other studies, it is important to reemphasize the potential for preexisting antibodies to bovine thrombin to cause immune-mediated coagulopathy. The availability of a readily available assay for antiplatelet antibodies has allowed improved understanding of the condition of heparin-induced thrombocytopenia; however, no readily available assay exists for antibodies to bovine thrombin. Furthermore, medical records do not always reliably document patient exposure to bovine thrombin, so many studies of this clinical problem depend on analysis of patients who have a high likelihood of exposure to bovine thrombin. Despite these obvious shortcomings in the data analysis, this study shows that a significant number of patients have antibodies to bovine thrombin up to 2 years after exposure. The fact that antibody titers were highly variable across the time periods and encompassed a more than 100-fold range (1.7-4.2 log units) is of concern since it is unknown whether a threshold exists where a certain antibody level increases the likelihood of development of a clinically relevant coagulopathy. As our understanding of the need to have maximized patient safety in every possible venue, this article makes the ongoing case for using recombinant thrombin products.

M. T. Watkins, MD

Postthrombotic vein wall remodeling: Preliminary observations
Deatrick KB, Elfline M, Baker N, et al (Univ of Michigan Health System, Ann Arbor)
J Vasc Surg 53:139-146, 2011

Background.—Postthrombotic syndrome is characterized by a fibrotic vein injury following deep vein thrombosis (DVT). We sought to quantify the change in vein wall thickness in patients who fail to resolve DVT by 6 months and whether there were differences in blood or plasma levels of inflammatory proteins associated with venous remodeling.

Methods.—Patients presenting with confirmed lower extremity DVT were prospectively recruited for this study. Duplex imaging of the lower extremity venous system was performed, and blood was collected at entrance and repeat evaluation with blood draw and ultrasound imaging at 1 and 6 months. DVT resolution and thickness of the vein wall was quantified by ultrasound imaging in each segment affected by thrombus, and a contralateral, unaffected vein wall served as a control. Gene and protein expression of inflammatory markers were examined from leukocytes and serum, respectively. Analysis of variance or Student t-tests were used, and a $P < .05$ was significant. N = 10 to 12 for all analyses.

Results.—Thirty-two patients (12 patients with DVT resolution at 6 months, 10 patients with persistent thrombus at 6 months, and 10 healthy controls) were compared. Both resolving and nonresolving DVT were associated with a 1.5- to 1.8-fold increased vein wall thickness at 6 months ($P = .008$) as compared with nonaffected vein wall segments. However, the thickness of the affected segments was 1.4-fold greater in patients who had total resolution of the DVT by 6 months than in patients who had persistent chronic thrombus 6 months after presentation ($P = .01$). There was a four- to five-fold increased level of matrix metalloproteinase-9 (MMP-9) antigen in thrombosed patients compared with nonthrombosed patient controls ($P < .05$), while Toll-like receptor-9 (TLR-9) gene expression was three-fold less than controls ($P < .05$) at enrollment. D-dimer and P-selectin were higher in thrombosed as compared to controls at diagnosis but not at 6 months. Both TLR-4 (marker of inflammation) and P-selectin gene expression were higher in leukocytes from patients with chronic DVT compared with those who resolved at 1 month after diagnosis ($P < .05$).

Conclusions.—This preliminary study suggests ongoing vein wall remodeling after DVT, measurable by ultrasound and associated with certain biomarkers. At 6 months, the vein wall is markedly thickened and directly correlates with resolution. This suggests that the vein wall response is initiated early following thrombus formation and persists even in the presence of total resolution.

▶ This article is extremely important because it provides data on ultrasound findings and serum markers of inflammation that may predict persistence of thrombosis and higher risk of postthrombotic syndrome. The rationale for these studies is based on the possibility that identification of patients at risk for postthrombotic syndrome might allow patients to be treated with more aggressive interventions such as pharmacomechanical thrombectomy. A crucial finding was that patients who resolved their deep vein thrombosis (DVT) had higher serum P-selectin at 1 month after enrollment, indicating that active thrombus metabolism is occurring in patients whose clot is resolving compared with those with a chronic thrombus. Importantly, most of the genetic and molecular markers of inflammation that differentiated clot resolvers versus nonresolvers were present at 1 month rather than 6 months. Most clinicians would be wary of undertaking pharmacomechanical thrombolysis at 6 months following DVT but not at 1 month. Thus an important missing bit of information from this article is clinical symptoms. If investigators of this important clinical problem were able to draw an association between early symptoms (or quality of life) and these molecular markers, a greater rationale for early pharmacomechanical thrombolysis could be made.

M. T. Watkins, MD

Relation of *Aspirin* Failure to Clinical Outcome and to Platelet Response to *Aspirin* in Patients With Acute Myocardial Infarction

Beigel R, Hod H, Fefer P, et al (Chaim Sheba Med Ctr, Tel-Hashomer, Israel; et al)
Am J Cardiol 107:339-342, 2011

Aspirin failure, defined as occurrence of an acute coronary syndrome despite aspirin use, has been associated with a higher cardiovascular risk profile and worse prognosis. Whether this phenomenon is a manifestation of patient characteristics or failure of adequate platelet inhibition by aspirin has never been studied. We evaluated 174 consecutive patients with acute myocardial infarction. Of them, 118 (68%) were aspirin naive and 56 (32%) were regarded as having aspirin failure. Platelet function was analyzed after ≥72 hours of aspirin therapy in all patients. Platelet reactivity was studied by light-transmitted aggregometry and under flow conditions. Six-month incidence of major adverse coronary events (death, recurrent acute coronary syndrome, and/or stroke) was determined. Those with aspirin failure were older (p = 0.002), more hypertensive (p <0.001), more hyperlipidemic (p <0.001), and more likely to have had a previous cardiovascular event and/or procedure (p <0.001). Cumulative 6-month major adverse coronary events were higher in the aspirinfailure group (14.3% vs 2.5% p <0.01). Patients with aspirin failure had lower arachidonic acid–induced platelet aggregation (32 ± 24 vs 45 ± 30, p = 0.003) after aspirin therapy compared to their aspirin-naive counterparts. However, this was not significant after adjusting for differences in baseline characteristics (p = 0.82). Similarly, there were no significant differences in adenosine diphosphate–induced platelet aggregation and platelet deposition under flow conditions. In conclusion, our results suggest that aspirin failure is merely a marker of higher-risk patient profiles and not a manifestation of inadequate platelet response to aspirin therapy.

▶ This intriguing article sought to understand whether the clinical definition of aspirin failure in patients suffering from an acute myocardial infarction was related to a primary defect in platelet aggregation. While there was evidence of reduced arachidonic acid–induced platelet aggregation, this was related primarily to underlying risk factors than an actual defect in the platelet response to aspirin therapy. The arachidonic acid response is often associated with alterations in membrane lipids; however, 63% of the aspirin failure patients were on a statin. It's not known from the study whether these patients were on adequate doses of statins or had an appropriate therapeutic response to statin therapy. Certainly we believe there are likely similar circumstances in patients with carotid restenosis or early vein graft failure. A number of clinical databases such as the private sector National Surgical Quality Improvement Program or the Vascular Study Group of New England used to study quality of care in surgical patients may be able to provide important information regarding the potential role of aspirin failure in patients following peripheral vascular interventions.

M. T. Watkins, MD

Resveratrol Reverses Endothelial Nitric-Oxide Synthase Uncoupling in Apolipoprotein E Knockout Mice
Xia N, Daiber A, Habermeier A, et al (Johannes Gutenberg Univ, Mainz, Germany; et al)
J Pharmacol Exp Ther 335:149-154, 2010

A crucial cause of the decreased bioactivity of nitric oxide (NO) in cardiovascular diseases is the uncoupling of the endothelial NO synthase (eNOS) caused by the oxidative stress-mediated deficiency of the NOS cofactor tetrahydrobiopterin (BH_4). The reversal of eNOS uncoupling might represent a novel therapeutic approach. The treatment of apolipoprotein E knockout (ApoE-KO) mice with resveratrol resulted in the up-regulation of superoxide dismutase (SOD) isoforms (SOD1–SOD3), glutathione peroxidase 1 (GPx1), and catalase and the down-regulation of NADPH oxidases NOX2 and NOX4 in the hearts of ApoE-KO mice. This was associated with reductions in superoxide, 3-nitrotyrosine, and malondialdehyde levels. In parallel, the cardiac expression of GTP cyclohydrolase 1 (GCH1), the rate-limiting enzyme in BH_4 biosynthesis, was enhanced by resveratrol. This enhancement was accompanied by an elevation in BH4 levels. Superoxide production from ApoE-KO mice hearts was reduced by the NOS inhibitor L-N^G-nitro-arginine methyl ester, indicating eNOS uncoupling in this pathological model. Resveratrol treatment resulted in a reversal of eNOS uncoupling. Treatment of human endothelial cells with resveratrol led to an up-regulation of SOD1, SOD2, SOD3, GPx1, catalase, and GCH1. Some of these effects were preventable with sirtinol, an inhibitor of the protein deacetylase sirtuin 1. In summary, resveratrol decreased superoxide production and enhanced the inactivation of reactive oxygen species. The resulting reduction in BH_4 oxidation, together with the enhanced biosynthesis of BH_4 by GCH1, probably was responsible for the reversal of eNOS uncoupling. This novel mechanism (reversal of eNOS uncoupling) might contribute to the protective effects of resveratrol.

▶ The ability of the enzyme endothelial nitric oxide synthase (eNOS) to produce NO is dependent on the presence of oxygen, arginine, and an enzymatic cofactor called tetrahydrobiopterin (BH_4). Deficiencies in NOS activity are believed to be associated with hypertension, atherosclerosis, and thrombotic events. This article provides mechanistic insight on how resveratrol, a polyphenol phytoalexin that is present in a variety of plant species and red wine, may reverse eNOS dysfunction. This of course has relevance to the theory as to why red wine appears to be protective against cardiovascular morbidity in select populations. The authors provide conclusive evidence that resveratrol induces the expression of antioxidant enzymes that reduce oxidative and nitrosative stress in cardiac tissue. Resveratrol also enhanced the expression of guanosine triphosphate cyclohydrolase 1, the rate-limiting enzyme in BH_4 biosynthesis. Thus resveratrol has multiple mechanistic effects, which can prevent eNOS dysfunction. The abstract does not do the whole substance of the article justice because hidden in the discussion part of the article is intriguing speculation that is data driven. The authors provide a supplemental figure in the original article demonstrating where they used a sirtuin 1 (SIRT1) inhibitor sirtinol and SIRT1 small interfering RNA to demonstrate that some of the effects of resveratrol on gene expression are indeed SIRT1 dependent. SIRT1 is a histone deacetylase SIRT1, which regulates a variety of cellular functions such as genome maintenance, longevity, and metabolism. It is highly likely that this also applies to the in vivo effect of resveratrol. There are many ways to induce SIRT1, which may be relevant to ischemia reperfusion in patients with cardiovascular disease or those require organ transplantation.

M. T. Watkins, MD

S-glutathionylation uncouples eNOS and regulates its cellular and vascular function
Chen C-A, Wang T-Y, Varadharaj S, et al (Ohio State Univ, Columbus)
Nature 468:1115-1118, 2010

Endothelial nitric oxide synthase (eNOS) is critical in the regulation of vascular function, and can generate both nitric oxide (NO) and superoxide ($O_2\bullet^-$), which are key mediators of cellular signalling. In the presence of Ca^{2+}/calmodulin, eNOS produces NO, endothelial-derived relaxing factor, from L-arginine (L-Arg) by means of electron transfer from NADPH through a flavin containing reductase domain to oxygen bound at the haem of an oxygenase domain, which also contains binding sites for tetrahydrobiopterin (BH4) and L-Arg. In the absence of BH4, NO synthesis is abrogated and instead $O_2\bullet^-$ is generated. While NOS dysfunction occurs in diseases with redox stress, BH_4 repletion only partly restores NOS activity and NOS-dependent vasodilation. This suggests that there is an as yet unidentified redox-regulated mechanism controlling NOS function. Protein thiols can undergo S-glutathionylation, a reversible protein modification involved in cellular signalling and adaptation. Under oxidative stress, S-glutathionylation occurs through thiol–disulphide exchange with oxidized glutathione or reaction of oxidant-induced protein thiyl radicals with reduced glutathione. Cysteine residues are critical for the maintenance of eNOS function; we therefore speculated that oxidative stress could alter eNOS activity through S-glutathionylation. Here we show that S-glutathionylation of eNOS reversibly decreases NOS activity with an increase in $O_2\bullet^-$ generation primarily from the reductase, in which two highly conserved cysteine residues are identified as sites of S-glutathionylation and found to be critical for redox-regulation of eNOS function. We show that eNOS Sglutathionylation in endothelial cells, with loss of NO and gain of $O_2\bullet^-$ generation, is associated with impaired endothelium-dependent vasodilation. In hypertensive vessels, eNOS S-glutathionylation is increased with impaired endothelium-dependent vasodilation that is restored by thiol-specific reducing agents, which reverse this S-glutathionylation. Thus, S-glutathionylation of eNOS is a pivotal switch providing redox regulation of cellular signalling, endothelial function and vascular tone.

▶ This is an important article because it sheds light on why the enzyme nitric oxide synthase (eNOS) has the potential to be both cytotoxic and cytoprotective. NOS is an enzyme responsible for synthesizing nitric oxide (NO), a vascular signaling molecule which is actually a gas. The Nobel Prize in Medicine was awarded to Furghott and Ignarro for their seminal description and elucidation of the nature of this molecule. While innumerable models of ischemia, reperfusion, and intimal hyperplasia have shown that administration of exogenous NO donors, and in some instances, NOS inhibitors can provide protection against vascular injury, the fate of endogenous NOS is not clearly known. This article shows that conditions of oxidative stress (inflammation and reperfusion injury) can result in uncoupling of NOS, so that the toxic reactive oxygen metabolite superoxide ion is produced instead of NO. These investigators identify a precise mechanism contributing to NOS uncoupling. They observed that oxidized glutathione induced a dose-dependent S-glutathionylation of human eNOS that was chemically reversed by reducing agents. This means that conditions that prevent oxidation of glutathione could also protect uncoupling of NOS and prevent tissue injury in a variety of conditions.

M. T. Watkins, MD

Tissue Characterization of In-Stent Neointima Using Intravascular Ultrasound Radiofrequency Data Analysis
Kang S-J, Mintz GS, Park D-W, et al (Univ of Ulsan College of Medicine, Seoul, Korea; Cardiovascular Res Foundation, NY)
Am J Cardiol 106:1561-1565, 2010

Using virtual histology and intravascular ultrasound (VH-IVUS), tissue characterization of restenotic in-stent neointima after drug-eluting stent (DES) and bare metal stent (BMS) implantation was assessed. VH-IVUS was performed in 117 lesions (70 treated with DESs and 47 treated with BMSs) with angiographic in-stent restenosis and intimal hyperplasia (IH) >50% of the stent area. The region of interest was placed between the luminal border and the inner border of the struts and tissue composition was reported as percentages of IH area (percent fibrous, percent fibrofatty, percent necrotic core, percent dense calcium) at the 2 sites of maximal percent IH and maximal percent necrotic core. Mean follow-up times between stent implantation and VH-IVUS study were 43.5 ± 33.8 months for BMS-treated lesions and 11.1 ± 7.8 months for DES-treated lesions (p < 0.001). The 2 groups had greater percent necrotic core and percent dense calcium at maximal percent IH and maximal percent necrotic core sites, especially in stents that had been implanted for longer periods. In conclusion, this VH-IVUS analysis showed that BMS- and DES-treated lesions develop in-stent necrotic core and dense calcium, suggesting the development of in-stent neoatherosclerosis.

▶ The major finding of this virtual histology/intravascular ultrasound assessment of in-stent restenotic lesions is that stents that have been implanted for 24 months or longer develop stenotic lesions that contain a necrotic core and dense calcium, suggestive of in-stent neoatherosclerosis. These findings are in contrast to histopathologic studies that have reported that the main components of restenotic tissue after drug-eluting stent or bare metal stent (BMS) implantation are proteoglycan-rich smooth muscle cells and fibrolipid regions.

Previously, BMSs had been associated with an early peak in intimal hyperplasia (IH), occurring 6 to 12 months after implantation, followed by regression of IH and a decrease in luminal narrowing. These authors point out that a longer-term follow-up study after BMS implantation has revealed a triphasic luminal response characterized by an early restenosis phase (within 6 months), an intermediate regression phase, and a late renarrowing phase (4 years), suggesting that in-stent restenosis may not be as stable as previously thought. The findings in this report are based on observations in the coronary circulation and need to be evaluated in the peripheral arena. These findings may mean that virtual histology and intravascular ultrasound examinations of in-stent restenosis should be considered as a routine component for the assessment of in-stent restenosis. The kind of novel secondary intervention for in-stent restenosis may be dictated by the findings from this kind of analysis. Calcified lesions might be better treated with repeat angioplasty/stenting, whereas fibromuscular lesions might be better addressed with photodynamic therapy or other novel therapeutic modalities.

M. T. Watkins, MD

Zoledronate Inhibits Intimal Hyperplasia in Balloon-injured Rat Carotid Artery
Wu L, Zhu L, Shi WH, et al (Huashan Hosp of Fudan Univ, Shanghai, China)
Eur J Vasc Endovasc Surg 41:288-293, 2011

Background and Objective.—Zoledronate has been reported to inhibit the proliferation, adhesion and migration of vascular smooth muscle cells. In the present study, we assessed whether systemic and local delivery of zoledronate would be sufficient to prevent intimal hyperplasia.

Methods.—Twenty-four male Sprague-Dawley rats were assigned into four groups: non-treated group, systemic zoledronate-treated group, local collagen-treated group and local zoledronate-treated group. All four groups underwent balloon injury to the right common carotid artery. The left uninjured carotid arteries of the non-treated group were considered as normal artery samples. Twenty-one days after arterial injury and treatment, the right and left common carotid arteries were fixed, sectioned, stained and measured by computer-aided image analysis.

Results.—At 3 weeks, there was a 59% reduction of the intima/media area ratio in the systemic zoledronate-treated group compared with the non-treated group ($P < 0.01$). There was an 87% reduction of the intima/media area ratio in the local zoledronate-treated group compared with the local collagen-treated group ($P < 0.01$).

Conclusions.—Both systemic and local delivery of zoledronate correspond to a significant reduction in intimal hyperplasia seen at 3 weeks.

▶ This article reflects a logical extension of the authors' previous in vitro studies where they established the novel concept that zoledronic acid has the ability to alter rat vascular smooth muscle cell proliferation, migration, and adhesion.

Those findings were seminal since prior to that article, the general concept in the scientific community was that zoledronate and bisphosphonates modulated vascular disease through their action on macrophages. It is clear from these studies where zoledronate was administered locally to balloon-injured arteries that zoledronate can modulate in vivo intimal hyperplasia in the short term (3 weeks). It remains to be determined that this action is entirely independent of macrophages since zoledronate could be modulating the local activity of macrophages in the arterial wall. If the inhibition of intimal hyperplasia was to occur in the absence of macrophages, our understanding of what cells are inactivated by zoledronate would be clearer. These findings are encouraging since zoledronate is already approved by the Food and Drug Administration for other uses. Long-term in vivo studies on the durability of this treatment are needed.

M. T. Watkins, MD

Mitochondrial Injury Underlies Hyporeactivity of Arterial Smooth Muscle in Severe Shock

Song R, Bian H, Wang X, et al (Southern Med Univ, Guangzhou, PR China)
Am J Hypertens 24:45-51, 2011

Background.—Our previous data showed membrane hyperpolarization of arteriolar smooth muscle cells (ASMCs) caused by adenosine triphosphate (ATP)—sensitive potassium channels (K_{ATP}) activation contributed to vascular hyporeactivity in shock. Despite supply of oxygen and nutrients, vascular hyporeactivity to vasoconstrictor agents still remains, which may result from low ATP level. The study was designed to investigate shock-induced mitochondrial changes of rat ASMCs in the genesis and treatment of hypotension in severe shock.

Methods.—The animals were divided into four groups: controls, hemorrhagic shock, CsA+shock (preadministration of cyclosporin A before bleeding), and ATR+CsA+shock (preadministration of atractyloside, followed by CsA and bleeding). ASMCs were isolated and the ultrastructure and function of ASMC mitochondria and the vasoresponsiveness to norepinephrine (NE) was measured on microcirculatory preparations.

Results.—Ultrastructurally, the hemorrhagic shock group showed swollen mitochondria with poorly defined cristae. In this group, the number of ASMCs with low mitochondrial membrane potential ($\Delta\psi_m$) was increased by 49.7%, and the intracellular ATP level was reduced by 82.1%, which led to activation of K_{ATP} plasma membrane channels with resultant ASMC hyperpolarization and low vasoreactivity. These changes were reduced in the CsA+shock group. When mitochondrial damage was aggravated by ATR in the ATR+CsA+shock group, the CsA did not protect. Compared to the shock group, vasoresponsiveness to NE was much improved in the CsA+shock group.

Conclusions.—Mitochondrial ASMC dysfunction is involved in the genesis of reduced vasoreactivity in severe shock. Mitochondrial protection may therefore be a new approach in the treatment of shock-induced hypotension.

▶ The authors describe the potential molecular basis for the lack of response to a routinely used vasopressor (norepinephrine) in a model of shock. This is a clinically relevant question, as it describes a commonly encountered scenario for patients with severe hemorrhage. The authors detail a sequence of cellular events that starts with the opening of the nonspecific mitochondrial permeability transition pore. This pore opening, which occurs during reperfusion (ie, the resuscitation after the shock), leads to influx of water molecules and resultant swelling. The authors demonstrate in a series of experiments, the architectural changes, altered membrane potential, and reduced adenosine triphosphate in the mitochondria after the onset of hemorrhage in their rat model of shock. This in turn is tied to a decreased influx of calcium and ultimately to impaired response of the arteriolar smooth muscle to norepinephrine. This report is interesting in its mechanistic description of the problem and in the demonstration of the role of cyclosporine, a clinically available drug, in reversing this dysfunction. It will be interesting to see follow-up work with cyclosporine given after the onset of hemorrhage (ischemia), conditions which more truthfully recapitulate clinical practice.

R. S. Crawford, MD

Vascular Endothelial Growth Factor-B Acts as a Coronary Growth Factor in Transgenic Rats Without Inducing Angiogenesis, Vascular Leak, or Inflammation

Bry M, Kivelä R, Holopainen T, et al (Univ of Helsinki and Helsinki Univ Central Hosp, Finland; et al)
Circulation 122:1725-1733, 2010

Background.—Vascular endothelial growth factor-B (VEGF-B) binds to VEGF receptor-1 and neuropilin-1 and is abundantly expressed in the heart, skeletal muscle, and brown fat. The biological function of VEGF-B is incompletely understood.

Methods and Results.—Unlike placenta growth factor, which binds to the same receptors, adeno-associated viral delivery of VEGF-B to mouse skeletal or heart muscle induced very little angiogenesis, vascular permeability, or inflammation. As previously reported for the VEGF-B$_{167}$ isoform, transgenic mice and rats expressing both isoforms of VEGF-B in the myocardium developed cardiac hypertrophy yet maintained systolic function. Deletion of the VEGF receptor-1 tyrosine kinase domain or the arterial endothelial Bmx tyrosine kinase inhibited hypertrophy, whereas loss of VEGF-B interaction with neuropilin-1 had no effect. Surprisingly, in rats, the heart-specific VEGF-B transgene induced impressive growth of the epicardial coronary vessels and their branches, with large arteries also seen deep inside the subendocardial myocardium. However, VEGF-B, unlike other VEGF family members, did not induce significant capillary angiogenesis, increased permeability, or inflammatory cell recruitment.

Conclusions.—VEGF-B appears to be a coronary growth factor in rats but not in mice. The signals for the VEGF-B—induced cardiac hypertrophy are mediated at least in part via the endothelium. Because cardiomyocyte damage in myocardial ischemia begins in the subendocardial myocardium, the VEGF-B—induced increased arterial supply to this area could have therapeutic potential in ischemic heart disease.

▶ Vascular endothelial growth factor (VEGF) has been well documented as a potent angiogenic growth factor. However, it also promotes inflammation and vascular leakage. In this study, the authors elucidate the functions of VEGF-B. VEGF-B binds to VEGF receptor-1 (VEGFR-1) and neuropilin-1, both of which are expressed in heart muscle. Transgenic mice and rats bearing different isoforms of VEGF-B were generated. Also, adenoassociated virus vectors with the VEGF-B genes were injected into skeletal muscle and myocardium of experimental animals. The main findings of this study were that VEGF-B induced a remarkable growth of the coronary vascular tree in the rat and promoted myocardial hypertrophy in both the mouse and rat. These arteries in the rat were nearly the caliber of epicardial coronary arteries. Unlike VEGF and placental growth factor, VEGF-B did not induce any inflammation or vascular permeability. Additionally, the authors found that deletion of the VEGFR-1 tyrosine kinase domain or the arterial Bmx tyrosine kinase attenuated the hypertrophic effects of VEGF-B. These results have potentially significant therapeutic applications in patients with myocardial ischemia.

R. S. Crawford, MD

2 Coronary Disease

Vital Exhaustion as a Risk Factor for Adverse Cardiac Events (from the Atherosclerosis Risk in Communities [ARIC] Study)
Williams JE, Mosley TH Jr, Kop WJ, et al (LaGrange College, GA; Univ of Mississippi Med Ctr, Jackson; Univ of Maryland School of Medicine, Baltimore; et al)
Am J Cardiol 105:1661-1665, 2010

Vital exhaustion, defined as excessive fatigue, feelings of demoralization, and increased irritability, has been identified as a risk factor for incident and recurrent cardiac events, but there are no population-based prospective studies of this association in US samples. We examined the predictive value of vital exhaustion for incident myocardial infarction or fatal coronary heart disease in middle-aged men and women in 4 US communities. Participants were 12,895 black or white men and women enrolled in the Atherosclerosis Risk In Communities (ARIC) study cohort and followed for the occurrence of cardiac morbidity and mortality from 1990 through 2002 (maximum follow-up 13.0 years). Vital exhaustion was assessed using the 21-item Maastricht Questionnaire and scores were partitioned into approximate quartiles for statistical analyses. High vital exhaustion (fourth quartile) predicted adverse cardiac events in age-, gender-, and race-center—adjusted analyses (1.69, 95% confidence interval 1.40 to 2.05) and in analyses further adjusted for educational level, body mass index, plasma low-density lipoprotein and high-density lipoprotein cholesterol levels, systolic and diastolic blood pressure levels, diabetes mellitus, cigarette smoking status, and pack-years of cigarette smoking (1.46, 95% confidence interval 1.20 to 1.79). Risk for adverse cardiac events increased monotonically from the first through the fourth quartile of vital exhaustion. Probabilities of adverse cardiac events over time were significantly higher in people with high vital exhaustion compared to those with low exhaustion (p = 0.002). In conclusion, vital exhaustion predicts long-term risk for adverse cardiac events in men and women, independent of established biomedical risk factors (Fig 1).

▶ Vital exhaustion is defined as a state of excessive fatigue, increased irritability, and demoralization. European studies have suggested a link between vital exhaustion and coronary heart disease. Vital exhaustion is closely linked to depression, and the 2 conditions share common characteristics such as irritability and fatigue. The study indicates that fatigue is a real and measurable risk factor for cardiovascular disease (Fig 1). Fatigue has also previously been

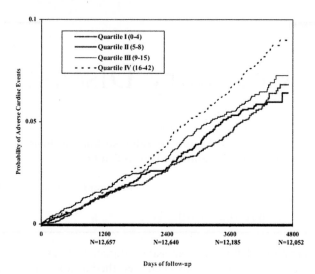

FIGURE 1.—Kaplan-Meier product limit estimate of the cumulative probability of adverse cardiac events by level of vital exhaustion (p = 0.01, 0.0005, 0.002 for differences between quartiles 4 and 3, quartiles 4 and 2, and quartiles 4 and 1, respectively). (Reprinted from the American Journal of Cardiology, Williams JE, Mosley TH Jr, Kop WJ, et al. Vital exhaustion as a risk factor for adverse cardiac events (from the Atherosclerosis Risk In Communities [ARIC] study). *Am J Cardiol.* 2010;105:1661-1665. Copyright 2010, with permission from Elsevier.)

associated with myocardial infarction (MI). This is especially so in women. Over 70% of women in a recent study reported unusual fatigue prior to MI with about 30% of men reporting fatigue preceding MI.[1] Other studies have also suggested an inverse relationship between exhaustion and social/economic status.[2] The Maastricht Questionnaire examines only the presence or absence of vital exhaustion but not the etiology. It is possible residual or unmeasured confounders, such as the underlying etiology of vital exhaustion, may be additive risk factors for cardiovascular events.

G. L. Moneta, MD

References

1. McSweeney JC, Cody M, O'Sullivan P, Elberson K, Moser DK, Garvin BJ. Women's early warning symptoms of acute myocardial infarction. *Circulation.* 2003; 108:2619-2623.
2. Schuitemaker GE, Dinant GJ, van der Pol GA, Appels A. Assessment of vital exhaustion and identification of subjects at increased risk of myocardial infarction in general practice. *Psychosomatics.* 2004;45:414-418.

Simultaneous Aortic and Coronary Assessment in Abdominal Aortic Aneurysm Patients by Thoraco-abdominal 64-Detector-row CT Angiography: Estimate of the Impact on Preoperative Management: A Pilot Study
Budde RPJ, Huo F, Cramer MJM, et al (Univ Med Ctr Utrecht, The Netherlands; Yantai Yuhuangding Hosp, China)
Eur J Vasc Endovasc Surg 40:196-201, 2010

Objectives.—To estimate the influence of information on the coronary arteries obtained from routine thoraco-abdominal CT angiography (CTA) on pre-operative clinical management in abdominal aortic aneurysm (AAA) patients.

Methods.—Twenty-eight AAA patients underwent pre-operative thoraco-abdominal electrocardiography (ECG)-gated 64-detector-row CTA to evaluate aortic pulsatility for prosthesis size matching. Retrospectively, the coronaries were reconstructed from the same data set and scored on a per segment basis for stenosis (0%, ≤50% or >50%) and grading confidence (poor, adequate or high). An experienced cardiologist was presented information on patient characteristics obtained from patient records and CTA findings. Suggested changes in European Society of Cardiology guidelines based patient management based on CTA information were scored.

Results.—On CTA, 17 patients (61%) had significant coronary disease (>50% stenosis) including left main ($n = 4$), single ($n = 7$) and multiple ($n = 6$) vessel disease. Grading confidence was adequate or high in 86% of proximal and middle segments. Based on CTA findings, patient management would have been changed in 4 out of the 28 patients (14%; 95% CI 1−27%) by adding coronary angiography ($n = 4$). In five patients who underwent coronary artery bypass grafting previously, CT did not change management but confirmed graft patency.

Conclusions.—Information on coronary pathology and coronary bypass graft patency can be readily obtained from thoraco-abdominal CTA and may alter pre-operative patient management, as shown in 14% of AAA patients in our study.

▶ Dedicated electrocardiogram-gated CT of the chest has been validated against coronary angiography for identifying coronary artery disease with 64-row detector scanners (sensitivity = 98%; specificity = 88%; and negative predictive value = 96%).[1] Coronary CT angiography (CTA) is useful in patients with a low to moderate pretest probability in which a negative study excludes coronary artery disease. However, a positive study only has a 50% to 60% likelihood of identifying clinically significant disease as determined by cardiac stress testing. All patients with aortic aneurysmal disease undergo CTA evaluation that typically includes both the chest and abdominal vessels. The authors used retrospective cardiac gating to evaluate the coronary artery vessels in patients undergoing thoracoabdominal CTA. Using these images, while not protocoled for specific coronary imaging, the proximal and middle coronary artery segments were visualized in 93% and 92%, respectively. The compromise in temporal resolution resulted in only 50% of distal beds being visualized. When compared with standard preoperative cardiac risk stratification, the thoracoabdominal CTA changed preoperative testing in 4 of 28 patients. This study does not change current preoperative risk assessment guidelines, but it is intuitive to review preoperative thoracoabdominal imaging for the assessment of coronary artery disease as part of the cardiac risk evaluation.

Z. M. Arthurs, MD

Reference

1. Stein PD, Yaekoub AY, Matta F, Sostman HD. 64-slice CT for diagnosis of coronary artery disease: a systematic review. *Am J Med.* 2008;121:715-725.

3 Epidemiology

Arterial stiffness predicts cardiovascular outcome in a low-to-moderate cardiovascular risk population: the EDIVA (*Estudo de DIstensibilidade VAscular*) project
Maldonado J, for the participants in the EDIVA Project (Faculdade de Medicina da Universidade de Lisboa, Penacova, Portugal)
J Hypertens 29:669-675, 2011

Background.—Pulse wave velocity (PWV) is a recognized marker of arterial stiffness, although little knowledge exists of their relationship to long-term cardiovascular risk in general populations.

Methods and Results.—A prospective, multicenter, observational study included 2200 Portuguese nationals (1290 men), aged between 18 and 91 years (mean 46.33 ± 13.76 years). They underwent clinical assessment and annual PWV measurement using a Complior device, and major adverse cardiovascular events (MACEs) — death, stroke, myocardial infarction, unstable angina, peripheral arterial disease, revascularization, or renal failure — were recorded. During a mean follow-up of 21.42 ± 10.76 months, there were 47 nonfatal MACEs (2.1% of the sample). PWV was significantly higher in individuals with events than in those without events (11.76 ± 2.13 vs. 10.01 ± 2.01 m/s, respectively, $P<0.001$). The study population was divided into two groups by PWV, classified as normal (PWV <95th percentile) or high (PWV >95th percentile), according to predefined criteria for normality. Cumulative event-free survival at 2 years was 99.3% in the normal PWV group and 95% in the high PWV group. The hazard ratio for MACE in the high PWV group was 9.901 [95% confidence interval (CI) $5.00-19.59$, $P<0.001$], and 4.832 (95% CI $2.35-9.94$, $P<0.001$) when adjusted for other risk factors. For absolute PWV, the adjusted hazard ratio (per 1 m/s change) was 1.316 (95% CI $1.13-1.53$, $P<0.001$).

Conclusion.—The results of the initial analysis of this study highlight the clinical relevance of PWV as a cardiovascular risk marker and demonstrate that PWV measurement can make an important contribution to assessment of cardiovascular prognosis (Fig 1).

▶ Arterial stiffness is thought to be a manifestation of early atherosclerosis and pulse wave velocity (PWV) measurements reflect arterial stiffness. PWV measurements are used to measure aortic distensibility. More distensible aortas are less stiff than less distensible aortas. PWV measurements, therefore, are increased in less distensible aortas. As decreased distensibility of the aorta may be a marker of atherosclerosis, patients with decreased aortic distensibility

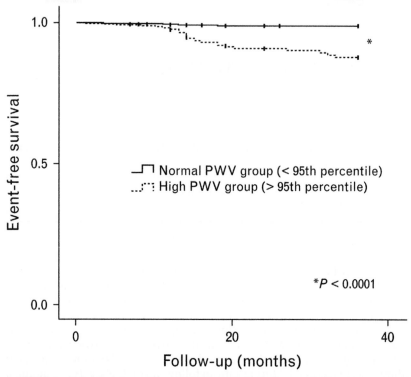

FIGURE 1.—Probability of event-free survival in the study population according to pulse wave velocity (normal PWV group: unbroken line vs. high PWV group: broken line). The difference between the groups was highly significant (P < 0.0001). (Reprinted from Maldonado J, for the participants in the EDIVA Project. Arterial stiffness predicts cardiovascular outcome in a low-to-moderate cardiovascular risk population: the EDIVA (*Estudo de DIstensibilidade VAscular*) project. *J Hypertens.* 2011;29:669-675, with permission from Wolters Kluwer Health Lippincott Williams & Wilkins.)

may be at increased risk of cardiovascular events. This study was designed to determine the relationship between PWV measurements as a reflection of arterial stiffness and long-term cardiovascular risk in the general population. PWV measurements were based on distance/time ratio in m/s with the pulse wave measured in the right carotid and right femoral artery. Normal PWV measurements were defined statistically according to the 95th percentile adjusted for sex and age calculated from a sample of 668 individuals with low cardiovascular risk and a mean age of 39.73 ± 15.6 years. Increasingly, investigators are evaluating arterial distensibility as a risk factor for clinical cardiovascular events. Previous investigations have shown that carotid femoral PWV is an excellent indicator of aortic stiffness and is related to cardiovascular mortality and morbidity in patients with diabetes, hypertension, or renal failure.[1,2] One of the goals of this study was to raise awareness of the concept of arterial distensibility as a cardiovascular risk factor (Fig 1). The authors hope to convince primary care physicians that PWV assessment can be useful in a therapeutic approach to modification of cardiovascular risk. Additional work, however, will clearly be required demonstrating modification of cardiovascular risk based on an assessment of PWV measurements that results in a decrease in clinical events.

G. L. Moneta, MD

References

1. Blacher J, Guerin AP, Pannier B, Marchais SJ, Safar ME, London GM. Impact of aortic stiffness on survival in end-stage renal disease. *Circulation.* 1999;99: 2434-2439.
2. Laurent S, Boutouyrie P, Asmar R, et al. Aortic stiffness is an independent predictor of all-cause and cardiovascular mortality in hypertensive patients. *Hypertension.* 2001;37:1236-1241.

Aspirin for Prevention of Cardiovascular Events in a General Population Screened for a Low Ankle Brachial Index: A Randomized Controlled Trial
Fowkes FGR, for the Aspirin for Asymptomatic Atherosclerosis Trialists (Univ of Edinburgh, Scotland; et al)
JAMA 303:841-848, 2010

Context.—A low ankle brachial index (ABI) indicates atherosclerosis and an increased risk of cardiovascular and cerebrovascular events. Screening for a low ABI can identify an asymptomatic higher risk group potentially amenable to preventive treatments.

Objective.—To determine the effectiveness of aspirin in preventing events in people with a low ABI identified on screening the general population.

Design, Setting, and Participants.—The Aspirin for Asymptomatic Atherosclerosis trial was an intention-to-treat double-blind randomized controlled trial conducted from April 1998 to October 2008, involving 28 980 men and women aged 50 to 75 years living in central Scotland, free of clinical cardiovascular disease, recruited from a community health registry, and had an ABI screening test. Of those, 3350 with a low ABI (≤ 0.95) were entered into the trial, which was powered to detect a 25% proportional risk reduction in events.

Interventions.—Once daily 100 mg aspirin (enteric coated) or placebo.

Main Outcome Measures.—The primary end point was a composite of initial fatal or nonfatal coronary event or stroke or revascularization. Two secondary end points were (1) all initial vascular events defined as a composite of a primary end point event or angina, intermittent claudication, or transient ischemic attack; and (2) all-cause mortality.

Results.—After a mean (SD) follow-up of 8.2 (1.6) years, 357 participants had a primary end point event (13.5 per 1000 person-years, 95% confidence interval [CI], 12.2-15.0). No statistically significant difference was found between groups (13.7 events per 1000 person-years in the aspirin group vs 13.3 in the placebo group; hazard ratio [HR], 1.03; 95% CI, 0.84-1.27). A vascular event comprising the secondary end point occurred in 578 participants (22.8 per 1000 person-years; 95% CI, 21.0-24.8) and no statistically significant difference between groups (22.8 events per 1000 person-years in the aspirin group vs 22.9 in the placebo group; HR, 1.00; 95% CI, 0.85-1.17). There was no significant difference in all-cause mortality between groups (176 vs 186 deaths, respectively; HR, 0.95; 95% CI, 0.77-1.16). An initial event of major hemorrhage requiring admission to hospital occurred in 34 participants (2.5 per 1000 person-years) in the aspirin group and 20 (1.5 per 1000 person-years) in the placebo group (HR, 1.71; 95% CI, 0.99-2.97).

Conclusion.—Among participants without clinical cardiovascular disease, identified with a low ABI based on screening a general population, the administration of aspirin compared with placebo did not result in a significant reduction in vascular events.

Trial Registration.—isrctn.org Identifier: ISRCTN66587262.

▶ A low ankle brachial index (ABI) is a marker of systemic atherosclerosis and is associated with coexisting cerebrovascular and coronary disease. In men with an ABI < 0.9, there is a 27% risk over 10 years of a major coronary event versus 9% in those with ABIs between 1.11 and 1.4. For women, the figures are 19% and 9%.[1] It is controversial whether a screening ABI should be performed in an asymptomatic patient, as there is minimal evidence for an effective intervention in asymptomatic individuals with a low ABI.[2] The authors therefore sought to determine the effectiveness of aspirin in preventing cardiovascular events in otherwise asymptomatic individuals found to have a low ABI. The results are from the Aspirin for Asymptomatic Atherosclerosis trial. This was an intention-to-treat, double-blind, randomized, controlled trial conducted between April 1998 and October 2008. It involved 28 980 men and women aged between 50 and 75 years who were free of clinical vascular disease. The trial suggests that ABI screening in individuals free of clinical cardiovascular disease is unlikely to be beneficial if the intervention for a low ABI is prophylactic aspirin (Fig 2 in the original article). It does not rule out the possibility that other therapies such as statins or perhaps different antiplatelet agents with less hemorrhagic risk might confer benefit. In practical terms, the authors note that the results indicate that somewhere between 500 and 600 people from the general population would need to be screened with ABI studies and treated with aspirin to prevent 1 major cardiovascular event over 8 years. It seems difficult to justify the resources required for such massive screening with such little return.

G. L. Moneta, MD

References

1. Fowkes FG, Murray GD, Butcher I, et al. Ankle brachial index combined with Framingham Risk Score to predict cardiovascular events and mortality: a meta-analysis. *JAMA.* 2008;300:197-208.
2. US Preventative Services Task Force, AHRQ. Publication No. 05-0583-A-EF. http//www.ahrg.gov/clinic.uspstf05/pad/padrs.htm.

Carotid Ultrasound Identifies High Risk Subclinical Atherosclerosis in Adults With Low Framingham Risk Scores

Eleid MF, Lester SJ, Wiedenbeck TL, et al (Mayo Clinic College of Medicine, Scottsdale, AZ)
J Am Soc Echocardiogr 23:802-808, 2010

Background.—Worldwide, cardiovascular (CV) disease remains the most common cause of morbidity and mortality. Although effective in predicting CV risk in select populations, the Framingham risk score (FRS) fails to identify many young individuals who experience premature CV events. Accordingly, the aim of this study was to determine the prevalence of high-risk carotid intima-media thickness (CIMT) or plaque, a marker of atherosclerosis and predictor of CV events, in young asymptomatic individuals with low and intermediate FRS (<2% annualized event rate) using the carotid ultrasound protocol recommended by the American Society of Echocardiography and the Society of Vascular Medicine.

Methods.—Individuals aged ≤ 65 years not taking statins and without diabetes mellitus or histories of coronary artery disease underwent CIMT and plaque examination for primary prevention. Clinical variables including lipid values, family history of premature coronary artery disease, and FRS and subsequent pharmacotherapy recommendations were retrospectively collected for statistical analysis.

Results.—Of 441 subjects (mean age, 49.7 ± 7.9 years), 184 (42%; 95% confidence interval, 37.3%-46.5%) had high-risk carotid ultrasound findings (CIMT ≥ 75th percentile adjusted for age, gender, and race or presence of plaque). Of those with the lowest FRS of ≤5% (n = 336) (mean age, 48.0 ± 7.6 years; mean FRS, 2.5 ± 1.5%), 127 (38%; 95% confidence interval, 32.6%-43.0%) had high-risk carotid ultrasound findings. For individuals with FRS ≤ 5% and high-risk carotid ultrasound findings (n = 127; mean age, 47.3 ± 8.1 years; mean FRS, 2.5 ± 1.5%), lipid-lowering therapy was recommended by their treating physicians in 77 (61%).

Conclusions.—Thirty-eight percent of asymptomatic young to middle-aged individuals with FRS ≤ 5% have abnormal carotid ultrasound findings associated with increased risk for CV events. Pharmacologic therapy for CV prevention was recommended in the majority of these individuals. The lack of radiation exposure, relatively low cost, and ability to detect early-stage atherosclerosis suggest that carotid ultrasound for CIMT and plaque detection should continue to be explored as a primary tool for CV risk stratification in young to middle-aged adults with low FRS.

▶ Presumably, clinical events induced by atherosclerotic disease are preceded by a period of asymptomatic atherosclerosis. Population-based algorithms such as the Framingham risk score (FRS) are recommended to identify at-risk individuals and determine aggressiveness of preventive therapy.[1] However, population-based risk algorithms do not quantify atherosclerosis but only provide a probability of cardiovascular events over a relatively short fixed period, usually

10 years or less. The FRS also does not incorporate family history, premature coronary artery disease, remote smoking history, impaired fasting glucose, triglyceride levels, or waist circumference in risk assessment. Test for subclinical atherosclerosis has therefore been recommended to add incremental information and provide more accurate risk stratification. In this study, the authors tested the hypothesis that patients with a low (< 5%) 10-year risk for a first cardiovascular event and intermediate (6%-20%) 10-year risk by FRS have increased cardiovascular risk as determined by abnormally thickened carotid intima-media thickness (IMT). The results of the study indicate disconnect between risk assessment by the FRS and carotid IMT. Studies have also found that high-risk carotid ultrasound findings influence physicians to prescribe aspirin or lipid-lowering therapies.[2,3] However, while physicians may make treatment decisions based on finding of increased carotid IMT, it appears that following changes in IMT to monitor effects of drug therapy will not reduce subsequent clinical events (see also the abstract by Costanzo et al in this issue of the journal). A practical point may be that carotid IMT can be used to identify patients at increased risk for cardiovascular events, but once treatment is initiated subsequent studies to monitor effectiveness of treatment may not be needed.

G. L. Moneta, MD

References

1. Expert Panel on Detection, Evaluation, and Treatment of High Blood Cholesterol in Adults. Executive summary of the third report of the National Cholesterol Education Program (NCEP) expert panel on detection, evaluation, and treatment of high blood cholesterol in adults (Adult Treatment Panel III). *JAMA.* 2001;285: 2486-2497.
2. Wyman RA, Gimelli G, McBride PE, Korcarz CE, Stein JH. Does detection of carotid plaque affect physician behavior or motivate patients? *Am Heart J.* 2007;154:1072-1077.
3. Korcarz CE, DeCara JM, Hirsch AT, et al. Ultrasound detection of increased carotid intima-media thickness and carotid plaque in an office practice setting: does it affect physician behavior or patient motivation? *J Am Soc Echocardiogr.* 2008;21:1156-1162.

Comparative Determinants of 4-Year Cardiovascular Event Rates in Stable Outpatients at Risk of or With Atherothrombosis
Bhatt DL, for the REACH Registry Investigators (Brigham and Women's Hosp, Boston, MA; et al)
JAMA 304:1350-1357, 2010

Context.—Clinicians and trialists have difficulty with identifying which patients are highest risk for cardiovascular events. Prior ischemic events, polyvascular disease, and diabetes mellitus have all been identified as predictors of ischemic events, but their comparative contributions to future risk remain unclear.

Objective.—To categorize the risk of cardiovascular events in stable outpatients with various initial manifestations of atherothrombosis using simple clinical descriptors.

Design, Setting, and Patients.—Outpatients with coronary artery disease, cerebrovascular disease, or peripheral arterial disease or with multiple risk factors for atherothrombosis were enrolled in the global Reduction of Atherothrombosis for Continued Health (REACH) Registry and were followed up for as long as 4 years. Patients from 3647 centers in 29 countries were enrolled between 2003 and 2004 and followed up until 2008. Final database lock was in April 2009.

Main Outcome Measures.—Rates of cardiovascular death, myocardial infarction, and stroke.

Results.—A total of 45 227 patients with baseline data were included in this 4-year analysis. During the follow-up period, a total of 5481 patients experienced at least 1 event, including 2315 with cardiovascular death, 1228 with myocardial infarction, 1898 with stroke, and 40 with both a myocardial infarction and stroke on the same day. Among patients with atherothrombosis, those with a prior history of ischemic events at baseline (n=21 890) had the highest rate of subsequent ischemic events (18.3%; 95% confidence interval [CI], 17.4%-19.1%); patients with stable coronary, cerebrovascular, or peripheral artery disease (n=15 264) had a lower risk (12.2%; 95% CI, 11.4%-12.9%); and patients without established atherothrombosis but with risk factors only (n=8073) had the lowest risk (9.1%; 95% CI, 8.3%-9.9%) (*P*<.001 for all comparisons). In addition, in multivariable modeling, the presence of diabetes (hazard ratio [HR], 1.44; 95% CI, 1.36-1.53; *P*<.001), an ischemic event in the previous year (HR, 1.71; 95% CI, 1.57-1.85; *P*<.001), and polyvascular disease (HR, 1.99; 95% CI, 1.78-2.24; *P*<.001) each were associated with a significantly higher risk of the primary end point.

Conclusion.—Clinical descriptors can assist clinicians in identifying high-risk patients within the broad range of risk for outpatients with atherothrombosis.

▶ Recent clinical trials evaluating pharmacologic agents in patients with stable atherosclerosis, diabetes mellitus, or acute coronary syndromes have reported event rates in placebo groups lower than initially projected.[1-3] It is clearly important to identify patients for trials who are at higher risk for cardiovascular events to increase likelihood that a particular therapy might demonstrate benefits. Clinicians also would like to know which patients with atherosclerosis have the highest risk. The Reduction of Atherothrombosis for Continued Health Registry is a data set comprising patients with various manifestations of atherosclerosis. Manifestations vary from asymptomatic adults with risk factors to patients with stable atherosclerosis to those with prior ischemic events. In this study, the authors analyze the effects of prior ischemic events, polyvascular disease, and diabetes mellitus with respect to comparative contributions to future cardiovascular risk. They sought to categorize the risk of cardiovascular events in stable outpatients with various initial manifestations of atherothrombosis using simple clinical descriptors. The data indicate that polyvascular disease and a history of ischemic events particularly in the last year are strongly associated with cardio-vascular death, myocardial infarction, and stroke. Most vascular surgical patients would fall into the high-risk groups. This perhaps explains in part the high mortality rates of vascular surgical patients over time and somewhat cynically may explain why vascular surgery patients tend to be repeat customers. Once a patient with vascular disease has a cardiovascular event, they are much more likely to have additional events.

G. L. Moneta, MD

References

1. Bhatt DL, Lincoff AM, Gibson CM, et al. Intravenous platelet blockade with can-grelor during PCI. *N Eng J Med*. 2009;361:2330-2341.
2. Sacco RL, Diener HC, Yusuf S, et al. Aspirin and extended-release dipyridamole versus clopidogrel for recurrent stroke. *N Eng J Med*. 2008;359:1238-1251.
3. Topol EG, Bousser MG, Fox KA, et al. Rimonabant for prevention of cardiovas-cular events (CRESCENDO): a randomised, multicentre, placebo-controlled trial. *Lancet*. 2010;376:517-523.

Comparison of Effects of Statin Use on Mortality in Patients With Peripheral Arterial Disease With Versus Without Elevated C-Reactive Protein and D-Dimer Levels

Vidula H, Tian L, Liu K, et al (Northwestern Univ Feinberg School of Medicine, Chicago, IL; Stanford Univ, Palo Alto, CA; et al)
Am J Cardiol 105:1348-1352, 2010

We determined whether statin use was associated with lower all-cause and cardiovascular disease (CVD) mortality in 579 participants with lower extremity peripheral arterial disease (PAD) according to the presence and absence of elevated C-reactive protein (CRP) and D-dimer levels. Statin use was determined at baseline and at each annual visit. The CRP and D-dimer levels were measured at baseline. The mean follow-up was 3.7 years. The analyses were adjusted for age, gender, race, co-morbidities, ankle brachial index, cholesterol, and other confounders. Of the 579 participants, 242 (42%) were taking a statin at baseline and 129 (22%) died during follow-up. Statin use was associated with lower all-cause mortality (hazard ratio 0.51, 95% confidence interval [CI] 0.30 to 0.86, p = 0.012) and CVD mortality (hazard ratio 0.36, 95% CI 0.14 to 0.89, p = 0.027) compared to statin nonuse. No statistically significant interac-tion was found for the baseline CRP or D-dimer level with the association of statin use and mortality. However, statin therapy was associated with significantly lower all-cause and total mortality only among participants with baseline CRP values greater than the median and not among those with CRP values less than the median (hazard ratio 0.44, 95% CI 0.23 to 0.88 vs hazard ratio 0.73, 95% CI 0.31 to 1.75 for all-cause mortality and hazard ratio 0.20, 95% CI 0.063 to 0.65 vs hazard ratio 0.59, 95% CI

0.093 to 3.79 for CVD mortality). In conclusion, among those with PAD, statin use was associated with lower all-cause and CVD mortality compared to no statin use. The favorable association of statin use with mortality was not influenced significantly by the baseline CRP or D-dimer level.

▶ Patients with peripheral arterial disease (PAD), both men and women, have increased levels of inflammatory biomarkers and D-dimer compared with those without PAD.[1] Such patients represent an ideal core to study associations between statin therapy, mortality, and biomarker levels. The author used patients with PAD participating in the Walking and Leg Circulation Studies 1 and 2.[2,3] The findings are consistent with the results of the Justification for the Use of Statins in Prevention: an Intervention Trial Evaluating Rosuvastatin (JUPITER) trial. JUPITER demonstrated reduced cardiovascular events in patients with relatively low cholesterol levels who had elevated C-reactive protein (CRP) levels. Patients in JUPITER did not have PAD, though all those in this trial, by definition, had PAD. The data here suggest that the relative benefit of statin therapy was somewhat greater in persons with CRP levels greater than median compared with those with CRP levels less than median. There was no association with D-dimer levels. Relative benefits of statin therapy in patients with high versus low CRP levels, however, were not statistically significant but may reflect insufficient power in the study. At this point, the study can be regarded as extending the results of JUPITER to patients with PAD and provides evidence for routine use of statin therapy in patients with PAD regardless of elevation or nonelevation of cholesterol levels.

G. L. Moneta, MD

References

1. McDermott MM, Guralnik JM, Corsi A, et al. Patterns of inflammation associated with peripheral arterial disease: the InCHIANTI study. *Am Heart J.* 2005;150: 276-281.
2. McDermott MM, Liu K, Greenland P, et al. Functional decline in peripheral arterial disease: associations with the ankle brachial index and leg symptoms. *JAMA.* 2004;292:453-461.
3. McDermott MM, Hoff F, Ferrucci L, et al. Lower extremity ischemia, calf skeletal muscle characteristics, and functional impairment in peripheral arterial disease. *J Am Geriatr Soc.* 2007;55:400-406.

Diabetes mellitus, fasting blood glucose concentration, and risk of vascular disease: a collaborative meta-analysis of 102 prospective studies
The Emerging Risk Factors Collaboration (Univ of Cambridge, UK; et al)
Lancet 375:2215-2222, 2010

Background.—Uncertainties persist about the magnitude of associations of diabetes mellitus and fasting glucose concentration with risk of coronary heart disease and major stroke subtypes. We aimed to quantify these associations for a wide range of circumstances.

Methods.—We undertook a meta-analysis of individual records of diabetes, fasting blood glucose concentration, and other risk factors in people without initial vascular disease from studies in the Emerging Risk Factors Collaboration. We combined within-study regressions that were adjusted for age, sex, smoking, systolic blood pressure, and bodymass index to calculate hazard ratios (HRs) for vascular disease.

Findings.—Analyses included data for 698 782 people (52 765 non-fatal or fatal vascular outcomes; 8·49 million person-years at risk) from 102 prospective studies. Adjusted HRs with diabetes were: 2·00 (95% CI 1·83—2·19) for coronary heart disease; 2·27 (1·95—2·65) for ischaemic stroke; 1·56 (1·19—2·05) for haemorrhagic stroke; 1·84 (1·59—2·13) for unclassified stroke; and 1·73 (1·51—1·98) for the aggregate of other vascular deaths. HRs did not change appreciably after further adjustment for lipid, inflammatory, or renal markers. HRs for coronary heart disease were higher in women than in men, at 40—59 years than at 70 years and older, and with fatal than with non-fatal disease. At an adult population-wide prevalence of 10%, diabetes was estimated to account for 11% (10—12%) of vascular deaths. Fasting blood glucose concentration was non-linearly related to vascular risk, with no significant associations between 3·90 mmol/L and 5·59 mmol/L. Compared with fasting blood glucose concentrations of 3·90—5·59 mmol/L, HRs for coronary heart disease were: 1·07 (0·97—1·18) for lower than 3·90 mmol/L; 1·11 (1·04—1·18) for 5·60—6·09 mmol/L; and 1·17 (1·08—1·26) for 6·10—6·99 mmol/L. In people without a history of diabetes, information about fasting blood glucose concentration or impaired fasting glucose status did not significantly improve metrics of vascular disease prediction when added to information about several conventional risk factors.

Interpretation.—Diabetes confers about a two-fold excess risk for a wide range of vascular diseases, independently from other conventional risk factors. In people without diabetes, fasting blood glucose concentration is modestly and nonlinearly associated with risk of vascular disease (Figs 1 and 2).

▶ By May 2010, the Emerging Risk Factors Collaboration from 121 prospective studies of vascular risk factors had secured individual records of 1.27 million adults. The studies from which the records were obtained did not select participants on the basis of previous vascular disease. The studies recorded case-specific vascular morbidity or mortality or both using well-defined criteria. All studies had accrued more than 1 year of follow-up. The authors used these data in an attempt to produce reliable estimates of the association of diabetes and fasting blood glucose concentrations with fatal or first ever nonfatal incident vascular disease (and deaths from other vascular disorders) under a wide range of conditions. There are a lot of numbers in this article. When one puts the numbers in a public health perspective, the analysis is quite sobering. The data suggest that 10% of vascular deaths in the populations of developed countries can be attributed to diabetes. This corresponds to an estimated 325 000 deaths per year just in developed countries. Because results do not change after adjustment for lipid, inflammatory,

	Number of cases	HR (95% CI)	I^2 (95% CI)
Coronary heart disease*	26505	2·00 (1·83-2·19)	64 (54-71)
Coronary death	11556	2·31 (2·05-2·60)	41 (24-54)
Non-fatal myocardial infarction	14741	1·82 (1·64-2·03)	37 (19-51)
Stroke subtypes*			
Ischaemic stroke	3799	2·27 (1·95-2·65)	1 (0-20)
Haemorrhagic stroke	1183	1·56 (1·19-2·05)	0 (0-26)
Unclassified stroke	4973	1·84 (1·59-2·13)	33 (12-48)
Other vascular deaths	3826	1·73 (1·51-1·98)	0 (0-26)

FIGURE 1.—Hazard ratios (HRs) for vascular outcomes in people with versus those without diabetes at baseline. Analyses were based on 530 083 participants. HRs were adjusted for age, smoking status, body-mass index, and systolic blood pressure, and, where appropriate, stratified by sex and trial arm. 208 coronary heart disease outcomes that contributed to the grand total could not contribute to the subtotals of coronary death or non-fatal myocardial infarction because there were fewer than 11 cases of these coronary disease subtypes in some studies. *Includes both fatal and non-fatal events. (Reprinted from The Lancet, The Emerging Risk Factors Collaboration. Diabetes mellitus, fasting blood glucose concentration, and risk of vascular disease: a collaborative meta-analysis of 102 prospective studies. *Lancet.* 2010;375: 2215-2222. Copyright 2010, with permission from Elsevier.)

A Coronary heart disease

	Number of participants	Number of cases	HR (95% CI)	Interaction p value
Sex				
Male	306533	20218	1·89 (1·73-2·06)	<0·0001
Female	223550	6287	2·59 (2·29-2·93)	
Age at survey				
40-59 years	410833	17686	2·51 (2·25-2·80)	<0·0001
60-69 years	75785	5045	2·01 (1·80-2·26)	
≥70 years	43465	3774	1·78 (1·54-2·05)	
Smoking status				
Other	343864	13702	2·35 (2·11-2·61)	<0·0001
Current	186219	12803	1·82 (1·65-2·00)	
BMI*				
Bottom third	176274	6701	2·30 (2·00-2·64)	0·0143
Middle third	176332	9103	2·45 (2·15-2·79)	
Top third	177477	10701	1·98 (1·76-2·21)	
Systolic blood pressure†				
Bottom third	183314	4915	2·85 (2·48-3·27)	<0·0001
Middle third	192622	9079	2·31 (2·05-2·60)	
Top third	154147	12511	1·97 (1·78-2·18)	

B Ischaemic stroke

	Number of participants	Number of cases	HR (95% CI)	Interaction p value
Sex				
Male	168191	2193	2·16 (1·84-2·52)	0·0089
Female	125571	1606	2·83 (2·35-3·40)	
Age at survey				
40-59 years	234263	1729	3·74 (3·06-4·58)	0·0001
60-69 years	38140	1134	2·06 (1·64-2·58)	
≥70 years	21359	936	1·80 (1·42-2·27)	
Smoking status				
Other	191125	2471	2·58 (2·19-3·05)	0·1355
Current	102637	1328	2·18 (1·76-2·69)	
BMI*				
Bottom third	110044	1149	1·90 (1·50-2·40)	0·0001
Middle third	97478	1163	2·28 (1·85-2·80)	
Top third	86240	1487	2·90 (2·49-3·37)	
Systolic blood pressure†				
Bottom third	113199	711	3·06 (2·33-4·01)	0·7275
Middle third	106966	1217	2·79 (2·23-3·49)	
Top third	73597	1871	2·49 (2·02-3·07)	

FIGURE 2.—Hazard ratios (HRs) for coronary heart disease and ischaemic stroke in people with versus those without diabetes at baseline, by individual characteristics HRs were adjusted as described in figure 1. BMI=body-mass index. *Bottom third=<23·8 kg/m² (mean 21·7 kg/m²); middle third=23·8-<27 kg/m² (mean 25·3 kg/m²); and top third=≥27 kg/m² (mean 30·7 kg/m²). †Bottom third=<123 mm Hg (mean 113 mm Hg); middle third=123-<141 mm Hg (mean 132 mm Hg); and top third=≥141 mm Hg (mean 157 mm Hg). (Reprinted from The Lancet, The Emerging Risk Factors Collaboration. Diabetes mellitus, fasting blood glucose concentration, and risk of vascular disease: a collaborative meta-analysis of 102 prospective studies. *Lancet.* 2010;375:2215-2222. Copyright 2010, with permission from Elsevier.)

or renal markers, the burden of diabetes in relationship to vascular deaths will continue to increase as diabetes prevalence continues to increase. This will happen even if there are decreases in the rates of cigarette smoking and improvement of treatment of other vascular risk factors. It is also important to note the increased burden of vascular disease in patients with modestly elevated blood glucose concentrations that do not meet the definition of diabetes mellitus. The ever-expanding obesity epidemic (no pun intended) is going to result in hundreds of thousands of diabetes-related deaths over the next decade.

G. L. Moneta, MD

Does Carotid Intima-Media Thickness Regression Predict Reduction of Cardiovascular Events? A Meta-Analysis of 41 Randomized Trials

Costanzo P, Perrone-Filardi P, Vassallo E, et al (Federico II Univ, Naples, Italy)

J Am Coll Cardiol 56:2006-2020, 2010

Objectives.—The purpose of this study was to verify whether intima-media thickness (IMT) regression is associated with reduced incidence of cardiovascular events.

Background.—Carotid IMT increase is associated with a raised risk of coronary heart disease (CHD) and cerebrovascular (CBV) events. However, it is undetermined whether favorable changes of IMT reflect prognostic benefits.

Methods.—The MEDLINE database and the Cochrane Database were searched for articles published until August 2009. All randomized trials assessing carotid IMT at baseline, at end of follow-up, and reporting clinical end points were included. A weighted random-effects meta-regression analysis was performed to test the relationship between mean and maximum IMT changes and outcomes. The influence of baseline patients' characteristics, cardiovascular risk profile, IMT at baseline, follow-up, and quality of the trials was also explored. Overall estimates of effect were calculated with a fixed-effects model, random-effects model, or Peto method.

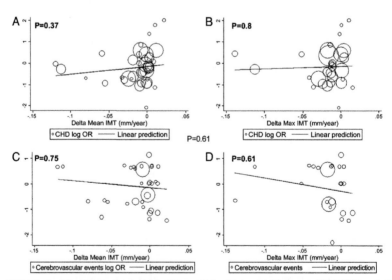

FIGURE 2.—Meta-Regression Analysis Between Delta Mean and Maximum IMT, CHD, and CBV Events. Meta-regression analysis between delta mean and maximum (max) intima-media thickness (IMT) for (A, B) coronary heart disease (CHD) events and (C, D) cerebrovascular (CBV) events. The log of odds ratios (ORs) is reported on the y-axis, and the covariate is reported on the x-axis. Bubble size for each study is proportional to the inverse of the variance. (Reprinted from the Journal of the American College of Cardiology, Costanzo P, Perrone-Filardi P, Vassallo E, et al. Does carotid intima-media thickness regression predict reduction of cardiovascular events? A meta-analysis of 41 randomized trials. *J Am Coll Cardiol.* 2010;56: 2006-2020. Copyright 2010, with permission from the American College of Cardiology Foundation.)

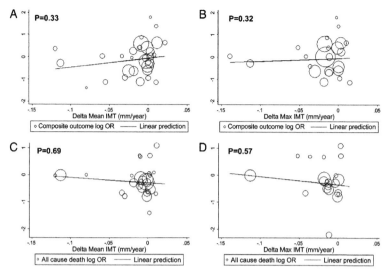

FIGURE 3.—Meta-Regression Analysis Between Delta Mean and Maximum IMT, Composite Outcome, and All-Cause Death. Meta-regression analysis between delta mean and maximum (max) intima-media thickness (IMT) for (**A, B**) composite outcome and (**C, D**) all-cause death. Log of odds ratios (OR) is reported on the y-axis, and the covariate is reported on the x-axis. Bubble size for each study is proportional to the inverse of the variance. (Reprinted from the Journal of the American College of Cardiology, Costanzo P, Perrone-Filardi P, Vassallo E, et al. Does carotid intima-media thickness regression predict reduction of cardiovascular events? A meta-analysis of 41 randomized trials. *J Am Coll Cardiol*. 2010;56:2006-2020. Copyright 2010, with permission from the American College of Cardiology Foundation.)

Results.—Forty-one trials enrolling 18,307 participants were included. Despite significant reduction in CHD, CBV events, and all-cause death induced by active treatments (for CHD events, odds ratio [OR]: 0.82, 95% confidence interval [CI]: 0.69 to 0.96, p = 0.02; for CBV events, OR: 0.71, 95% CI: 0.51 to 1.00, p = 0.05; and for all-cause death, OR: 0.71, 95% CI: 0.53 to 0.96, p = 0.03), there was no significant relationship between IMT regression and CHD events (Tau 0.91, p = 0.37), CBV events (Tau −0.32, p = 0.75), and all-cause death (Tau −0.41, p = 0.69). In addition, subjects' baseline characteristics, cardiovascular risk profile, IMT at baseline, follow-up, and quality of the trials did not significantly influence the association between IMT changes and clinical outcomes.

Conclusions.—Regression or slowed progression of carotid IMT, induced by cardiovascular drug therapies, do not reflect reduction in cardiovascular events (Figs 2 and 3).

▶ Carotid intima-media thickness (IMT) predicts cardiovascular events. Predictions are more robust for cerebral compared with coronary events.[1] IMT is an attractive biomarker potentially useful as a therapeutic target in subjects at increased cardiovascular risk. IMT is, in fact, considered a manifestation of subclinical atherosclerosis and has been included in the list of organ-damaged conditions in European hypertension guidelines and in the European prevention guidelines.[2,3] IMT changes, either regression or slowing of progression, have been used as surrogate clinical end points in randomized clinical studies of lipid-lowering agents, antihypertensive agents, oral antidiabetic agents, and antioxidant drugs, in subjects at intermediate to high cardiovascular risk. Information verifying whether the changes in IMT were associated with consistent changes in cardiovascular risk profile would be relevant for interpretation of IMT variations and surrogate clinical end points and for identifying therapeutic targets for cardiovascular therapies. The principle finding of the study is that carotid IMT changes do not correlate with changes in major cardiovascular events that are induced by drug treatments in subjects at intermediate to high cardiovascular risk (Figs 2 and 3). The US Preventative Task Force also recognizes uncertainty of the correlation of IMT changes with clinical events.[4] It is conceivable that there are many determinants of IMT that may reduce the clinical strength and statistical significance of IMT changes and their ability to predict cardiovascular outcomes in comparison to more direct atherosclerotic risk factors. It may also be that atherosclerosis in the carotid artery is not generally representative of the atherosclerotic process throughout the body. Atherosclerotic plaques in the carotid artery tend to grow longitudinally at twice the rate that they grow in thickness. Therefore, IMT may be a less sensitive measure of plaque evolution than total plaque burden.[5] The bottom line, however, is that while IMT increase indicates increased cardiovascular risk, changes in IMT induced by drug therapy do not appear to reflect improved clinical outcome.

G. L. Moneta, MD

References

1. Lorenz MW, Markus HS, Bots ML, Rosvall M, Sitzer M. Prediction of clinical cardiovascular events with carotid intima-media thickness: a systematic review and meta-analysis. *Circulation.* 2007;115:459-467.
2. Manciag G, De Backer G, Dominiczak A, et al. 2007 Guidelines for the management of arterial hypertension: The Task Force for the Management of Arterial Hypertension of the European Society of Hypertension (ESH) and of the European Society of Cardiology (ESC). *Eur Heart J.* 2007;28:1462-1536.
3. Fourth Joint Task Force of the European Society of Cardiology and other societies on cardiovascular disease prevention in clinical practice. European guidelines on cardiovascular disease prevention in clinical practice. *Eur J Cardiovasc Prev Rehab.* 2007;14:E1-E40.
4. Helfand M, Buckley DI, Freeman M, et al. Emerging risk factors for coronary heart disease: a summary of systematic reviews conducted for the U.S. Preventive Services Task Force. *Ann Intern Med.* 2009;151:496-507.
5. Mackinnon AD, Jerrard-Dunne P, Sitzer M, Buehler A, von Kegler S, Markus HS. Rates and determinants of site-specific progression of carotid artery intima-media thickness: the carotid atherosclerosis progression study. *Stroke.* 2004;35:2150-2154.

Process of Care Partly Explains the Variation in Mortality Between Hospitals After Peripheral Vascular Surgery

Hoeks SE, Scholte op Reimer WJM, Lingsma HF, et al (Erasmus Med Ctr, Rotterdam, The Netherlands; Hogeschool van Amsterdam, The Netherlands; et al)

Eur J Vasc Endovasc Surg 40:147-154, 2010

Objectives.—The aim of this study is to investigate whether variation in mortality at hospital level reflects differences in quality of care of peripheral vascular surgery patients.

Design.—Observational study.

Materials.—In 11 hospitals in the Netherlands, 711 consecutive vascular surgery patients were enrolled.

Methods.—Multilevel logistic regression models were used to relate patient characteristics, structure and process of care to mortality at 1 year. The models were constructed by consecutively adding age, sex and Lee index, then remaining risk factors, followed by structural measures for quality of care and finally, selected process of care parameters.

Results.—Total 1-year mortality was 11%, ranging from 6% to 26% in different hospitals. Large differences in patient characteristics and quality indicators were observed between hospitals (e.g., age >70 years: 28−58%; beta-blocker therapy: 39−87%). Adjusted analyses showed that a large part of variation in mortality was explained by age, sex and the Lee index (Akaike's information criterion (AIC) = 59, $p < 0.001$). Another substantial part of the variation was explained by process of care (AIC = 5, $p = 0.001$).

Conclusions.—Differences between hospitals exist in patient characteristics, structure of care, process of care and mortality. Even after adjusting for the patient population at risk, a substantial part of the variation in mortality can be explained by differences in process measures of quality of care.

► This timely study evaluated the variation in mortality at 11 hospitals in the Netherlands to see if this is a reflection of quality of care in vascular surgery patients. The Donabedian paradigm based on a 3-component (structure, process, and outcome) approach to assessing quality of care was used. The 11 hospitals were divided into 3 clusters based on the percentage of patients who were dead at 1 year. Short-term (30-day), 1-year, and 3-year mortalities were evaluated, and 1-year all-cause mortality was chosen as the primary end point. Variation in patient characteristics based on comorbid conditions and the Lee index (open surgical procedures, ischemic heart disease, history of congestive heart failure, history of cerebrovascular disease, diabetes mellitus, and renal insufficiency) varied among the tertiles of hospitals as would be expected (all were statistically significant except for age > 70 years, history of angina pectoris, myocardial infarction, and heart failure). Of these variables, age, sex, and the Lee index explained the majority of variation in mortality. Using multilevel stepwise logistic regression, process of care, which was based on the American College of Cardiology and the American Heart Association guidelines for perioperative care, explained a large part of the variation in mortality as well ($P = .001$). These findings held true when the dependent variable of the logistic regression was changed to 30-day mortality. The authors found significant differences in obtaining the recommended noninvasive cardiac testing (only 21% were performed) as well as variation in the tertiles regarding the use of β-blockers (52%-34%) and statins (60%-48%).

Obviously, this study is important to identify that process of care is an important factor in patient outcomes in vascular surgery, and as more quality improvement programs develop (ie, National Surgical Quality Improvement Program, the Vascular Study Group of New England, etc), factors will be identified in our specialty to improve quality of care. As more pay for performance initiatives are enacted, it will be in our best interest to identify means of improving process of care to improve patient outcomes.

N. Singh, MD

4 Vascular Laboratory and Imaging

Comparison of indirect radiation dose estimates with directly measured radiation dose for patients and operators during complex endovascular procedures
Panuccio G, Greenberg RK, Wunderle K, et al (Cleveland Clinic Foundation, OH)
J Vasc Surg 53:885-894, 2011

Background.—A great deal of attention has been directed at the necessity and potential for deleterious outcomes as a result of radiation exposure during diagnostic evaluations and interventional procedures. We embarked on this study in an attempt to accurately determine the amount of radiation exposure given to patients undergoing complex endovascular aortic repair. These measured doses were then correlated with radiation dose estimates provided by the imaging equipment manufacturers that are typically used for documentation and analysis of radiation-induced risk.

Methods.—Consecutive patients undergoing endovascular thoracoabdominal aneurysm (eTAAA) repair were prospectively studied with respect to radiation dose. Indirect parameters as cumulative air kerma (CAK), kerma area product (KAP), and fluoroscopy time (FT) were recorded concurrently with direct measurements of dose (peak skin dose [PSD]) and radiation exposure patterns using radiochromatic film placed in the back of the patient during the procedure. Simultaneously, operator exposure was determined using high-sensitivity electronic dosimeters. Correlation between the indirect and direct parameters was calculated. The observed radiation exposure pattern was reproduced in phantoms with over 200 dosimeters located in mock organs, and effective dose has been calculated in an in vitro study. Scatter plots were used to evaluate the relationship between continuous variables and Pearson coefficients.

Results.—eTAAA repair was performed in 54 patients over 5 months, of which 47 had the repair limited to the thoracoabdominal segment. Clinical follow-up was complete in 98% of the patients. No patients had evidence of radiation-induced skin injury. CAK exceeded 15 Gy in 3 patients (the Joint Commission on Accreditation of Healthcare Organizations [JCAHO] threshold for sentinel events); however, the direct measurements were well below 15 Gy in all patients. PSD was measured by quantifying the exposure of the radiochromatic film. PSD correlated weakly with FT but better with CAK and KAP ($r = 0.55$, 0.80, and 0.76, respectively). The following formula provides the best estimate of actual PSD $= 0.677 + 0.257$ CAK. The average effective dose was 119.68 mSv (for type II or III eTAAA) and 76.46 mSv (type IV eTAAA). The operator effective dose averaged 0.17 mSv/case and correlated best with the KAP ($r = 0.82$, $P < .0001$).

Conclusion.—FT cannot be used to estimate PSD, and CAK and KAP represent poor surrogate markers for JCAHO-defined sentinel events. Even when directly measured PSDs were used, there was a poor correlation with clinical event (no skin injuries with an average PSD >2 Gy). The effective radiation dose of an eTAAA is equivalent to two preoperative computed tomography scans. The maximal operator exposure is 50 mSv/year, thus, a single operator could perform up to 294 eTAAA procedures annually before reaching the recommended maximum operator dose.

▶ Intraoperative radiation safety is an incredibly important aspect of our profession that we are all responsible for. This article by Panuccio et al serves to bring this issue to the forefront for us and force us to address the realities and limitations of this challenge. The group from the Cleveland Clinic chose to determine the amount of radiation exposure given to patients undergoing complex endovascular aortic repair. These measured doses were then correlated with radiation dose estimates. They found that among 54 patients undergoing endovascular thoracoabdominal aortic aneurysm repair (eTAAA), none had any evidence of radiation-induced skin injury. They also found poor correlation between fluoroscopy time and that other measures, cumulative air kerma, and kerma area product represented poor surrogate markers for the Joint Commission on Accreditation of Healthcare Organizations defined sentinel events. Lastly, they found the effective radiation dose of an eTAAA is equivalent to 2 preoperative CT scans. According to radiation safety standards, this would mean that a single operator could perform up to 294 eTAAA annually.

While demonstrating the radiation safety of eTAAA, this article also emphasizes that it is optimal to minimize the peak skin dose in any 1 region by optimizing the beam collimation, reduction of the milliampere, fewer fluoroscopy pulses, and acquisition images coupled with frequent changes in the pattern of the radiation field by altering the tube angle. The authors state that clearly efforts must be made to decrease procedural doses. They point out, however, that the bulk of exposure (over time) for patients undergoing endovascular aneurysm repair resides within the multiple CT scans used to assess aneurysms preoperatively and postoperatively. Lastly, this article points out that in addition to increasing the safety of endovascular procedures for the patient, we need to minimize operator radiation doses. This requires vigilance on the point of the surgical leaders to make sure that all members of the operative team appropriately wear their radiation dosimeters, lead aprons, and thyroid shields. Education in radiation safety measures and refresher training for those individuals exceeding 30% of the recommended International Commission on Radiological Protection limit are mandatory. Finally, additional protective measures include the use of ceiling-mounted mobile shields and a lead skirt on the table and its shoulder attachment to reduce the amount of scattered radiation exposure to the team.

D. L. Gillespie, MD, RVT

Detecting traumatic internal carotid artery dissection using transcranial Doppler in head-injured patients
Bouzat P, Francony G, Brun J, et al (Albert Michallon Hosp, Grenoble, France)
Intensive Care Med 36:1514-1520, 2010

Purpose.—The early diagnosis of traumatic internal carotid artery dissection (TICAD) is essential for initiating appropriate treatment and improving outcome. We searched for criteria from transcranial Doppler (TCD) measurements on admission that could be associated with subsequent TICAD diagnosis in patients with traumatic brain injury (TBI).

Methods.—We conducted a retrospective 1:4 matched (age, mean arterial blood pressure) cohort study of 11 TBI patients with TICAD and absent or mild brain lesions on initial CT scan, 22 TBI controls with comparable brain CT scan lesions (controls 1), and 22 TBI controls with more severe brain CT scan lesions (controls 2) on admission. TCD measurements were obtained on admission from both middle cerebral arteries (MCA). All patients had subsequent CT angiography to diagnose TICAD.

Results.—A >25% asymmetry in the systolic blood flow velocity between the two MCA was found in 9/11 patients with TICAD versus 0/22 in controls 1 and 5/22 in controls 2 ($p < 0.01$). The combination of this asymmetry with an ipsilateral pulsatility index ≤ 0.80 was found in 9/11 patients with TICAD versus none in the two groups of controls ($p < 0.01$).

Conclusions.—Our results suggest that significant asymmetry in the systolic blood flow velocity between the MCAs and a reduced ipsilateral pulsatility index could be criteria from TCD measurements associated with the occurrence of TICAD in head-injured patients. If prospectively validated, these findings could be incorporated in screening protocols for TICAD in patients with TBI.

▶ Traumatic internal carotid artery dissection (TICAD) is an important cause of stroke in young people accounting for 20% of all strokes in younger patients.[1,2] Diagnosis of TICAD may be delayed because of concurrent facial and cranial injuries with symptoms presenting as unexpected neurologic deficits up to 1 week post injury. In many institutions, computed tomographic angiography (CTA) is used as a screening modality for TICAD. Transcranial Doppler (TCD) studies are also frequently used in the monitoring of patients with head injury. There have been 2 case reports that have suggested asymmetric mean blood flow velocities between middle cerebral arteries, as determined TCD may be helpful in diagnosis of TICAD.[3,4] The authors of this article routinely perform TCD measurements on all patients admitted to their emergency room for head injury. Using this material they conducted a retrospective matched cohort study in search for TCD abnormalities in patients in whom TICAD was subsequently confirmed by CTA. In many centers, CTA is routinely used to screen for carotid dissection in at-risk trauma patients and screening for traumatic brain injury with TCD may not be applicable in such centers. However, CTAs can sometimes be difficult to interpret when evaluating for carotid dissection. The study suggests that TCD may be an important adjunctive test to confirm the suspicion of TICAD in cases where CTA is not clearly diagnostic. The number of patients is small in this series, and confirmatory studies will be required. The data are, however, interesting and suggest potential expanded application of TCD technology.

G. L. Moneta, MD

References

1. Arthurs ZM, Starnes BW. Blunt carotid and vertebral artery injuries. *Injury.* 2008; 39:1232-1241.
2. Menon RK, Norris JW. Cervical arterial dissection: current concepts. *Ann N Y Acad Sci.* 2008;1142:200-217.
3. Achtereekte HA, van der Kruijk RA, Hekster RE, Keunen RW. Diagnosis of traumatic carotid artery dissection by transcranial Doppler ultrasound: case report and review of the literature. *Surg Neurol.* 1994;42:240-244.
4. Romner B, Sjöholm H, Brandt L. Transcranial Doppler sonography, angiography and SPECT measurements in traumatic carotid artery dissection. *Acta Neurochir (Wien).* 1994;126:185-191.

Radiologic Importance of a High-Resistive Vertebral Artery Doppler Waveform on Carotid Duplex Ultrasonography

Kim ESH, Thompson M, Nacion KM, et al (Cleveland Clinic, OH)
J Ultrasound Med 29:1161-1165, 2010

Objective.—The appearance of the vertebral artery (VA) waveform on a pulsed Doppler examination performed during standard carotid duplex ultrasonography (CDU) may suggest vertebrobasilar disease. We sought to determine the radiographic importance of high-resistive (HR) pulsed Doppler VA waveforms seen on CDU.

Methods.—The Noninvasive Vascular Laboratory database was queried for CDU studies noting the HR VA Doppler signal. Studies with unilateral or bilateral HR and antegrade VA waveforms with correlative neuroimaging studies within 60 days were included. Imaging reports were reviewed to determine the following: (1) a normal VA; (2) at least moderate distal VA or basilar artery (BA) stenosis, occlusion, or dissection; (3) a congenitally diminutive VA; or (4) other abnormalities.

Results.—Of 1338 studies with 1 or more HR VA waveforms, 79 studies met all inclusion criteria (n = 157 arteries) and had adequate correlative neuroimaging. There were 90 HR VAs, and HR waveforms were equally distributed between right and left sides. The mean peak systolic velocity of HR versus low-resistive (LR) VAs was 51.7 versus 63.6 cm/s ($P = .04$); the mean end-diastolic velocity of HR versus LR VAs was 4.6 versus 17.3 cm/s ($P < .001$); and the resistive index of HR versus LR VAs was 0.92 versus 0.73 ($P < .001$). Of all HR VAs, 18.9% were normal; 38.9% had distal vertebrobasilar stenosis or occlusion; 35.6% were congenitally diminutive; and 6.7% had other abnormalities (proximal stenosis, excessive tortuosity, fibromuscular dysplasia, and BA hypoplasia).

Conclusions.—The finding of an HR spectral Doppler signal in the VA was associated with major vertebrobasilar disease (46% of cases) and should prompt additional neuroimaging in the appropriate clinical situation (Table 2).

▶ During the performance of duplex ultrasonography for carotid artery disease, the vertebral arteries are usually also routinely examined. However, in most centers, examination of the vertebral arteries is limited and generally confined to determining the direction of blood flow in the vertebral artery. However, it is also possible to obtain qualitative analysis of Doppler spectral waveform characteristics. A normal vertebral artery has flow throughout diastole as it feeds the low-resistance circulatory bed of the brain. A loss of diastolic flow theoretically indicates advanced occlusive distal vertebrobasilar disease through the creation of increased resistance to circulation (Fig 1 in the original article). The authors sought to determine associations with high resistance pulse Doppler vertebral artery waveforms visualized on color duplex ultrasound. This is the largest correlative study of neuroimaging with Doppler waveform of the V2 segment of the vertebral artery. One wonders about the high false-positive rate of 18.9% in this study. This may relate to lack of a single standard neuroimaging comparator or the fact that the vertebral artery waveforms were only qualitatively assessed as either being high resistance or low resistance. However, when others compared vertebral arteries with an end-diastolic velocity of 0 to those with an end-diastolic velocity greater than 0, but still considered high resistance, those with end-diastolic velocities of 0 were no more likely to have significant vertebral artery disease on neuroimaging than those with higher end-diastolic velocities (Table 2). The article is valuable in that it gives those of us who read ultrasound

TABLE 2.—Radiographic Correlations of HR VA Doppler Signals

Parameter	Normal, n (%)	Congenitally Diminutive, n (%)	Vertebrobasilar Occlusive Disease, n (%)[a]	Other Abnormalities, n (%)[b]	Overall P
LR (n = 67)	46 (68.7)	3 (4.5)	10 (14.9)	8 (11.9)	<.001
HR (n = 90)	17 (18.9)	32 (35.6)	35 (38.9)	6 (6.7)	
EDV 0 cm/s (n = 51)	9 (17.6)	18 (35.3)	23 (45.1)	1 (1.96)	.13
EDV >0 cm/s (n = 38)	8 (21.1)	14 (36.8)	11 (29.0)	5 (13.2)	

Findings of vertebrobasilar neuroimaging by EDV on CDU. High-resistive VAs with an EDV of 0 (no flow at end diastole) were no more likely to have significant vertebrobasilar disease than those with an EDV of greater than 0 cm/s (mean EDV for HR VAs with an EDV >0 cm/s, 10.8 cm/s; P not significant).
[a]Includes at least moderate distal VA or BA stenosis, occlusion, or dissection.
[b]Includes proximal stenosis, excessive tortuosity, fibromuscular dysplasia, and BA hypoplasia.

studies of the extracranial cerebrovascular arteries an idea of the distribution of abnormalities producing high resistance vertebral artery waveforms.

G. L. Moneta, MD

Arterial imaging in patients with lower extremity ischemia and diabetes mellitus
Pomposelli F (Beth Israel Deaconess Med Ctr, Boston, MA)
J Vasc Surg 52:81S-91S, 2010

Precise, comprehensive imaging of the arterial circulation is the cornerstone of successful revascularization of the ischemic extremity in patients with diabetes mellitus. Arterial imaging is challenging in these patients because the disease is often multisegmental with a predilection for the distal tibial and peroneal arteries. Occlusive lesions and the arterial wall itself are often calcified and patients presenting with ischemic complications frequently have underlying renal insufficiency. Intra-arterial digital subtraction angiography (DSA), contrast enhanced magnetic resonance angiography (MRA), and more recently, computerized tomographic angiography (CTA) have been used as imaging modalities in lower extremity ischemia. Each has specific advantages and shortcomings in this patient population, which will be summarized and contrasted in this review. DSA is an invasive technique most often performed from a femoral arterial puncture and requires the injection of arterial contrast, which can occasionally cause allergic reactions. In patients with pre-existing renal insufficiency, contrast infusion can result in worsening renal failure; although usually self-limited, it may occasionally require hemodialysis, especially in patients with diabetes. However, DSA provides the highest degree of spatial resolution and image quality. It is also the only modality in which the diagnosis and treatment of arterial disease can be performed simultaneously. MRA is noninvasive, and when enhanced with gadolinium contrast injection provides arterial images of comparable quality to DSA and in some circumstances may uncover distal arterial targets not visualized on DSA. However, spatial resolution is inferior to DSA and erroneous interpretations due to acquisition artifacts are common. Specialized equipment and imaging techniques are necessary to minimize their occurrence in the distal lower extremity. In addition, due to the risk of inducing nephrogenic systemic fibrosis, gadolinium-enhanced MRA cannot be used in patients with renal insufficiency. CTA is noninvasive and rapidly performed, with better spatial resolution than MRA, but requires the largest volume of contrast infusion, exposes patients to high-doses of radiation, and is subject to interpretive error due to reconstruction artifacts especially in heavily calcified arteries, limiting its usefulness in many patients with diabetes. For patients in whom the planned intervention is a surgical bypass, DSA and MRA will provide high quality images of the lower extremity arterial anatomy. For patients in whom a catheter-based intervention is the likely treatment, a diagnostic DSA immediately followed

TABLE.—Advantages and Disadvantages of DSA, CTA, and MRA for Lower Extremity Arterial Imaging

Modality	Advantages	Disadvantages
DSA	Best resolution Combines diagnosis and treatment "gold standard"	Invasive, radiation exposure Access complications Adverse reactions to contrast Allergic reactions Contrast nephropathy
MRA	Noninvasive, no radiation Images not obscured by calcium Can image arteries not seen on DSA	Inferior spatial resolution Long acquisition times Acquisition artifacts NSF
CTA	Noninvasive Excellent spatial resolution Rapid image acquisition time Multiple reconstruction techniques	Obscured by calcium Highest contrast volume Adverse reactions to contrast Radiation exposure Imaging artifacts

CTA, Computed tomography angiography; DSA, digital subtraction angiography; MRA, magnetic resonance angiography; NSF, nephrogenic systemic fibrosis.

by a catheter-based treatment in the same procedure is the preferred approach. In patients with pre-existing renal dysfunction, in which gadolinium-enhanced MRA is contraindicated, DSA or CTA can be performed. However, patients should have an infusion of intravenous normal saline solution or sodium bicarbonate before the procedure to reduce the incidence of contrast-induced nephropathy (Table).

▶ This is an excellent review of imaging the lower extremity of ischemic limbs in patients with diabetes mellitus. The review discusses the various modalities of imaging, with their advantages and disadvantages. Specifically, digital subtraction angiography, contrast-enhanced magnetic resonance angiography, and computerized tomographic angiography are delineated in detail. For any vascular specialist who evaluates and treats lower extremity ischemia, specifically in patients with diabetes, this review provides a comprehensive review on imaging that is essential for the understanding of when and why to use different techniques of imaging the arterial system. The review covers the important reasons for using each test, indicating how the test works, which vessels are particularly visualized with that particular imaging modality, and importantly, the potential adverse events that can occur and which every practitioner either ordering or performing the examination should be aware of. The Table in the review summarizes the various imaging modalities, outlining the advantages and disadvantages for each.

J. D. Raffetto, MD

5 Perioperative Considerations

Risk factors and outcome of new-onset cardiac arrhythmias in vascular surgery patients

Winkel TA, Schouten O, Hoeks SE, et al (Dept of Vascular Surgery, Erasmus MC, Rotterdam, The Netherlands; Reinier de Graaf Hosp, Delft, The Netherlands; et al)

Am Heart J 159:1108-1115, 2010

Background.—The pathophysiology of new-onset cardiac arrhythmias is complex and may bring about severe cardiovascular complications. The relevance of perioperative arrhythmias during vascular surgery has not been investigated. The aim of this study was to assess risk factors and prognosis of new-onset arrhythmias during vascular surgery.

Methods.—A total of 513 vascular surgery patients, without a history of arrhythmias, were included. Cardiac risk factors, inflammatory status, and left ventricular function (LVF; N-terminal pro−B-type natriuretic peptide and echocardiography) were assessed. Continuous electrocardiography (ECG) recordings for 72 hours were used to identify ischemia and new-onset arrhythmias: atrial fibrillation, sustained ventricular tachycardia, supraventricular tachycardia, and ventricular fibrillation. Logistic regression analysis was applied to identify preoperative risk factors for arrhythmias. Cox regression analysis assessed the impact of arrhythmias on cardiovascular event-free survival during 1.7 years.

Results.—New-onset arrhythmias occurred in 55 (11%) of 513 patients: atrial fibrillation, ventricular tachycardia, supraventricular tachycardia, and ventricular fibrillation occurred in 4%, 7%, 1%, and 0.2%, respectively. Continuous ECG showed myocardial ischemia and arrhythmias in 17 (3%) of 513 patients. Arrhythmia was preceded by ischemia in 10 of 55 cases. Increased age and reduced LVF were risk factors for the development of arrhythmias. Multivariate analysis showed that perioperative arrhythmias were associated with long-term cardiovascular events, irrespective of the presence of perioperative ischemia (hazard ratio 2.2, 95% CI 1.3-3.8, $P = .004$).

Conclusion.—New-onset perioperative arrhythmias are common after vascular surgery. The elderly and patients with reduced LVF show arrhythmias. Perioperative continuous ECG monitoring helps to identify this high-risk group at increased risk of cardiovascular events and death.

▶ More than 30 years ago, Goldman[1] published a prospective series on patients undergoing major noncardiac surgery and only 4% developed postoperative supraventricular arrhythmias. One conclusion was that postoperative supraventricular arrhythmias were often transient and the most important thing was to correct the cause of the arrhythmia. We now know that cardiac arrhythmias occurring postoperatively are associated with increased hospital stay and higher cardiac morbidity and mortality and can be seen in up to 20% of patients undergoing noncardiac surgery.[2,3] The risk of cardiovascular events is also especially elevated in noncardiac vascular surgical patients.[4] Patients undergoing noncardiac surgery who have postoperative cardiac arrhythmias have primarily atrial arrhythmias that originate within the first few postoperative days. Many events are asymptomatic and often transient and unpredictable, suggesting that true prevalence may be underestimated in clinical practice. The number of each type of arrhythmia occurring in this study did not permit meaningful subset analysis. The association of arrhythmias with older age and preoperative decreased left ventricular function is not all that surprising but has some implications. Currently, many vascular surgical patients are routinely subjected to telemetry monitoring. Given the number of arrhythmias identified in this study, the current data may question the use of such a blanket policy for patients without known preoperative left ventricular dysfunction.

G. L. Moneta, MD

References

1. Goldman L. Supraventricular tachyarrhythmias in hospitalized adults after surgery. Clinical correlates in patients over 40 years of age after major noncardiac surgery. *Chest.* 1978;73:450-454.
2. Brathwaite D, Weissman C. The new onset of atrial arrhythmias following major noncardiothoracic surgery is associated with increased mortality. *Chest.* 1998;114: 462-468.
3. Walsh SR, Tang T, Wijewardena C, Yarham SI, Boyle JR, Gaunt ME. Postoperative arrhythmias in general surgical patients. *Ann R Coll Surg Engl.* 2007;89: 91-95.
4. Schouten O, Bax JJ, Poldermans D. Preoperative cardiac risk assessment in vascular surgery patients: seeing beyond the perioperative period. *Eur Heart J.* 2008;29:283-284.

A statewide consortium of surgical care: A longitudinal investigation of vascular operative procedures at 16 hospitals
Henke PK, Kubus J, Englesbe MJ, et al (Univ of Michigan, Ann Arbor)
Surgery 148:883-892, 2010

Background.—Regional surgical quality improvement consortiums are becoming more common. Herein we have reported the effectiveness of a statewide consortium focusing on open vascular operative procedures.

Methods.—The statewide Michigan Surgical Quality Consortium was established in 2005 with 16 hospitals that report cases of vascular open operative intervention, in a sampling manner consistent with the private sector National Surgical Quality Improvement Program. Data are abstracted by onsite trained nurses using defined and validated pre-, peri-, and postoperative variables with 30-day follow-up. Outpatient and emergent cases were excluded. We compared outcomes over the course of the consortium (era I, April 2005—March 2007; era II, April 2007—March 2008) via univariate and multivariate techniques.

Results.—Era I ($n = 2,453$) and era II ($n = 3,409$) cases were similar in age (mean, 68 years), gender (61% male), relative value units (mean, 21), and distribution of Current Procedural Terminology codes. Duration of stay and operative time decreased by 15% and 11%, respectively, when comparing era I with era II ($P < .001$). Mortality at 30 days was not different between eras I and II (2.7% vs 2.5%; $P =$ NS), but morbidity was decreased (15.8% vs 13.8%; $P = .02$). Specific decreases were noted in sepsis and pulmonary, but not cardiac or renal, complications. When evaluating both eras, modifiable variables (able to be altered by the surgeon) for morbidity included increased length of operation (odds ratio [OR], 1.004; 95% confidence interval [CI], 1.003—1.005; $P < .0001$), hypertension (OR, 1.46; 95% CI, 1.03—2.1; $P = .03$), and blood transfusion (OR, 2.8; 95% CI, 2.04—3.88; $P < .0001$). However, anemic patients (11%; hematocrit <30) who were transfused were less likely to suffer morbidity (OR, 56; 95% CI, 0.47—0.67; $P < .0001$) than those transfused who were not anemic. The absolute 2% reduction in complications led to a $172 cost savings for the payers per patient in era II compared with era I.

Conclusion.—A statewide quality-of-care consortium with timely feed-back of data was associated with decreased morbidity over a relatively short follow-up period in vascular patients. Focusing on best processes in real-world practice, such as appropriate transfusion and length of oper-ation, may further improve vascular surgical outcomes.

▶ Morbidity of vascular surgery can be reduced from proper application of endoluminal techniques. Many patients with vascular disease, given the limits of technology, still, however, require major open procedures. With the publica-tion of the Institute of Medicine's landmark report, *To Err is Human*, in 1999, there has been increased emphasis on identifying processes to improve outcomes and quality of care. There has also been increased oversight from both government and nongovernmental quality organizations. These include both national bodies such as the National Surgical Quality Improvement Program (NSQIP) and more regional quality of care consortiums. In Michigan, there is a statewide volunteer group of hospitals called the Michigan Surgical Quality Consortium (MSQC). These are primarily nonteaching hospitals that use the NSQIP data abstraction and reporting format. MSQC feeds back infor-mation to individual hospitals regarding their hospital morbidity and mortality data. There are quarterly conferences that review evidence-based practices, such as venous thromboembolism prophylaxis, pulmonary complications, and transfusions. In this study, the authors sought to determine whether improvements in morbidity or mortality have occurred since the inception of the MSQC program. The study indicates that a statewide surgical hospital consortium using the NSQIP platform can produce significant but modest decreases in morbidity over a relatively short time. This decrease in morbidity translated into a significant projected cost savings, despite the fact the cost of NSQIP is about $135 000. Financial support of MSQC, a pay-for-participation system, is primarily provided by the Blues of Michigan. There is currently an effort to establish regional vascular consortiums nationwide. The cost of collecting and analyzing this type of data is not insignificant, and perhaps efforts should be made for these regional consortiums to be supported by insurance companies rather than individual physicians and hospitals.

G. L. Moneta, MD

Bleeding Complications With Dual Antiplatelet Therapy Among Patients With Stable Vascular Disease or Risk Factors for Vascular Disease: Results From the Clopidogrel for High Atherothrombotic Risk and Ischemic Stabilization, Management, and Avoidance (CHARISMA) Trial
Berger PB, for the CHARISMA Investigators (Ctr for Clinical Studies, Geisinger Clinic, Danville, PA; et al)
Circulation 121:2575-2583, 2010

Background.—Uncertainty exists about the frequency, correlates, and clinical significance of bleeding with dual antiplatelet therapy (DAPT), particularly over an extended period in a stable population. We sought to determine the frequency and time course of bleeding with DAPT in patients with established vascular disease or risk factors only; identify correlates of bleeding; and determine whether bleeding is associated with mortality.

Methods and Results.—We analyzed 15 603 patients enrolled in the Clopidogrel for High Atherothrombotic Risk and Ischemic Stabilization, Management, and Avoidance (CHARISMA) trial, a double-blind, placebo-controlled, randomized trial comparing long-term clopidogrel 75 mg/d versus placebo; all patients received aspirin (75 to 162 mg) daily. Patients had either established stable vascular disease or multiple risk factors for vascular disease without established disease. Median follow-up was 28 months. Bleeding was assessed with the use of the Global Utilization of Streptokinase and t-PA for Occluded Coronary Arteries (GUSTO) criteria. Severe bleeding occurred in 1.7% of the clopidogrel group versus 1.3% on placebo ($P=0.087$); moderate bleeding occurred in 2.1% versus 1.3%, respectively ($P<0.001$). The risk of bleeding was greatest the first year. Patients without moderate or severe bleeding during the first year were no more likely than placebo-treated patients to have bleeding thereafter. The frequency of bleeding was similar in patients with established disease and risk factors only. In multivariable analysis, the relationship between moderate bleeding and all-cause mortality was strong (hazard ratio, 2.55; 95% confidence interval, 1.71 to 3.80; *P*<0.0001), along with myocardial infarction (hazard ratio, 2.92; 95% confidence interval, 2.04 to 4.18; *P*<0.0001) and stroke (hazard ratio, 4.20; 95% confidence interval, 3.05 to 5.77; *P*<0.0001). *Conclusions.*—In CHARISMA, there was an increased risk of bleeding with long-term clopidogrel. The incremental risk of bleeding was greatest in the first year and similar thereafter. Moderate bleeding was strongly associated with mortality.

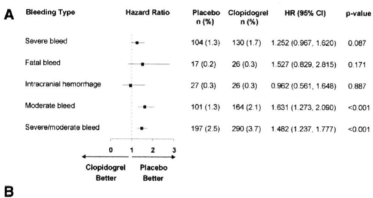

FIGURE 1.—A, Frequency and types of bleeding among the 15 603 patients enrolled in CHARISMA. Bleeding rates were cumulative Kaplan-Meier estimates. HRs and their 95% CIs were measured by Cox proportional hazard models. *P* values were calculated with log-rank tests. B, Frequency and types of bleeding in patients with established vascular disease (symptomatic) and risk factors without established vascular disease (asymptomatic). Bleeding rates were cumulative Kaplan-Meier estimates. HRs, their 95% CIs, and *P* values for interaction of baseline vascular disease state and treatment effect were measured by Cox proportional hazard models. (Reprinted from Berger PB, for the CHARISMA Investigators. Bleeding complications with dual antiplatelet therapy among patients with stable vascular disease or risk factors for vascular disease: results from the clopidogrel for high atherothrombotic risk and ischemic stabilization, management, and avoidance (CHARISMA) trial. *Circulation.* 2010;121:2575-2583.)

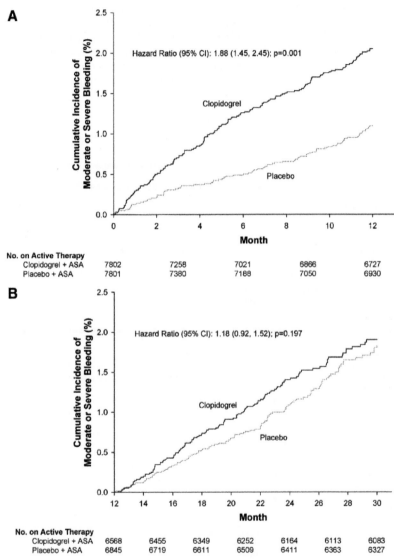

A

Hazard Ratio (95% CI): 1.88 (1.45, 2.45); p=0.001

Clopidogrel

Placebo

No. on Active Therapy					
Clopidogrel + ASA	7802	7258	7021	6866	6727
Placebo + ASA	7801	7380	7188	7050	6930

B

Hazard Ratio (95% CI): 1.18 (0.92, 1.52); p=0.197

Clopidogrel

Placebo

No. on Active Therapy						
Clopidogrel + ASA	6568	6455	6349	6252	6164	6113	6083
Placebo + ASA	6845	6719	6611	6509	6411	6363	6327

FIGURE 2.—Kaplan-Meier curves for moderate or severe bleeding. A, Kaplan-Meier curves for moderate or severe bleeding in the first year. B, Kaplan-Meier curves for moderate or severe bleeding after the first year in patients who did not have moderate or severe bleeding during the first year. ASA indicates acetylsalicylic acid. (Reprinted from Berger PB, for the CHARISMA Investigators. Bleeding complications with dual antiplatelet therapy among patients with stable vascular disease or risk factors for vascular disease: results from the clopidogrel for high atherothrombotic risk and ischemic stabilization, management, and avoidance (CHARISMA) trial. *Circulation.* 2010;121:2575-2583.)

Clinical Trial Registration.—URL: http://www.clinicaltrials.gov. Unique identifier: NCT00050817 (Figs 1 and 2).

▶ It is known that dual antiplatelet therapy using clopidogrel and aspirin is effective in reducing thrombotic events in patients with acute coronary syndromes and those undergoing placement of both bare and drug-eluting coronary stents. In the original Clopidogrel for High Atherothrombotic Risk and Ischemic Stabilization, Management, and Avoidance (CHARISMA) study on a background of aspirin therapy, clopidogrel was compared with placebo for a median of 28 months for ability to reduce thrombotic events. On this background of aspirin therapy, clopidogrel did not reduce thrombotic events in the overall study population.[1] However, in patients with stable vascular disease, clopidogrel in addition to aspirin led to a 12% relative decrease in cardiovascular death, myocardial infarction, or stroke versus those who were treated for risk factors only where there was a 20% increase in these events.[2] Because the source of this increased risk in patients with risk factors may only be bleeding, the authors sought to determine if bleeding risk was sufficiently high to argue against dual antiplatelet therapy even in patients with stable vascular disease, who appear to benefit from dual antiplatelet therapy. Results here, however, did not confirm the idea that excess bleeding in lower risk patients explained greater mortality with use of dual antiplatelet therapy in at-risk patients only. For the vascular surgeon who frequently treats his or her patient with dual antiplatelet therapy, the bottom line is that such therapy will be associated with a risk of moderate or severe bleeding of approximately 4% and that this risk is greatest in the first year of therapy (Figs 1 and 2). In addition, further analysis of the CHARISMA trial has indicated that in dual antiplatelet therapy, lower dose aspirin administered with clopidogrel has a lower risk of bleeding than higher doses of aspirin.[3] Overall, dual antiplatelet therapy administered to patients with established vascular disease lowers risk of future cardiovascular events with a small, but measurable, increased risk of bleeding that, if it occurs, will adversely affect mortality.

G. L. Moneta, MD

References

1. Bhatt DL, Fox KA, Hacke W, et al. Clopidogrel and aspirin versus aspirin alone for the prevention of atherothrombotic events. *N Engl J Med.* 2006;354:1706-1717.
2. Bhatt DL, Flather MD, Hacke W, et al. Patients with prior myocardial infarction, stroke, or symptomatic peripheral arterial disease in the CHARISMA trial. *J Am Coll Cardiol.* 2007;49:1982-1988.
3. Steinhubl SR, Bhatt DL, Brennan DM, et al. Aspirin to prevent cardiovascular disease: the association of aspirin dose and clopidogrel with thrombosis and bleeding. *Ann Intern Med.* 2009;150:379-386.

Changes in Red Blood Cell Transfusion Practice during the Turn of the Millennium: A Retrospective Analysis of Adult Patients Undergoing Elective Open Abdominal Aortic Aneurysm Repair Using the Mayo Database

Long TR, Curry TB, Stemmann JL, et al (Mayo Clinic, Rochester, MN)
Ann Vasc Surg 24:447-454, 2010

Background.—Significant changes in perioperative red blood cell (RBC) transfusion practice during the past two decades have been reported but similar data are not available for patients undergoing abdominal aortic aneurysm (AAA) surgery.

Methods.—Adult patients who had undergone primary, elective, open AAA repair were stratified into one of two transfusion-related groups: early practice (1980—1982) or late practice (2003—2006). RBC transfusion and hemoglobin concentration (Hb) were analyzed as a continuous variable and compared between groups with use of the rank sum test. Perioperative complications were compared between groups with Fisher's exact test. Data were age adjusted, and analyses were corrected for multiple comparisons.

Results.—Compared with the early practice group, patients in the late practice group had significantly lower intraoperative (mean 10 ± 1.4 vs. 11.5 ± 1.5 g/dL), postoperative (11.9 ± 1.4 vs. 13.4 ± 1.5 g/dL), and discharge Hbs (mean 10.8 ± 1.2 vs. 12.5 ± 1.5 g/dL) ($p < 0.0001$ for each variable). Patients in the late practice group were significantly less likely to receive intraoperative allogenic transfusions (46% vs. 99%, $p < 0.0001$). Additionally, significantly fewer total allogenic units of RBCs per patient were transfused in the late practice group (mean 1.7 vs. 4.3, $p < 0.0001$). Intraoperative autotransfusions were used in 97% of the late practice patients but in none of the early practice patients ($p < 0.0001$). In the late practice group, 119 patients (40%) experienced a major perioperative morbidity or mortality event compared with 106 patients (35%) in the early practice group ($p = 0.27$).

Conclusion.—In this retrospective analysis, we observed significantly lower perioperative Hb, fewer allogenic RBC transfusions, and more autotransfusions in open AAA repairs done in 2003—2006 versus those done in 1980—1982. Additionally, late transfusion practice patients were older and had more comorbid diseases. Despite these observations, no significant differences in perioperative morbidity or mortality were observed between groups.

▶ The average cost of transfusion of a red blood cell (RBC) unit is $153.68, and there are 14 million units of RBCs transfused annually in the United States.[1] Changes in transfusion practice over the last decade include decreases in hematrocrit and hemoglobin threshold levels for transfusion and a decrease in the number of allogenic RBC units transfused during major surgery. The authors previously reported lower hemoglobin levels in patients undergoing major spine operations that did not seem to result in any significant change in perioperative morbidity or mortality.[2] There is currently enthusiasm for reducing the number of transfused units because of cost and reported increased morbidity and mortality and infectious complications with increased transfusions. The authors sought to determine whether changes in transfusion practice during a 2-decade study had any impact on perioperative morbidity and mortality in patients undergoing open elective abdominal aortic aneurysm (AAA) repair. They could not demonstrate any difference in the 2 time periods. RBC transfusion is associated with worsening of outcomes in cardiac surgery patients and in patients experiencing acute coronary syndrome.[3,4] However, a randomized trial in critically ill patients comparing liberal versus conservative RBC transfusion found no difference in survival with the 2 treatment strategies.[5] This study also found no difference in major morbidity or mortality in patients undergoing AAA repair with respect to a changing transfusion policy using more conservative thresholds for transfusion. However, the patients did no worse and given the expense incurred with each unit transfused, a more conservative policy for patients undergoing open AAA repair is at least indicated financially if not medically.

G. L. Moneta, MD

References

1. Sullivan NT, Cotten R, Read EJ, Wallace EL. Blood collection and transfusion in the United States in 2001. *Transfusion.* 2007;47:385-394.
2. Wass CT, Long TR, Faust RJ, Yaszemski MJ, Joyner MJ. Changes in red blood cell transfusion practice during the past two decades: a retrospective analysis, with the Mayo database, of adult patients undergoing major spine surgery. *Transfusion.* 2007;47:1022-1027.
3. Murphy GJ, Reeves BC, Rogers CA, Rizvi SI, Culliford L, Angelini GD. Increased mortality, postoperative morbidity, and cost after red blood cell transfusion in patients having cardiac surgery. *Circulation.* 2007;116:2544-2552.
4. Rao SV, Jollis JG, Harrington RA, et al. Relationship of blood transfusion and clinical outcomes in patients with acute coronary syndromes. *JAMA.* 2004;292:1555-1562.
5. Hébert PC, Wells G, Blajchman MA, et al. A multicenter, randomized, controlled clinical trial of transfusion requirements in critical care. Transfusion Requirements in Critical Care Investigators, Canadian Critical Care Trials Group. *N Engl J Med.* 1999;340:409-417.

Cost-effectiveness analysis of general anaesthesia *versus* local anaesthesia for carotid surgery (GALA Trial)
Gomes M, the GALA Collaborative Group (Univ of York, UK; et al)
Br J Surg 97:1218-1225, 2010

Background.—Health outcomes and costs are both important when deciding whether general (GA) or local (LA) anaesthesia should be used during carotid endarterectomy. The aim of this study was to assess the cost-effectiveness of carotid endarterectomy under LA or GA in patients with symptomatic or asymptomatic carotid stenosis for whom surgery was advised.

Methods.—Using patient-level data from a large, multinational, randomized controlled trial (GALA Trial) time free from stroke, myocardial infarction or death, and costs incurred were evaluated. The cost-effectiveness outcome was incremental cost per day free from an event, within a time horizon of 30 days.

Results.—A patient undergoing carotid endarterectomy under LA incurred fewer costs (mean difference £178) and had a slightly longer event-free survival (difference 0·16 days, but the 95 per cent confidence limits around this estimate were wide) compared with a patient who had GA. Existing uncertainty did not have a significant impact on the decision to adopt LA, over a wide range of willingness-to-pay values.

Conclusion.—If cost-effectiveness was considered in the decision to adopt GA or LA for carotid endarterectomy, given the evidence provided by this study, LA is likely to be the favoured treatment for patients for whom either anaesthetic approach is clinically appropriate.

▶ Studies have indicated that carotid endarectomy (CEA) is cost-effective relative to medical management in treatment of both symptomatic and asymptomatic patients with significant internal carotid artery occlusive disease.[1,2]

CEA also appears to be more cost-effective than carotid angioplasty.[3] The General Anaesthetic versus Local Anaesthetic for carotid surgery (GALA) Trial was a large international randomized trial conducted in 95 centers and 24 countries with 3526 subjects that compared general and local anesthesia for CEA. The trial primarily focused on odds of stroke and death with general versus local anesthesia and found no clear difference in perioperative events when CEA was performed with local versus general anesthesia. In this secondary analysis, the authors sought to determine cost-effectiveness of CEA under general versus local anesthesia in patients with symptomatic or asymptomatic carotid stenosis. Unfortunately, the cost data here are 7 to 8 years old, and it should be noted that the median length of hospital stay in this trial for patients undergoing CEA, with either local or general anesthesia, was 6 days, an extraordinarily long time by North American standards. It is, therefore, very unlikely that one can extrapolate this data beyond the United Kingdom or Europe. The conclusion that local anesthesia is more cost-effective than general anesthesia based on this data is likely suspect in 2010. The data cannot be used to justify one form of anesthetic over another for performance of CEA. Surgeons and anesthesiologists should continue to use the anesthetic technique that they are most comfortable with as clinical end points appear to be the same with local and general anesthesia as indicated in the original GALA Trial.

G. L. Moneta, MD

References

1. Cronenwett JL, Birkmeyer JD, Nackman GB, et al. Cost-effectiveness of carotid endarterectomy in asymptomatic patients. *J Vasc Surg.* 1997;25:298-309.
2. Henricksson M, Lundgren F, Carlsson P. Cost-effectiveness of endarterectomy in patients with asymptomatic carotid artery stenosis. *Br J Surg.* 2008;95:714-720.
3. Kilaru S, Korn P, Kasirajan K, et al. Is carotid angioplasty and stenting more cost effective than carotid endarterectomy? *J Vasc Surg.* 2003;37:331-339.

Effect of early plasma transfusion on mortality in patients with ruptured abdominal aortic aneurysm
Mell MW, O'Neil AS, Callcut RA, et al (Stanford Univ, CA; Univ of Wisconsin, Madison)
Surgery 148:955-962, 2010

Background.—The ratio of red blood cell (PRBC) transfusion to plasma (FFP) transfusion (PRBC:FFP ratio) has been shown to impact survival in trauma patients with massive hemorrhage. The purpose of this study was to determine the effect of the PRBC:FFP ratio on mortality for patients with massive hemorrhage after ruptured abdominal aortic aneurysm (RAAA).

Methods.—A retrospective review was performed of patients undergoing emergent open RAAA repair from January 1987 to December 2007. Patients with massive hemorrhage ($\geq$10 units of blood products transfused prior to conclusion of the operation) were included. The effects of patient demographics, admission vital signs, laboratory values, perioperative variables, amount of blood products transfused, and the PRBC:FFP ratio on 30-day mortality were analyzed by multivariate analysis.

Results.—One hundred and twenty-eight of the 168 (76%) patients undergoing repair for RAAA received at least 10 units of blood products within the peri-operative period. Mean age was 73.1 ± 9.1 years, and 109 (85%) were men. Thirty-day mortality was 22.6% (29/128), including 11 intra-operative deaths. By multivariate analysis, 30-day mortality was markedly lower (15% vs 39%; $P < .03$) for patients transfused at a PRBC:FFP ratio $\leq$2:1 (HIGH FFP group) compared with those transfused at a ratio of >2:1 (LOW FFP), and the likelihood of death was more than 4-fold greater in the LOW FFP group (odds ratio 4.23; 95% confidence interval, 1.2–14.49). Patients in the HIGH FFP group had a significantly lower incidence of colon ischemia than those in the LOW FFP group (22.4% vs 41.1%; $P = .004$).

Conclusion.—For RAAA patients requiring massive transfusion, more equivalent transfusion of PRBC to FFP (HIGH FFP) was independently associated with lower 30-day mortality. The lower incidence of colonic ischemia in the HIGH FFP group may suggest an additional benefit of early plasma transfusion that could translate into further mortality reduction. Analysis from this study suggests the potential feasibility for a more standardized protocol of initial resuscitation for these patients, and prospective studies are warranted to determine the optimum PRBC:FFP ratio in RAAA patients.

▶ There are a number of factors known to influence survival after ruptured abdominal aortic aneurysm (AAA). Adverse predictors include advanced age, preoperative shock, poor intraoperative hemodynamics, oliguria, and postoperative complications. Improved outcomes have been associated with increased surgeon volume and specialty training. Researchers in resuscitation research have recently focused on types and amounts of blood products administered with respect to mortality after massive hemorrhage from trauma. It appears in patients with trauma who require at least 10 units of blood products in < 24 hours that mortality can be decreased with increased administration of fresh frozen plasma (FFP) and decreased administration of packed red blood cells (PRBCs). A PRBC to FFP ratio of < 2:1 seems to be associated with the greatest decrease in mortality after trauma.[1] The authors hypothesized that this should logically extend to patients with ruptured AAA who require massive transfusion. The very-low overall 30-day mortality of 22.6% in a group of patients undergoing open repair of a ruptured AAA is exemplary. While this low mortality rate likely suggests some referral bias and transfer of patients to a regional center, the results are nonetheless excellent. The clear benefit in this study and in the trauma literature of a higher ratio of transfusion of FFP to PRBC in patients with massive hemorrhage strongly argues for a standardized protocol of resuscitation of patients with ruptured AAA, whereas avoidance of coagulopathy or minimizing coagulopathy would appear to be an obvious potential benefit of increased use of FFP during the resuscitation of the AAA patient. It also appears from the authors' data that a reduction in colon ischemia may be an additional benefit of more liberal use of FFP during massive transfusion of the patient with ruptured AAA.

G. L. Moneta, MD

Reference

1. Holcomb JB, Wade CE, Michalek JE, et al. Increased plasma and platelet to red blood cell ratios improves outcome in 466 massively transfused civilian trauma patients. *Ann Surg.* 2008;248:447-458.

Randomized Controlled Trial of Dual Antiplatelet Therapy in Patients Undergoing Surgery for Critical Limb Ischemia
Burdess A, Nimmo AF, Garden OJ, et al (The Univ of Edinburgh, UK; et al)
Ann Surg 252:37-42, 2010

Background and Objective.—Patients with critical limb ischemia have a perioperative cardiovascular morbidity comparable to patients with acute coronary syndromes. We hypothesized that perioperative dual antiplatelet therapy would improve biomarkers of atherothrombosis without causing unacceptable bleeding in patients undergoing surgery for critical limb ischemia.

Methods.—In a double-blind randomized controlled trial, 108 patients undergoing infrainguinal revascularization or amputation for critical limb ischemia were maintained on aspirin (75 mg daily) and randomized to clopidogrel (600 mg prior to surgery, and 75 mg daily for 3 days; n = 50) or matched placebo (n = 58). Platelet activation and myocardial injury were assessed by flow cytometry and plasma troponin concentrations, respectively.

Results.—Clopidogrel reduced platelet-monocyte aggregation before surgery (38%−30%; $P = 0.007$). This was sustained in the postoperative period ($P = 0.0019$). There were 18 troponin-positive events (8 [16.0%] clopidogrel vs. 10 [17.2%] placebo; relative risk [RR]: 0.93, 95% confidence interval [CI]: 0.39−2.17; $P = 0.86$). Half of troponin-positive events occurred preoperatively with clopidogrel causing a greater decline in troponin concentrations ($P < 0.001$). There was no increase in major life-threatening bleeding (7 [14%] vs. 6 [10%]; RR: 1.4, 95% CI: 0.49−3.76; $P = 0.56$) or minor bleeding (17 [34%] vs. 12 [21%]; RR 1.64, 95% CI: 0.87−3.1; $P = 0.12$), although blood transfusions were increased (28% vs. 12.6%, RR: 2.3, 95% CI: 1.0−5.29; $P = 0.037$).

Conclusions.—In patients with critical limb ischemia, perioperative dual antiplatelet therapy reduces biomarkers of atherothrombosis without causing unacceptable bleeding. Large-scale randomized controlled trials are needed to establish whether dual antiplatelet therapy improves clinical outcome in high-risk patients undergoing vascular surgery.

▶ Myocardial injury is common following vascular surgery with reported incidences between 8% and 40%. It is known that in patients with vascular disease, use of clopidogrel has a moderate additional secondary preventative effect to that of aspirin for prevention of cardiovascular end points.[1,2] In addition, the combination of aspirin and clopidogrel reduces recurrent ischemic events in patients with acute coronary syndrome. The authors reasoned that given the benefits of dual antiplatelet therapy noted above, it would be reasonable to postulate that dual antiplatelet therapy may have benefit in patients undergoing vascular surgery. The hypothesis was that the perioperative dual antiplatelet therapy would improve biomarkers of atherothrombosis in patients undergoing surgery for critical limb ischemia without causing unacceptable bleeding intra- and postoperatively. Although the study was underpowered to detect a difference in clinical events, the authors were able to demonstrate improvements in biomarkers of platelet activation and myocardial injury without an increase in bleeding complications. It is of interest that many troponin-positive events occurred before surgery. This suggests that silent preoperative myocardial injury is more common than previously suspected in patients with critical limb ischemia. The study indicates potential benefits of dual antiplatelet therapy in the perioperative period in patients with critical limb ischemia. Whether these improvements in surrogate biomarkers translate into clinical benefit remains to be established.

G. L. Moneta, MD

References

1. Bhatt DL, Fox KA, Hacke W, et al. Clopidogrel and aspirin versus aspirin alone for the prevention of atherothrombotic events. *N Engl J Med.* 2006;354:1706-1717.
2. Yusuf S, Zhao F, Mehta SR, et al. Effects of clopidogrel in addition to aspirin in patients with acute coronary syndromes without ST-segment elevation. *N Engl J Med.* 2001;345:494-502.

Relation between Preoperative and Intraoperative New Wall Motion Abnormalities in Vascular Surgery Patients: A Transesophageal Echocardiographic Study

Galal W, Hoeks SE, Flu WJ, et al (Erasmus Univ Med Ctr, Rotterdam, the Netherlands; et al)
Anesthesiology 112:557-566, 2010

Background.—Coronary revascularization of the suspected culprit coronary lesion assessed by preoperative stress testing is not associated with improved outcome in vascular surgery patients.

Methods.—Fifty-four major vascular surgery patients underwent preoperative dobutamine echocardiography and intraoperative transesophageal echocardiography. The locations of left ventricular rest wall motion abnormalities and new wall motion abnormalities (NWMAs) were scored using a seven-wall model. During 30-day follow-up, postoperative cardiac troponin release, myocardial infarction, and cardiac death were noted.

Results.—Rest wall motion abnormalities were noted by dobutamine echocardiography in 17 patients (31%), and transesophageal echocardiography was noted in 16 (30%). NWMAs were induced during dobutamine echocardiography in 17 patients (31%), whereas NWMAs were observed by transesophageal echocardiography in 23 (43%), κ value = 0.65. Although preoperative and intraoperative rest wall motion abnormalities showed an excellent agreement for the location (κ value = 0.92), the agreement for preoperative and intraoperative NWMAs in different locations was poor (κ value = 0.26—0.44). The composite cardiac endpoint occurred in 14 patients (26%).

Conclusions.—There was a poor correlation between the locations of preoperatively assessed stress-induced NWMAs by dobutamine echocardiography and those observed intraoperatively using transesophageal echocardiography. However, the composite endpoint of outcome was met more frequently in relation with intraoperative NWMAs.

▶ Patients with vascular surgery are at increased risk for developing adverse cardiac outcomes postoperatively. However, prophylactic coronary artery vascularization of suspected culprit coronary artery lesions assessed by preoperative testing is not associated with improved outcome following vascular surgical procedures.[1] Intraoperative transesophageal echocardiography (TEE) can detect regional wall motion abnormalities (WMAs) in patients undergoing major noncardiac surgery. However, it is unclear whether new WMAs (NWMAs) detected intraoperatively with TEE actually correlate with abnormalities detected preoperatively with noninvasive stress testing. The author sought to determine whether WMAs identified with dobutamine echocardiography correlate with those observed intraoperatively with TEE.

Reproducibility of WMAs at different perioperative times was not achievable in this study. The suggestion therefore is that optimized medical therapy remains superior over invasive interventions focused on preoperative detection of culprit lesions. In this series, there were no cardiac deaths or postoperative myocardial infarctions in patients without intraoperative NWMAs. The data therefore suggest patients with intraoperative NWMAs detected by TEE are perhaps the highest risk group for perioperative significant cardiac events. They demand the most careful assiduous perioperative management of cardiac parameters.

G. L. Moneta, MD

Reference

1. McFalls EO, Ward HB, Moritz TE, et al. Coronary-artery revascularization before elective major vascular surgery. *N Engl J Med.* 2004;351:2795-2804.

Risk of Surgery Following Recent Myocardial Infarction
Livhits M, Ko CY, Leonardi MJ, et al (David Geffen School of Medicine at UCLA; et al)
Ann Surg 253:857-864, 2011

Objective.—We aimed to assess the impact of recent myocardial infarction (MI) on outcomes after subsequent surgery in the contemporary clinical setting.

Background.—Prior work shows that a history of a recent MI is a risk factor for complications following noncardiac surgery. However, this data does not reflect current advances in clinical management.

Methods.—Using the California Patient Discharge Database, we retrospectively analyzed patients undergoing hip surgery, cholecystectomy, colectomy, elective abdominal aortic aneurysm repair, and lower extremity amputation from 1999 to 2004 (n = 563,842). Postoperative 30-day MI rate, 30-day mortality, and 1-year mortality were compared for patients with and without a recent MI using univariate analyses and multivariate logistic regression. Relative risks (RR) with 95% confidence intervals were estimated using bootstrapping with 1000 repetitions.

Results.—Postoperative MI rate for the recent MI cohort decreased substantially as the length of time from MI to operation increased (0–30 days = 32.8%, 31–60 days = 18.7%, 61–90 days = 8.4%, and 91–180 days = 5.9%), as did 30-day mortality (0–30 days = 14.2%, 31–60 days = 11.5%, 61–90 days = 10.5%, and 91–180 days = 9.9%). MI within 30 days of an operation was associated with a higher risk of postoperative MI (RR range = 9.98–44.29 for the 5 procedures), 30-day mortality (RR range, 1.83–3.84), and 1-year mortality (RR range, 1.56–3.14).

Conclusions.—A recent MI remains a significant risk factor for postoperative MI and mortality following surgery. Strategies such as delaying elective operations for at least 8 weeks and medical optimization should be considered (Fig 1).

▶ The American College of Cardiology and the American Heart Association recommend a waiting period of 4 to 6 weeks after a myocardial infarction

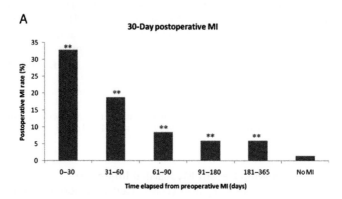

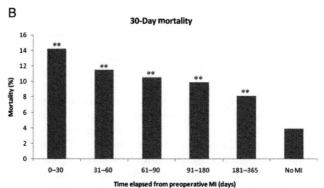

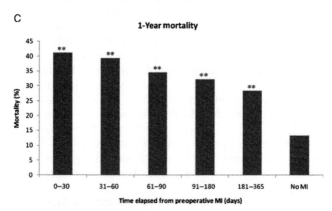

FIGURE 1.—Postoperative Outcomes By Time Elapsed From Recent Myocardial Infarction for All Operations. **A,** 30-Day postoperative myocardial infarction (MI) rate by time elapsed from recent MI for all operations. **P < 0.001 (compared with patients with no recent MI). **B,** 30-day mortality rate by time elapsed from recent myocardial infarction (MI) for all operations. **P < 0.001 (compared with patients with no recent MI). **C,** 1-year mortality rate by time elapsed from recent myocardial infarction (MI) for all operations. **P < 0.001 (compared with patients with no recent MI). (Reprinted from Livhits M, Ko CY, Leonardi MJ, et al. Risk of surgery following recent myocardial infarction. *Ann Surg.* 2011;253:857-864, with permission from Lippincott Williams & Wilkins.)

(MI) before elective surgery. This recommendation, however, is based on relatively low-quality evidence.[1] There are in fact no large contemporary studies assessing risk of surgery for patients with a history of recent MI. Recent advances in reducing operative complications, such as enhanced preoperative screening, better clinical optimization, improved intraoperative monitoring, and more frequent use of β-blockers and statin medications may reduce postoperative morbidity and mortality in patients with cardiac risk factors. Such advances, in fact, may also reduce risk of a subsequent MI in a patient with a recent MI undergoing elective surgery. By examining 5 common noncardiac operations (hip surgery, colectomy, cholecystectomy, abdominal aortic aneurysm repair, and amputation), the authors sought to determine whether a recent MI remains a risk factor for poor postoperative outcomes and whether that risk can be lessened by time elapsed from the MI. The data indicate a recent MI remains a significant risk factor for postoperative MI and mortality. Surprisingly, increased risk of postoperative MI following a recent MI appears greater for nonvascular operations. Perhaps patients undergoing vascular procedures have better perioperative optimization because of greater awareness of their risk factors for cardiac complications. It would be useful in future studies to examine clinical factors, such as β-blocker therapy, blood pressure control, and statin use, and their effects on postoperative MI rate in the patient undergoing elective surgery following a recent MI. Clearly, the bottom line is to wait as long as possible after an MI before proceeding with elective surgery. The most benefit is achieved after waiting 2 months following an MI.

G. L. Moneta, MD

Reference

1. Fleisher LA, Beckman JA, Brown KA, et al. ACC/AHA 2007 guidelines on perioperative cardiovascular evaluation and care for noncardiac surgery: a report of the American College of Cardiology/American Heart Association Task Force on Practice Guidelines (Writing Committee to Revise the 2002 Guidelines on Perioperative Cardiovascular Evaluation for Noncardiac Surgery): developed in collaboration with the American Society of Echocardiography, American Society of Nuclear Cardiology, Heart Rhythm Society, Society of Cardiovascular Anesthesiologists, Society for Cardiovascular Angiography and Interventions, Society for Vascular Medicine and Biology, and Society for Vascular Surgery. *Circulation.* 2007;116: e418-e499.

Statins and All-Cause Mortality in High-Risk Primary Prevention: A Meta-analysis of 11 Randomized Controlled Trials Involving 65 229 Participants

Ray KK, Seshasai SRK, Erqou S, et al (Univ of Cambridge, England; et al)
Arch Intern Med 170:1024-1031, 2010

Background.—Statins have been shown to reduce the risk of all-cause mortality among individuals with clinical history of coronary heart disease. However, it remains uncertain whether statins have similar mortality benefit in a high-risk primary prevention setting. Notably, all systematic reviews to date included trials that in part incorporated participants with prior cardiovascular disease (CVD) at baseline. Our objective was to reliably determine if statin therapy reduces all-cause mortality among intermediate to high-risk individuals without a history of CVD.

Data Sources.—Trials were identified through computerized literature searches of MEDLINE and Cochrane databases (January 1970-May 2009) using terms related to statins, clinical trials, and cardiovascular end points and through bibliographies of retrieved studies.

Study Selection.—Prospective, randomized controlled trials of statin therapy performed in individuals free from CVD at baseline and that reported details, or could supply data, on all-cause mortality.

Data Extraction.—Relevant data including the number of patients randomized, mean duration of follow-up, and the number of incident deaths were obtained from the principal publication or by correspondence with the investigators.

Data Synthesis.—Data were combined from 11 studies and effect estimates were pooled using a random-effects model meta-analysis, with heterogeneity assessed with the I^2 statistic. Data were available on 65 229 participants followed for approximately 244 000 person-years, during which 2793 deaths occurred. The use of statins in this high-risk primary prevention setting was not associated with a statistically significant reduction (risk ratio, 0.91; 95% confidence interval, 0.83-1.01) in the risk of all-cause mortality. There was no statistical evidence of heterogeneity among studies (I^2=23%; 95% confidence interval, 0%-61% [*P*=.23]).

Conclusion.—This literature-based meta-analysis did not find evidence for the benefit of statin therapy on all-cause mortality in a high-risk primary prevention set-up.

▶ This meta-analysis has enormous implications for patients, physicians, and the pharmaceutical industry. Three quarters of patients who take statins take them for primary prevention. Depending on perspective, the study has enormous implications for expenditures (from payers perspective) or revenue (from industry perspective). An editorial in the same issue of *Archives of Internal Medicine*, by Dr Green, points out that advocates for lipid-lowering therapy for primary prevention of cardiovascular disease feel benefit would likely accrue over a longer time of observation. Skeptics, on the other hand, postulate little incremental benefit will accrue later.[1] Dr Green points out that Josh Billings once said, "It ain't what folks don't know that's the problem, it's what they know that ain't so that is the problem." Accompanying meta-analysis of Ray et al is another article in the same issue of *Archives of Internal Medicine* entitled Cholesterol Lowering, Cardiovascular Diseases, and the Rosuvastatin-JUPITER Controversy, A Critical Reappraisal, by de Lorgeril M.[2] In this accompanying article, the authors point out that the Justification for the Use of Statins in Primary Prevention: An Intervention Trial Evaluating Rosuvastatin (JUPITER) trial is the only trial that has shown benefit for primary prevention with statins. These authors are highly critical of the JUPITER trial in terms of industry control industry-performed statistical analysis conflicts of interest of the authors and premature ending of the trial. All of these facets combine, in their opinion, to make the JUPITER trial results highly suspect. It may be statins for primary prevention of cardiovascular disease in patients at risk is not the home run everyone believes it is. When used for primary prevention, the only beneficiaries of statin therapy may be the pharmaceutical industry and their stockholders.

G. L. Moneta, MD

References

1. Green LA. Cholesterol-lowering therapy for primary prevention: still much we don't know. *Arch Intern Med.* 2010;170:1007-1008.
2. de Lorgeril M, Salen P, Abramson J, et al. Cholesterol lowering, cardiovascular diseases, and the rosuvastatin-JUPITER controversy, a critical reappraisal. *Arch Intern Med.* 2010;170:1032-1036.

Symptomatic perioperative venous thromboembolism is a frequent complication in patients with a history of deep vein thrombosis
Liem TK, Huynh TM, Moseley SE, et al (Oregon Health & Science Univ, Portland)
J Vasc Surg 52:651-657, 2010

Objectives.—Patients who undergo surgery are at risk for venous thromboembolism (VTE), and a history of prior deep vein thrombosis (DVT) increases that risk. This study determined the incidence and risk factors for symptomatic perioperative VTE in patients with a prior diagnosis of DVT.

Methods.—All lower extremity DVTs, diagnosed between January 2002 and December 2006, were identified through a vascular database. Patients who had subsequent surgery were reviewed. The following data were evaluated: location of DVT, time interval between DVT and surgery, type of surgery, common clinical VTE risk factors, postoperative venous duplex scans, computed tomography (CT) scans of the chest, and ventilation-perfusion scans.

Results.—A total of 372 patients with prior DVT underwent 1081 subsequent surgical procedures. One hundred nine patients undergoing 211 procedures had a follow-up venous duplex scan within 30 days after surgery. Of them, 46% received an inferior vena caval (IVC) filter, and pulmonary emboli were diagnosed in 3 patients (<1%). Overall, 24% of the patients developed DVT extension or new-site DVT in the perioperative period. The median time interval between the original DVT and surgery was 1.5 weeks in patients with DVT recurrence and 4 weeks in patients without recurrence ($P = .22$, Mann–Whitney). High-risk surgeries were associated with a >three-fold increased risk for recurrence, when compared with low-risk procedures (34% vs 11%; $P = .009$, χ^2). Perioperative VTE recurrence was not influenced by the location of the original thrombus or other VTE risk factors.

Conclusion.—In patients with prior DVT, perioperative symptomatic recurrence is common and is associated with high-risk procedures. A longer time interval between a DVT episode and subsequent surgery may decrease the risk of recurrence, but large clinical trials are needed to confirm this. Further prospective evaluations are needed to identify and treat patients at greatest risk for recurrence.

▶ The risk of venous thromboembolism (VTE) is increased in patients who undergo high-risk surgical procedures, such as abdominal cancer operations or total hip arthroplasty or total knee arthroplasty. It is reasoned that a previous deep venous thrombosis (DVT) or pulmonary embolism is a likely risk factor for subsequent recurrence of VTE around the time of a major operation. This study was designed to determine the incidence of perioperative VTE recurrence in patients with a history of lower extremity DVT. In addition, the authors sought to make some recommendation on appropriate timing for surgery after an initial episode of VTE. The authors found that the median time interval between previous DVT and a new DVT following operative intervention was 1.5 weeks for those developing recurrent DVT following operation. For those who did not have VTE recurrence following operation, the median time interval between initial DVT and operation was 4 weeks. While these data were not statistically significant, reflecting small numbers of patients in the study, it is consistent with the American College of Chest Physicians guidelines, indicating patients operated within 3 months of their original DVT are at high risk for recurrence. Only after 12 months following DVT, the risk of perioperative recurrence of VTE is considered low. The main points, therefore, are to defer elective surgery as long as possible in patients with a DVT within the last year. When deferring the operation is not possible, enhanced perioperative prophylactic measures for prevention of DVT are indicated.

G. L. Moneta, MD

The Impact of Platelet Transfusion in Massively Transfused Trauma Patients

Inaba K, Lustenberger T, Rhee P, et al (Los Angeles County and Univ of Southern California Med Ctr, CA; Univ of Arizona, Tuscon; et al)
J Am Coll Surg 211:573-579, 2010

Background.—The impact of platelet transfusion in trauma patients undergoing a massive transfusion (MT) was evaluated.

Study Design.—The Institutional Trauma Registry and Blood Bank Database at a Level I trauma center was used to identify all patients requiring an MT (≥10 packed red blood cells [PRBC] within 24 hours of admission). Mortality was evaluated according to 4 apheresis platelet (aPLT):PRBC ratios: Low ratio (<1:18), medium ratio (≥1:18 and <1:12), high ratio (≥1:12 and <1:6), and highest ratio (≥1:6).

Results.—Of 32,289 trauma patients, a total of 657 (2.0%) required an MT. At 24 hours, 171 patients (26.0%) received a low ratio, 77 (11.7%)

a medium ratio, 249 (37.9%) a high ratio, and 160 (24.4%) the highest ratio of aPLT:PRBC. After correcting for differences between groups, the mortality at 24 hours increased in a stepwise fashion with decreasing aPLT:PRBC ratio. Using the highest ratio group as a reference, the adjusted relative risk of death was 1.67 (adjusted p = 0.054) for the high ratio group, 2.28 (adjusted p = 0.013) for the medium ratio group, and 5.51 (adjusted p < 0.001) for the low ratio group. A similar stepwise increase in mortality with decreasing platelet ratio was observed at 12 hours after admission and for overall survival to discharge. After stepwise logistic regression, a high aPLT:PRBC ratio (adjusted p < 0.001) was independently associated with improved survival at 24 hours.

Conclusions.—For injured patients requiring a massive transfusion, as the apheresis platelet-to-red cell ratio increased, a stepwise improvement in survival was seen. Prospective evaluation of the role of platelet transfusion in massively transfused patients is warranted.

▶ There is increased emphasis on aggressive blood component therapy in the massively bleeding patient. Data suggest that improved survival for patients requiring massive transfusion when there is increased use of fresh frozen plasma (FFP) as reflected in ratios approaching 1:1 for administration of FFP and packed red blood cells. Another blood component that is often replaced in massively bleeding patients is platelets. While there is accumulating evidence supporting the use of increased amounts of FFP in the resuscitation of the massively bleeding patient, relatively little data are available to guide transfusion of platelets in the patients undergoing massive transfusion. Component therapy has long been standard for blood banks. Perhaps, unfortunately, this has resulted in individual judgments of how best to resuscitate the massively bleeding patient. Emerging data suggest that predetermined ratios of component therapy can lead to improved survival. In this study, as the platelet-to-red blood cell (RBC) ratio approached 1:6, improvement in survival was seen. While the magnitude of improvement in survival exerted by platelet transfusion in the massively bleeding injured patient was not as strong as that for plasma transfusion, the effect was clear in this study and independently associated of units of FFP transfusion. Additional work is needed, but it appears that platelet transfusion in the massively bleeding patient may be best guided by a ratio of platelets to RBCs transfused. This is opposed to guiding platelet transfusion by platelet count itself. Obviously, we can't directly extrapolate these data to the massively bleeding vascular surgical patient, such as those with ruptured aortic aneurysm, but also given the data presented by Mell et al,[1] it seems likely the massively bleeding vascular surgical patient should be treated in a similar manner as the injured patient undergoing massive transfusion.

G. L. Moneta, MD

Reference

1. Mell MW, O'Neil AS, Callcut RA, et al. Effect of early plasma transfusion on mortality in patients with ruptured abdominal aortic aneurysm. *Surgery.* 2010; 148:955-962.

Timing of Pre-Operative Beta-Blocker Treatment in Vascular Surgery Patients: Influence on Post-Operative Outcome

Flu W-J, van Kuijk J-P, Chonchol M, et al (Erasmus Med Ctr, Rotterdam, the Netherlands; Univ of Colorado Denver Health Sciences Centre, Aurora; et al)
J Am Coll Cardiol 56:1922-1929, 2010

Objectives.—This study evaluated timing of β-blocker initiation before surgery and its relationship with: 1) pre-operative heart rate and high-sensitivity C-reactive-protein (hs-CRP) levels; and 2) post-operative outcome.

Background.—Perioperative guidelines recommend β-blocker initiation days to weeks before surgery, on the basis of expert opinions.

Methods.—In 940 vascular surgery patients, pre-operative heart rate and hs-CRP levels were recorded, next to timing of β-blocker initiation before surgery (0 to 1, >1 to 4, >4 weeks). Pre- and post-operative troponin-T measurements and electrocardiograms were performed routinely. End points were 30-day cardiac events (composite of myocardial infarction and cardiac mortality) and long-term mortality. Multivariate regression analyses, adjusted for cardiac risk factors, evaluated the relation between duration of β-blocker treatment and outcome.

Results.—The β-blockers were initiated 0 to 1, >1 to 4, and >4 weeks before surgery in 158 (17%), 393 (42%), and 389 (41%) patients, respectively. Median heart rate at baseline was 74 ($\pm$17) beats/min, 70 ($\pm$16) beats/min, and 66 ($\pm$15) beats/min (p < 0.001; comparing treatment initiation >1 with <1 week pre-operatively), and hs-CRP was 4.9 ($\pm$7.5) mg/l, 4.1 ($\pm$.6.0) mg/l, and 4.5 ($\pm$6.3) mg/l (p = 0.782), respectively. Treatment initiated >1 to 4 or >4 weeks before surgery was associated with a lower incidence of 30-day cardiac events (odds ratio: 0.46, 95% confidence interval [CI]: 0.27 to 0.76, odds ratio: 0.48, 95% CI: 0.29 to 0.79) and long-term mortality (hazard ratio: 0.52, 95% CI: 0.21 to 0.67, hazard ratio: 0.50, 95% CI: 0.25 to 0.71) compared with treatment initiated <1 week pre-operatively.

Conclusions.—Our results indicate that β-blocker treatment initiated >1 week before surgery is associated with lower pre-operative heart rate and improved outcome, compared with treatment initiated <1 week pre-operatively. No reduction of median hs-CRP levels was observed in patients receiving β-blocker treatment >1 week compared with patients in whom treatment was initiated between 0 and 1 week before surgery (Fig 2, Table 2).

▶ Most randomized controlled trials and observational studies indicate a favorable effect on cardiovascular outcome for vascular surgery patients with perioperative β-blocker therapy. Benefit in perioperative outcomes may be secondary to heart rate control, reduction of systolic pressure, reduction in ventricular contractility, or antiarrhythmic properties of β-blockers. β-blockers may prevent plaque rupture in coronary arteries by reducing mechanical stress on the coronary plaques.[1] β-blockers also may decrease circulating levels of

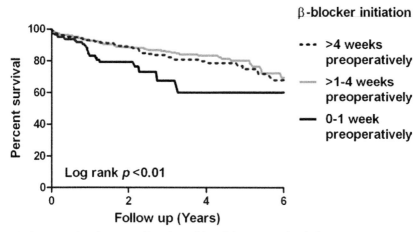

FIGURE 2.—Cumulative Long-Term Survival Stratified to Timing of β-Blocker Initiation. Log-rank p value: comparison of groups >1 to 4 weeks and >4 weeks with group 0 to 1 week. (Reprinted from the Journal of the American College of Cardiology, Flu W-J, van Kuijk J-P, Chonchol M, et al. Timing of Pre-operative beta-blocker treatment in vascular surgery patients: influence on post-operative outcome. *J Am Coll Cardiol*. 2010;56:1922-1929. Copyright 2010, with permission from the American College of Cardiology Foundation.)

TABLE 2.—Timing of β-Blocker Initiation Before Surgery and Post-Operative Outcome

	Timing of β-Blocker Initiation Before Surgery			
Post-Operative Outcome	0−1 Week (n = 158)	>1−4 Weeks (n = 393)	>4 Weeks (n = 389)	p Value*
30-day outcome				
Troponin-T release	40 (25)	54 (14)	56 (14)	0.032
Mortality	6 (4)	8 (2)	11 (3)	0.495
Stroke	3 (19)	2 (0.5)	2 (0.5)	0.021
Cardiovascular events	42 (27)	58 (15)	62 (16)	<0.001
Long-term outcome				
Mortality	30 (19)	55 (14)	57 (15)	0.039

Values are n (%).
*p value: comparison of groups >1 to 4 weeks and >4 weeks taken together with group 0 to 1 week.

C-reactive protein and therefore may stabilize coronary plaques through anti-inflammatory mechanisms.[2] Prior to this study, the duration of β-blocker treatment before vascular surgery and its effect on cardiovascular outcome in vascular surgical patients have not been specifically studied. The data in this article indicate that there are short-term (Table 2) and long-term (Fig 2) advantages to initiating β-blocker therapy more than 1 week preoperatively in patients undergoing vascular surgery. A number of questions do remain. Could one prescribe higher β-blocker doses to achieve more rapid heart rate control and then be able to routinely start treatment < 1 week preoperatively? Or will more aggressive up-titration of β-blocker therapy perhaps lead to potential overdosing of the drug and more side effects? Indeed, the Perioperative

Ischemic Evaluation trial suggested that higher β-blocker doses without up-titration in surgical patients can lead to increased incidence of bradycardia, hypertension, and stroke. Clearly, trying to initiate β-blocker therapy with monitoring and up-titration of therapy in less than a week would pose logistical difficulties. Another question is whether to use perioperative beta blockers in β-blocker—naive patients who require urgent vascular surgery. What this trial tells us is that in elective cases of vascular surgery, one should start β-blockers more than 1 week prior to surgery. What to do with β-blocker—naive patients who require urgent operation remains an open question as does how rapidly can β-blockers be safely introduced to the preoperative vascular surgery patient.

G. L. Moneta, MD

References

1. López-Sendón J, Swedberg K, McMurray J, et al. Expert consensus document on beta-adrenergic receptor blockers. *Eur Heart J.* 2004;25:1341-1362.
2. Jenkins NP, Keevil BG, Hutchinson IV, Brooks NH. Beta-blockers are associated with lower C-reactive protein concentrations in patients with coronary artery disease. *Am J Med.* 2002;112:269-274.

6 Grafts and Graft Complications

Open Repair for Ruptured Abdominal Aortic Aneurysm and the Risk of Spinal Cord Ischemia: Review of the Literature and Risk-factor Analysis
Peppelenbosch AG, Windsant ICV, Jacobs MJ, et al (Maastricht Univ Med Centre, The Netherlands)
Eur J Vasc Endovasc Surg 40:589-595, 2010

Objectives.—Spinal cord ischemia after open surgical repair for rAAA is a rare event. We estimated the current incidence and tried to identify risk factors. We also report a new case.

Methods.—Group A consisted of 10 reports on open repair for rAAA from 1980 until 2009. Only series of ≥100 patients were considered to estimate the incidence. Thirty three case reports from 1956 until 2009 were identified (group B). Case reports from group B were not encountered in group A. Group B patients were stratified according to the type of neurological deficit as described by Gloviczki (type I complete infarction and type II infarction of the anterior two third).

Results.—Group A consisted of 1438 patients. In group A 86% were male with a mean age of 72.1 years. The incidence of post-operative paraplegia was 1.2% (range 0−2.8%). In-hospital mortality was 46.9%. Of the 33 patients of group B were 86% male with a mean age of 68.0 years. Most patients developed a type I (42%) or type II (33%) deficit. In-hospital mortality was 51.6%. No significant differences between different types were encountered.

Conclusion.—Spinal cord ischemia after ruptured AAA is a rare complication with an incidence of 1.2% (range 0−2.8%) (Table 1).

▶ The purpose of this report was to identify the incidence of spinal cord ischemia (SCI) after open repair of ruptured abdominal aortic aneurysms (AAAs). SCI after any repair of infrarenal aortic pathology is a rare event, but these authors, respected in previous works regarding the management of ruptured AAAs, have done a thorough evaluation of the literature and shown that the incidence of SCI after open repair is 1.2% (range, 0%-2.8%). What I found most interesting about this article was a revisiting of the classification of ischemic neurological injuries according to Gloviczki et al (Table 1).[1] The clinical presentation of neurological deficit is variable according to the site of ischemic injury. These authors found after detailed analysis that most patients presenting with SCI after open

TABLE 1.—Classification of Ischemic Neurological Injuries According to Gloviczki et al[3]

Type	Site of Ischemia	Clinical Presentation of Neurological Deficit
I	Complete infarction of the distal spinal cord and conus	Bilateral flaccid paraplegia and sensory loss; bowel and bladder dysfunction
II	Infarction of the anterior two thirds of the spinal cord (anterior spinal artery syndrome)	Bilateral flaccid paraplegia and loss of pain and temperature sensation; intact proprioception and vibration sense
III	Infarction of the lumbosacral roots with or without patchy infarcts in the cord	Bilateral asymmetric paraparesis with or without bowel and bladder incontinence
IV	Unilateral lumbosacral plexus infarction	Same as above; preservation of paraspinal muscle innervation on EMG
V	Segmental infarction of the spinal cord	Bilateral spastic paraplegia with sensory loss.
VI	Infarction of the posterior third of the spinal cord (posterior spinal artery syndrome)	Intact motor function. Loss of proprioception and vibration sense

Editor's Note: Please refer to original journal article for full references.

repair of ruptured AAA (75%) had either type I or type II. Future reports detailing SCI should include this important classification.

B. W. Starnes, MD

Reference

1. Gloviczki P, Cross SA, Stanson AW, et al. Ischemic injury to the spinal cord or lumbosacral plexus after aorto-iliac reconstruction. *Am J Surg.* 1991;162:131-136.

Aspirin Plus Clopidogrel Versus Aspirin Alone After Coronary Artery Bypass Grafting: The Clopidogrel After Surgery for Coronary Artery Disease (CASCADE) Trial

Kulik A, Le May MR, Voisine P, et al (Boca Raton Regional Hosp, FL; Univ of Ottawa Heart Inst, Ontario, Canada; Hôpital Laval, Quebec, Canada; et al)
Circulation 122:2680-2687, 2010

Background.—Clopidogrel inhibits intimal hyperplasia in animal studies and therefore may reduce saphenous vein graft (SVG) intimal hyperplasia after coronary artery bypass grafting. The Clopidogrel After Surgery for Coronary Artery DiseasE (CASCADE) study was undertaken to evaluate whether the addition of clopidogrel to aspirin inhibits SVG disease after coronary artery bypass grafting, as assessed at 1 year by intravascular ultrasound.

Methods and Results.—In this double-blind phase II trial, 113 patients undergoing coronary artery bypass grafting with SVGs were randomized to receive aspirin 162 mg plus clopidogrel 75 mg daily or aspirin 162 mg plus placebo daily for 1 year. The primary outcome was SVG intimal hyperplasia (mean intimal area) as determined by intravascular ultrasound at 1 year. Secondary outcomes were graft patency, major adverse cardiovascular events, and major bleeding. One-year intravascular ultrasound and coronary angiography were performed in 92 patients (81.4%). At 1 year, SVG intimal area did not differ significantly between the 2 groups (4.1 ± 2.0 versus 4.5 ± 2.1 mm^2, aspirin-clopidogrel versus aspirin-placebo, P=0.44). Overall 1-year graft patency was 95.2% in the aspirin-clopidogrel group compared with 95.5% in the aspirin-placebo group (P=0.90), and SVG patency was 94.3% in the aspirin-clopidogrel group versus 93.2% in the aspirin-placebo group (P=0.69). Freedom from major adverse cardiovascular events at 1 year was 92.9 ± 3.4% in the aspirin-clopidogrel group and 91.1 ± 3.8% in the aspirin-placebo group (P=0.76). The incidence of major bleeding at 1 year was similar for the 2 groups (1.8% versus 0%, aspirin-clopidogrel versus aspirin-placebo, P=0.50).

Conclusions.—Compared with aspirin monotherapy, the combination of aspirin plus clopidogrel did not significantly reduce the process of SVG intimal hyperplasia 1 year after coronary artery bypass grafting (Fig 1).

▶ Up to 20% of saphenous vein grafts may occlude within the first year after coronary artery bypass surgery.[1,2] Intimal hyperplasia is a primary means of saphenous vein graft failure both in the coronary and peripheral circulation. This process is, at least in part, platelet mediated. In both animal models and in vitro experiments, clopidogrel has been shown to inhibit intimal proliferation and smooth muscle hyperplasia, whereas aspirin apparently does not inhibit intimal hyperplasia.[3] This was the first study to determine whether clopidogrel

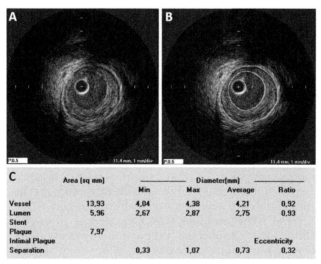

FIGURE 1.—IVUS image of an SVG 1 year after coronary artery bypass graft surgery (A). Manual planimetric measurements (B) were performed to identify the vessel area (green outer outline, also known as the external elastic lamina area) and lumen area (yellow inner outline). Subtraction of the lumen area from the vessel area determines the plaque area, which represents vein graft intimal hyperplasia (C). Min indicates minimum; Max, maximum. For interpretation of the references to color in this figure legend, the reader is referred to web version of this article. (Reprinted from Kulik A, Le May MR, Voisine P, et al. Aspirin plus clopidogrel versus aspirin alone after coronary artery bypass grafting: the clopidogrel after surgery for coronary artery disease (CASCADE) trial. *Circulation.* 2010;122:2680-2687, with permission from American Heart Association, Inc.)

inhibited saphenous vein graft intimal hyperplasia or improved angiographic graft patency following saphenous vein grafting. Results were based primarily on intravascular ultrasound imaging 1 year following coronary artery bypass graft (CABG) (Fig 1). Whereas the Clopidogrel in Unstable Angina to Prevent Recurrent Events (CURE) trial demonstrated that dual antiplatelet therapy reduced adverse outcomes in patients presenting with acute coronary syndrome who ultimately underwent CABG, that benefit appeared to be primarily ascribed to the preoperative portion of the patient's course. The coronary and peripheral circulations are obviously different, but the intimal hyperplasia process that affects saphenous vein grafts seems similar in the 2 circulations. This study does not provide evidence that the addition of clopidogrel to aspirin reduces initial hyperplasia or improves graft patency.

G. L. Moneta, MD

References

1. Desai ND, Cohen EA, Naylor CD, Fremes SE. A randomized comparison of radial-artery and saphenous-vein coronary bypass grafts. *N Engl J Med.* 2004; 351:2302-2309.
2. Alexander JH, Hafley G, Harrington RA, et al. Efficacy and safety of edifoligide, an E2F transcription factor decoy, for prevention of vein graft failure following coronary artery bypass graft surgery: PREVENT IV: a randomized controlled trial. *JAMA.* 2005;294:2446-2454.
3. Herbert JM, Dol F, Bernat A, Falotico R, Lalé A, Savi P. The antiaggregating and antithrombotic activity of clopidogrel is potentiated by aspirin in several experimental models in the rabbit. *Thromb Haemost.* 1998;80:512-518.

Long-Term Results of Endoscopic Versus Open Saphenous Vein Harvest for Lower Extremity Bypass
Julliard W, Katzen J, Nabozny M, et al (Univ of Rochester Med Ctr, NY)
Ann Vasc Surg 25:101-107, 2011

Background.—Endoscopic saphenous vein harvest (EVH) has been shown to lower wound infection rates and cost compared with conventional harvest, although long-term patency data are lacking. A small series of studies has recently suggested that patency is inferior to conventionally harvested vein technique, and we thus sought to explore this question by reviewing our cumulative experience with this technique.

Methods.—The short- and long-term outcomes of all lower extremity bypasses (LEBPs) using saphenous vein at one institution over a period of 8.5 years were retrospectively reviewed.

Results.—A total of 363 patients averaging 67 ± 24 to 100 years of age had undergone LEBP and had charts available for review. Of these 363 patients, 170 underwent EVH (90% using a noninsufflation technique) and 193 conventional (by means of continuous or skip incisions); 48% of patients reported tissue loss and no differences in indication for surgery were noted between groups. Mean follow-up was 35.1 (range: <1-105) months. Primary patency rates were worse in the EVH group as compared with conventional at six (63.3% ± 4.0% vs. 77.3% ± 3.3%), 12 (50.4% ± 4.2% vs. 73.7% ± 3.6%), and 36 (42.2% ± 4.5% vs. 59.1% ± 4.9%) months (all $p < 0.001$), although these differences were largely limited to patients with limb-threat and diabetes. However, limb salvage and survival, were identical between groups. Contrary to previous experience, there were no differences in length of stay or wound complication rates.

Conclusions.—The overall results of this study show an inferior long-term patency rate for endoscopically harvested saphenous vein after LEBP in our series as a whole, and do not confirm the short-term benefit previously shown in a selected cohort. These differences were, however, minimal or absent in patients with claudication or absence of diabetes, and EVH may continue to play a role in these cases (Figs 1 and 2).

▶ For lower extremity bypass surgery, greater saphenous veins are traditionally harvested with direct visualization of the vein through a long continuous incision or numerous shorter incisions along the length of the vein. Older case series suggested high rates of wound complications with open harvest of the greater saphenous vein.[1] Early case series of endoscopic vein harvest demonstrated similar patency of lower extremity bypasses with decreased wound complications in patients operated with endoscopic vein harvest versus open

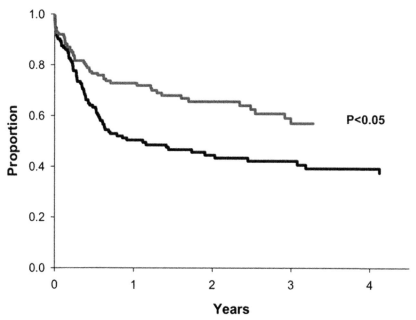

FIGURE 1.—Comparison of primary patency between vein grafts harvested using endoscopic (black) and open (green) techniques ($p < 0.05$). The standard errors do not exceed 10% at any time point. For interpretation of the references to color in this figure legend, the reader is referred to web version of this article. (Reprinted from Julliard W, Katzen J, Nabozny M, et al. Long-term results of endoscopic versus open saphenous vein harvest for lower extremity bypass. *Ann Vasc Surg.* 2011;25:101-107, with permission from Annals of Vascular Surgery Inc.)

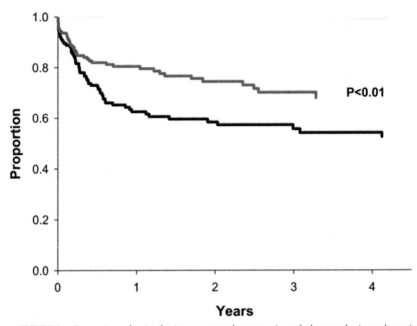

FIGURE 2.—Comparison of assisted primary patency between vein grafts harvested using endoscopic (black) and open (green) techniques ($p < 0.01$). The standard errors do not exceed 10% at any time point. For interpretation of the references to color in this figure legend, the reader is referred to web version of this article. (Reprinted from Julliard W, Katzen J, Nabozny M, et al. Long-term results of endoscopic versus open saphenous vein harvest for lower extremity bypass. *Ann Vasc Surg.* 2011;25:101-107, with permission from Annals of Vascular Surgery Inc.)

vein harvest.[2,3] A more recent series, however, demonstrated decreased graft patency after endoscopic vein harvest without improvement in wound complications in patients undergoing lower extremity bypass.[4] In addition, a large series of patients undergoing coronary artery bypass grafting (CABG) with endoscopic vein harvest showed decreased graft patency and decreased survival rates when compared with those patients undergoing CABG with open harvest of the greater saphenous vein.[5] Based on these more recent series, the authors thought to explore their results of lower extremity vein bypass with endoscopic vein harvest or open vein harvest over an 8.5-year period. The results of the study show overall inferior long-term patency for endoscopically harvested saphenous veins used in lower extremity bypass (Figs 1 and 2). The results do not confirm previously reported short-term benefits with the procedure. These authors were among the first to report a potential benefit of endoscopically harvested veins in the performance of lower extremity bypass. They are to be congratulated for the courage to reanalyze their data and to report updated results that are in conflict with their earlier observations.

The results of this study may be caused by many factors. The authors sometimes use endoscopic techniques below the knee, which may lead to inferior results. In addition, preoperative vein mapping with marking the course of the greater saphenous vein on the skin may result in decreased wound complications and less undermining of flaps in the current series compared with earlier series. The authors found little patency differences between endoscopic and open harvest in patients treated with claudication and in patients who are not diabetic. Therefore, there may be reason not to completely abandon endoscopic vein harvest but rather to restrict the technique to patients treated for claudication who are not diabetic and to limit the endoscopic harvest to the above-knee portion of the saphenous vein.

G. L. Moneta, MD

References

1. Kent KC, Bartek S, Kuntz KM, Anninos E, Skillman JJ. Prospective study of wound complications in continuous infrainguinal incisions after lower limb arterial reconstruction: incidence, risk factors, and cost. *Surgery.* 1996;119:378-383.
2. Jordan WD Jr, Alcocer F, Voellinger DC, Wirthlin DJ. The durability of endoscopic saphenous vein grafts: a 5-year observational study. *J Vas Surg.* 2001;34:434-439.
3. Illig KA, Rhodes JM, Sternbach Y, Shortell CK, Davies MG, Green RM. Reduction in wound morbidity rates following endoscopic saphenous vein harvest. *Ann Vasc Surg.* 2001;15:104-109.
4. Pullatt R, Brothers TE, Robison JG, Elliott BM. Compromised bypass graft outcomes after minimal-incision vein harvest. *J Vasc Surg.* 2006;44:289-295.
5. Lopes RD, Hafley GE, Allen KB, et al. Endoscopic versus open vein-graft harvesting in coronary-artery bypass surgery. *N Engl J Med.* 2009;361:235-244.

7 Aortic Aneurysm

Rupture Rates of Small Abdominal Aortic Aneurysms: A Systematic Review of the Literature
Powell JT, Gotensparre SM, Sweeting MJ, et al (Imperial College London, UK; Inst of Public Health, Cambridge, UK; et al)
Eur J Vasc Endovasc Surg 41:2-10, 2011

Background.—Small aneurysms of the abdominal aorta (3.0–5.5 cm in diameter) often are managed by regular surveillance, rather than surgery, because the risk of surgery is considered to outweigh the risk of aneurysm rupture. The risk of small aneurysm rupture is considered to be low. The purpose of this review is to summarise the reported estimates of small aneurysm rupture rates.

Methods and Findings.—We conducted a systematic review of the literature published before 2010 and identified 54 potentially eligible reports. Detailed review of these studies showed that both ascertainment of rupture, patient follow-up and causes of death were poorly reported: diagnostic criteria for rupture were never reported. There were only 14 studies from which rupture rates (as ruptures per 100 person-years) were available. These 14 published studies included 9779 patients (89% male) over the time period 1976–2006 but only 7 of these studies provided rupture rates specifically for the diameter range 3.0–5.5 cm, which ranged from 0 to 1.61 ruptures per 100 person-years.

Conclusions.—Rupture rates of small abdominal aortic aneurysms would appear to be low, but most studies have been poorly reported and did not have clear ascertainment and diagnostic criteria for aneurysm rupture (Fig 2).

▶ It is widely known that the larger an aortic aneurysm becomes, the higher the rate of rupture over time. What is NOT well known is the rupture rate for small aneurysms between 3.0 and 5.5 cm in diameter. Powell et al, in this well-conducted systematic review of the literature, have now provided us with the best information to date, albeit poor in quality, on this subject matter.

Over a 30-year period, a total of 10 160 studies were reviewed. Of these, only 14 studies provided rupture rates (as ruptures per 100 person-years) after analysis of 9779 patients (89% male). These 14 studies were published between 1991 and 2008 and included 4 randomized trials. Rupture rates for aneurysms in the diameter range of 3.0 to 5.5 cm could only be estimated from 7 studies, with rupture rates estimated as varying from 0 to 1.61 ruptures/100 person-years.[1-7] Two studies estimated the rupture rate to be greater than 1 rupture/100

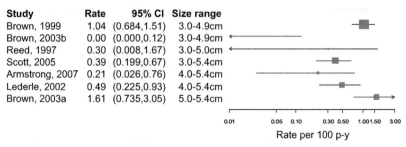

Study	Rate	95% CI	Size range
Brown, 1999	1.04	(0.684,1.51)	3.0-4.9cm
Brown, 2003b	0.00	(0.000,0.12)	3.0-4.9cm
Reed, 1997	0.30	(0.008,1.67)	3.0-5.0cm
Scott, 2005	0.39	(0.199,0.67)	3.0-5.4cm
Armstrong, 2007	0.21	(0.026,0.76)	4.0-5.4cm
Lederle, 2002	0.49	(0.225,0.93)	4.0-5.4cm
Brown, 2003a	1.61	(0.735,3.05)	5.0-5.4cm

Rate per 100 p-y

FIGURE 2.—Rupture rates (per 100 person-years) for small abdominal aortic aneurysm in each study, reporting conditional follow-up to 5.5 cm threshold, sorted by reported size range: total 5934 patients. Aneurysms reaching >5.5 cm have been excluded. These studies are depicted in order of increasing aneurysm size range but the distribution of diameters within these size ranges is not available. (Reprinted from Powell JT, Gotensparre SM, Sweeting MJ, et al. Rupture rates of small abdominal aortic aneurysms: a systematic review of the literature. *Eur J Vasc Endovasc Surg.* 2011;41:2-10. Copyright 2011, with permission from European Society for Vascular Surgery.)

person-years, whereas the point estimates for the remaining 5 studies were all below 0.5 ruptures/100 person-years. It was therefore decided because of large heterogeneity ($I^2 = 0.89$) that a formal synthesis of the results (ie, meta-analysis) was not appropriate (Fig 2).

We may never know the true rupture rate for aortic aneurysms of small diameter, but this is as close as we have come. Rupture rates for small abdominal aortic aneurysms appear to be low. Professor Janet T. Powell and her colleagues are to be congratulated on this well-conducted systematic review.

B. W. Starnes, MD

References

1. Lederle FA, Wilson SE, Johnson GR, et al. Immediate repair compared with surveillance of small abdominal aortic aneurysms. *N Eng J Med.* 2002;346: 1437-1444.
2. Brown LC, Powell JT. Risk factors for aneurysm rupture in patients kept under ultrasound surveillance. UK Small Aneurysm Trial Participants. *Ann Surg.* 1999; 230:289-296.
3. Brown PM, Zelt DT, Sobolev B. The risk of rupture in untreated aneurysms: the impact of size, gender, and expansion rate. *J Vasc Surg.* 2003;37:280-284.
4. Scott RAP, Kim LG, Ashton HA. Assessment of the criteria for elective surgery in screen-detected abdominal aortic aneurysms. *J Med Screen.* 2005;12:150-154.
5. Brown PM, Sobolev B, Zelt DT. Selective management of abdominal aortic aneurysms smaller than 5.0 cm in a prospective sizing program with gender-specific analysis. *J Vasc Surg.* 2003;38:762-765.
6. Reed WW, Hallett JW Jr, Damiano MA, Ballard DJ. Learning from the last ultrasound. A population-based study of patients with abdominal aortic aneurysm. *Arch Intern Med.* 1997;157:2064-2068.
7. Armstrong PA, Back MR, Bandyk DF, et al. Optimizing compliance, efficiency, and safety during surveillance of small abdominal aortic aneurysms. *J Vasc Surg.* 2007; 46:190-195.

The Incidence of Spinal Cord Ischaemia Following Thoracic and Thoracoabdominal Aortic Endovascular Intervention

Drinkwater SL, On behalf of the Regional Vascular Unit, St Mary's Hospital, Imperial College NHS Trust (St Mary's Hosp, London, UK; et al)
Eur J Vasc Endovasc Surg 40:729-735, 2010

Objectives.—To determine the incidence and risk factors for spinal cord ischaemia (SCI) following thoracic and thoracoabdominal aortic intervention.

Methods.—A prospective database of all thoracic and thoracoabdominal aortic interventions between 2001 and 2009 was used to investigate the incidence of SCI. All elective and emergency cases for all indications were included. Logistic regression was used to investigate which factors were associated with SCI.

Results.—235 patients underwent thoracic aortic stent grafting; 111(47%) thoracic aortic stent-grafts alone, with an additional 14(6%) branched or fenestrated thoracic grafts, 30(13%) arch hybrid procedures and 80(34%) visceral hybrid surgical and endovascular procedures. The global incidence of SCI for all procedures was 23/235 (9.8%) and this included emergency indications (ruptured TAAA and acute complex dissections) but the incidence varied considerably between types of procedures. Of the 23 cases, death occurred in 4 patients but recovery of function was seen in 6. Thus, permanent paraplegia occurred in 13/235 (5.5%) patients. Of the nine pre-specified factors investigated for association with SCI, only percentage of aortic coverage was significantly associated with the incidence of SCI; adjusted odds ratio per 10% increase in aorta covered = 1.78[95% CI 1.18−2.71], $p = 0.007$. The procedures in patients who developed SCI took longer (463.5 versus 307.2 minutes) and utilised more stents (4 versus 2).

Conclusion.—SCI following thoracic and thoracoabdominal aortic endovascular intervention is associated with the proportion of aorta covered. The degree of risk varies between different types of procedure and this should be carefully considered in both selection and consenting of patients (Fig 1).

▶ What is the most feared complication of thoracic and thoracoabdominal endovascular intervention? Paraplegia. In fact, many patients in my practice have stated that they would rather die than be paraplegic. This is yet another single-institution report, like many others before it, that attempts to identify those risk factors associated with the development of spinal cord injury (SCI) after thoracic and thoracoabdominal endovascular intervention. The overall rate of paraplegia in this study was 9.8%, which included emergency indications (ruptured thoracoabdominal aortic aneurysms and complex dissections).

Although this study has many weaknesses, there are many lessons to be learned here. First and foremost is that length of aortic coverage directly correlates with the development of SCI. We have learned this already from other studies, but these authors used the percentage of aorta covered instead of

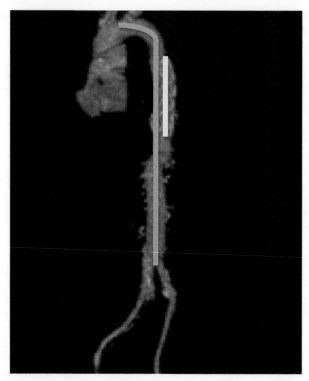

FIGURE 1.—Image of aorta showing measurements taken of length of aorta from brachiocephalic origin to iliac bifurcation and stent length. (Reprinted from Drinkwater SL, On behalf of the Regional Vascular Unit, St Mary's Hospital, Imperial College NHS Trust. The incidence of Spinal Cord Ischaemia Following Thoracic and Thoracoabdominal Aortic Endovascular Intervention. *Eur J Vasc Endovasc Surg.* 2010;40:729-735. Copyright 2010, with permission from the European Society for Vascular Surgery.

absolute distance and calculated this by measuring along the centerline from the origin of the left subclavian artery to the aortic bifurcation (the authors incorrectly refer to the aortic bifurcation in Fig 1 as the iliac bifurcation) and dividing this value into the total length of actual graft coverage (Fig 1). The shortest amount of aortic coverage by stent that developed SCI was 55% or (274 mm).

The authors then further subdivided patients into distinct categories of repair and found that the highest rate of SCI occurred with visceral hybrid procedures following in decreasing order by arch hybrid, fenestrated/branched graft, and finally simple endovascular thoracic aortic repair.

This series consisting of 235 patients is one of the first to suggest that the use of spinal drains had no impact on the rate of SCI and actually had an increased risk of SCI, even after adjustment for confounding variables such as urgency, indication, and procedure type. A noted weakness of this study, however, is that there is no record or analysis of the impact of hypotension at any time during the hospitalization after thoracic endovascular repair. The authors advocate on multiple occasions the use of adjunctive measures including maintenance of

MAPS > 80 mm Hg and yet give us no information on the impact of this strategy on subsequent neurologic outcomes.

B. W. Starnes, MD

Outcome in cirrhotic patients after elective surgical repair of infrarenal aortic aneurysm
Marrocco-Trischitta MM, Kahlberg A, Astore D, et al (San Raffaele Scientific Inst, Milan, Italy)
J Vasc Surg 53:906-911, 2011

Objective.—Abdominal surgery in patients with advanced liver disease has been reported to be associated with high morbidity and mortality rates. However, the surgical risk of infrarenal abdominal aortic aneurysm (AAA) repair in cirrhotics remains ill-defined. We reviewed our experience to investigate the predictors of the outcome in cirrhotic patients after elective AAA open repair.

Methods.—Between January 2001 and March 2006, 1189 patients underwent elective open repair of infrarenal AAA and 24 (2%) had a biopsy-proven cirrhosis (23 male, 1 female; mean age, 68 ± 7 years). The latter were retrospectively stratified according to the Child-Turcotte-Pugh (CTP) score and the Model for End-Stage Liver Disease (MELD) score. Operative variables, perioperative complications, and survival were recorded and compared with those of 48 concurrent noncirrhotic controls matched (2:1) by gender, age, aneurysm size, preoperative glomerular filtration rate, and type of reconstruction. The effect of CTP and MELD scores on midterm survival was investigated in cirrhotics with the Kaplan-Meier log-rank method.

Results.—No intraoperative or 30-day deaths were recorded. No significant differences in terms of major perioperative complications were observed between cirrhotic patients and controls. Operative time and intraoperative blood transfusion requirement were significantly higher in cirrhotics (162 ± 49 vs 132 ± 39 minutes; $P = .007$ and 273 ± 364 vs 84 ± 183 mL; $P = .040$, respectively). Hospital length of stay was nearly doubled in cirrhotic patients (11.0 ± 2.8 vs 5.8 ± 1.5 days; $P < .0001$). Twenty-two cirrhotic patients were classified as CTP A and two as CTP B. Median MELD score was 8 (range, 6-14). CTP class B was associated with higher intraoperative blood transfusion requirement (941 ± 54 vs 213 ± 314 mL; $P = .029$). At a mean follow-up of 30.7 ± 22.1 months, five deaths were recorded in cirrhotics, and three in controls. Actuarial survival at 2 years was 77.4% in cirrhotics and 97.8% in controls (log-rank test, $P = .026$). Both CTP B patients died within 6 months. CTP class B and a MELD score ≥10 were associated with reduced midterm survival rates (log-rank test, $P < .0001$ and $P = .021$, respectively).

Conclusions.—In our experience, elective AAA open repair in relatively compensated cirrhotics was safely performed with an acceptable increase of the magnitude of the operation. However, the reduced life expectancy of cirrhotics with a MELD score ≥10 suggests that such a procedure may not be warranted in this subgroup of patients.

▶ Cirrhosis is a major cause of morbidity and mortality in the United States and worldwide, and affected patients are increasing in number because of the widespread hepatitis C virus—related liver disease and alcohol abuse. As a result of the ongoing improvements and innovations in medical therapy, the cirrhotic population is expected to age; therefore, the association of advanced liver disease and abdominal aortic aneurysm (AAA) will become more common. In this retrospective review, the authors report on their experience performing elective AAA repair in 24 patients with biopsy-proven cirrhosis of the liver. They stratified patients according to the Child-Turcotte-Pugh (CTP) score and the Model for End-Stage Liver Disease (MELD) score and compared outcomes with 48 concurrent noncirrhotic controls matched (2:1) by sex, age, aneurysm size, preoperative glomerular filtration rate, and type of reconstruction. The effect of CTP and MELD scores on midterm survival was investigated in cirrhotic patients.

The authors report no intraoperative or 30-day deaths and no significant differences in terms of major perioperative complications between cirrhotic patients and controls. They did find operating time and intraoperative blood transfusion requirement were significantly higher in cirrhotic patients. They found hospital length of stay was nearly doubled in cirrhotic patients. Cirrhosis in 22 patients was classified as CTP A and in 2 as CTP B. Median MELD score was 8. At a mean follow-up of 30.7 ± 22.1 months, 5 deaths were recorded in cirrhotic patients, and 3 in controls. Actuarial survival rate at 2 years was 77.4% in cirrhotic patients and 97.8% in controls (log-rank test, $P = .026$). Both CTP B patients died within 6 months. CTP class B and a MELD score > 10 were associated with reduced midterm survival rates.

In short, the authors report that in those patients where you can identify as having cirrhosis that have low MELD scores and are well compensated, the overall morbidity and mortality are minimally increased. This of course assumes that you can identify patients at risk for cirrhosis if information on hepatitis C status or alcohol consumption is available. The well-compensated cirrhotic patient who ends up undergoing open operation is at high risk for increased morbidity and mortality. Treatment by open or endovascular methods may not matter. In short, surgeons should avoid operating on patients with cirrhosis if possible, as their overall survival is compromised. As the authors state, their data confirm that patients with a MELD score > 10 have a much lower expected survival rate at a midterm follow-up because of causes unrelated to their aneurysm. As a consequence, elective surgical repair of asymptomatic AAA does not appear warranted in this subgroup of patients. Rather, cirrhotic patients with a MELD score > 10 would probably be better treated conservatively, as also previously recommended by other authors regarding patients with large AAA associated with serious comorbidities.

D. L. Gillespie, MD, RVT

Analysis of risk factors for abdominal aortic aneurysm in a cohort of more than 3 million individuals
Kent KC, Zwolak RM, Egorova NN, et al (Society for Vascular Surgery, Chicago; IL; Mount Sinai School of Medicine, NY)
J Vasc Surg 52:539-548, 2010

Background.—Abdominal aortic aneurysm (AAA) disease is an insidious condition with an 85% chance of death after rupture. Ultrasound screening can reduce mortality, but its use is advocated only for a limited subset of the population at risk.

Methods.—We used data from a retrospective cohort of 3.1 million patients who completed a medical and lifestyle questionnaire and were evaluated by ultrasound imaging for the presence of AAA by Life Line Screening in 2003 to 2008. Risk factors associated with AAA were identified using multivariable logistic regression analysis.

Results.—We observed a positive association with increasing years of smoking and cigarettes smoked and a negative association with smoking cessation. Excess weight was associated with increased risk, whereas exercise and consumption of nuts, vegetables, and fruits were associated with reduced risk. Blacks, Hispanics, and Asians had lower risk of AAA than whites and Native Americans. Well-known risk factors were reaffirmed, including male gender, age, family history, and cardiovascular disease. A predictive scoring system was created that identifies aneurysms more efficiently than current criteria and includes women, nonsmokers, and individuals aged <65 years. Using this model on national statistics of risk factors prevalence, we estimated 1.1 million AAAs in the United States, of which 569,000 are among women, nonsmokers, and individuals aged <65 years.

Conclusions.—Smoking cessation and a healthy lifestyle are associated with lower risk of AAA. We estimated that about half of the patients with AAA disease are not eligible for screening under current guidelines. We have created a high-yield screening algorithm that expands the target population for screening by including at-risk individuals not identified with existing screening criteria (Figs 2A, B and C).

▶ Screening for abdominal aortic aneurysms has been recommended by the United States Preventative Services Task Force (USPSTF), but only for men aged 65 to 75 years with a history of smoking. However, about one-third of ruptured aneurysms and 41% of aortic aneurysm deaths are in women. Also, 22% of aneurysm-related deaths occur in nonsmokers.[1,2] The data here are important in that they address the limitations of the USPSTF position. However, Dr Michael Lilly notes in an accompanying commentary to the article that the lifestyle and demographic data reported here are unconfirmed, nonvalidated, and self-reported by a self-selected population of people sufficiently motivated by health concerns to pay for an out-of-pocket health screening. It is unlikely the USPSTF will change its position based on this type of data. Nevertheless, the data are consistent with what most vascular surgeons would believe. As an

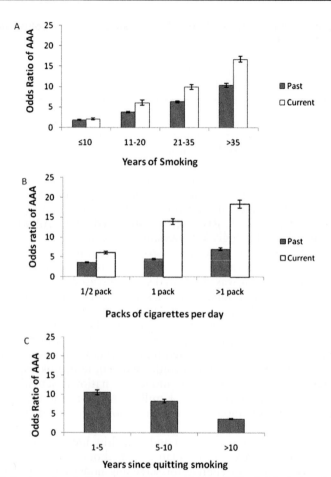

FIGURE 2.—Age-adjusted effects of lifestyle characteristics and risk of abdominal aortic aneurysm (*AAA*) in the Life Line Screening cohort are shown for (**A**) smoking duration, (**B**) number of cigarettes smoked per day, (**C**) time elapsed since quitting, Reference groups are once per month or less for food consumption and no smokers for all smoking variables. *Meats: Processed and red meats. The *vertical error bars* show 95% confidence intervals. (Reprinted from Kent KC, Zwolak RM, Egorova NN, et al. Analysis of risk factors for abdominal aortic aneurysm in a cohort of more than 3 million individuals. *J Vasc Surg.* 2010;52:539-548. Copyright 2010, with permission from the Society for Vascular Surgery.)

aside, it is nice to see that the authors found a negative association of abdominal aortic aneurysm risk with duration of smoking abstinence (Fig 2A-C). This is not something that I was previously aware of.

G. L. Moneta, MD

References

1. Mureebe L, Egorova N, Giacovelli JK, Gelijns A, Kent KC, McKinsey JF. National trends in the repair of ruptured abdominal aortic aneurysms. *J Vasc Surg.* 2008;48: 1101-1107.

2. Kung H-C, Hoyert DL, Xu J, Murphy SL. Deaths: final data for 2005. *Natl Vital Stat Rep.* 2008;56:1-120.

Association Between Aneurysm Shoulder Stress and Abdominal Aortic Aneurysm Expansion: A Longitudinal Follow-Up Study

Li Z-Y, Sadat U, U-King-Im J, et al (Southeast Univ, Nanjing, China; Cambridge Univ Hosps Foundation Trust, UK)
Circulation 122:1815-1822, 2010

Background.—Aneurysm expansion rate is an important indicator of the potential risk of abdominal aortic aneurysm (AAA) rupture. Stress within the AAA wall is also thought to be a trigger for its rupture. However, the association between aneurysm wall stresses and expansion of AAA is unclear.

Methods and Results.—Forty-four patients with AAAs were included in this longitudinal follow-up study. They were assessed by serial abdominal ultrasonography and computed tomography scans if a critical size was reached or a rapid expansion occurred. Patient-specific 3-dimensional AAA geometries were reconstructed from the follow-up computed tomography images. Structural analysis was performed to calculate the wall stresses of the AAA models at both baseline and final visit. A nonlinear large-strain finite element method was used to compute the wall-stress distribution. The relationship between wall stresses and expansion rate was investigated. Slowly and rapidly expanding aneurysms had comparable baseline maximum diameters (median, 4.35 cm [interquartile range, 4.12 to 5.0 cm] versus 4.6 cm [interquartile range, 4.2 to 5.0 cm]; $P=0.32$). Rapidly expanding AAAs had significantly higher shoulder stresses than slowly expanding AAAs (median, 300 kPa [interquartile range, 280 to 320 kPa] versus 225 kPa [interquartile range, 211 to 249 kPa]; $P=0.0001$). A good correlation between shoulder stress at baseline and expansion rate was found ($r=0.71$; $P=0.0001$).

Conclusion.—A higher shoulder stress was found to have an association with a rapidly expanding AAA. Therefore, it may be useful for estimating the expansion of AAAs and improve risk stratification of patients with AAAs (Fig 1).

▶ From a biomechanical perspective, aortic aneurysm rupture can be seen as an example of structural failure when mechanical stresses acting on a weakened aortic wall exceed local mechanical failure strength. These forces include blood pressure and wall shear stress. Wall stress may be caused by an influence of several concomitant factors including aneurysm shape, biochemical composition of the aneurysm wall, characteristic and shape of intraluminal thrombus, eccentricity of the aneurysm, and interaction between solid domains and fluid. While rupture of an aneurysm is determined by the balance between wall stress and wall strength, it is not possible currently to measure in vivo wall strength (Fig 1). However, changes in wall stresses may be useful in identifying

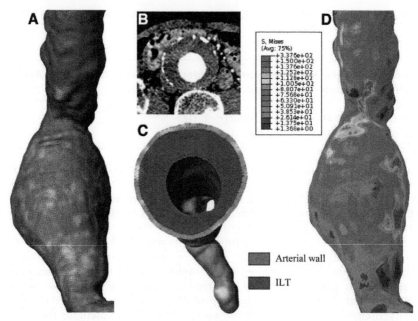

FIGURE 1.—Reconstruction of 3D AAA model based on CT and computed wall stress distributions. A, Three-dimensional AAA model and mesh; B, axial CT slice; C, cross-section of AAA model showing the AAA components (ILT, arterial wall, and lumen); D, 3D stress contours showing von Mises stress distribution. High stresses can often be found at the shoulder region. (Reprinted from Li Z-Y, Sadat U, U-King-Im J, et al. Association between aneurysm shoulder stress and abdominal aortic aneurysm expansion: a longitudinal follow-up study. *Circulation*. 2010;122:1815-1822, with permission from American Heart Association, Inc.)

abdominal aortic aneurysm (AAA) stability. Currently follow-up protocols for unoperated AAA are based primarily on the diameter of the aneurysm. The Society for Vascular Surgery uses AAA diameter as the primary criterion for determining follow-up intervals for unoperated AAAs. It is known that some small aneurysms rupture under observation. The data suggest extending aneurysm surveillance to include measurement of shoulder stress as well as aneurysm diameter would allow determination of which AAA should be repaired at relatively smaller diameters and which small aneurysms should be followed with closer follow-up intervals than currently recommended. At some point, this type of approach to risk stratification of aneurysm rupture will need to be incorporated into our clinical algorithms.

G. L. Moneta, MD

Association Between Serum Lipoproteins and Abdominal Aortic Aneurysm

Golledge J, van Bockxmeer F, Jamrozik K, et al (James Cook Univ School of Medicine, Townsville, Queensland, Australia; Univ of Western Australia School of Pathology and Laboratory Medicine, Fremantle, Australia; Univ of Adelaide School of Population Health and Clinical Practice, South Australia, Australia; et al)
Am J Cardiol 105:1480-1484, 2010

The importance of dyslipidemia in the etiology of abdominal aortic aneurysm (AAA) is poorly defined, in part because previous association analyses have often not considered the use of current lipid-modifying medications. Medications targeted at altering the concentrations of circulating lipids have an established role in occlusive atherosclerosis but are of unknown value in the primary prevention of AAA. We examined the association between fasting serum levels of triglycerides low- and high-density lipoprotein and the presence of an AAA in a cohort of 3,327 men aged 65 to 83 years. The analyses were adjusted for established risk factors of AAA and the prescription of lipid-modifying agents using multiple logistic regression analysis. Of the 3,327 men, 1,043 (31%) were receiving lipid-modifying therapy at the fasting lipid measurement. The lipid-modifying therapy was statins in most cases (n = 1,023). The serum high-density lipoprotein concentrations were lower in patients with AAAs. The serum high-density lipoprotein concentration was independently associated with a reduced risk of having an AAA in men not receiving current lipid-modifying therapy (odds ratio 0.72, 95% confidence interval 0.56 to 0.93 per 0.4-mM increase) and in the total cohort (odds ratio 0.76, 95% confidence interval 0.63 to 0.91 per 0.4-mM increase, adjusted for lipid-modifying therapy). The concentrations of low-density lipoprotein and triglycerides were not associated with the presence of AAAs. In conclusion, high-density lipoprotein appeared to be the most important lipid in predicting the risk of AAA development, with potential value as a therapeutic target. Current cardiovascular strategies aimed at lowering low-density lipoprotein might not have any effect on the prevention of AAAs.

▶ The relationship between dyslipidemia and development of abdominal aortic aneurysm (AAA) is unclear. Some studies have reported an association between low-density lipoprotein or high-density lipoprotein (HDL) and AAA; others have found no association. Previous studies have not used consistent definitions of dyslipidemia, have not stratified the current use of lipid-modifying medications, and often have not adjusted for other determinants of AAA. The result has been confusion regarding the role of dyslipidemia in the development of AAA. The authors have demonstrated a consistent association between a low serum HDL concentration and the presence of AAA in a population prone to aortic dilatation. The fact that the association was present in subgroups not receiving lipid-modifying medications and in men after adjusting for other risk factors, including lipid-modifying medications, is evidence that modification of HDL levels may be among an increasing number of potential therapeutic targets in the prevention or medical management of AAAs.

G. L. Moneta, MD

Meta-analysis of postoperative mortality after elective repair of abdominal aortic aneurysms detected by screening
Lindholt JS, Norman PE (Viborg Hosp, Denmark; Univ of Western Australia, Perth, Australia)
Br J Surg 98:619-622, 2011

Background.—The aim of this study was to compare the mortality rate within 30 days of elective surgery for abdominal aortic aneurysm (AAA) in men randomized to an invitation for ultrasound screening with that of men in the control group, whose aneurysms were detected incidentally.

Methods.—Relevant reports from randomized trials of screening were identified through a systematic search of MEDLINE. Four relevant trials were identified, and supplemented with data from the Viborg Vascular screening trial. Data were updated in two studies. Meta-analysis was undertaken with effects calculated as a fixed odds ratio (OR) with 95 per cent confidence interval. Heterogeneity between the studies was assessed by the χ^2 test.

Results.—There were 25 deaths (2.9 per cent) following elective surgery in 858 men invited for screening compared with 21 (5.5 per cent) of 383 in the control group (OR 0.49, 0.27 to 0.88). There were 18 deaths (2.4 per cent) following elective surgery for 747 screen-detected AAAs compared with 28 (6.1 per cent) following elective repair of 459 incidentally detected aneurysms (OR 0.37, 0.20 to 0.68).

Conclusion.—The offer of screening identifies men whose early survival following elective AAA repair is better than that of men with an AAA detected incidentally.

▶ An incidentally detected abdominal aortic aneurysm (AAA) occurs in the setting of evaluation for another medical problem. AAAs detected with screening are those found in patients without an ongoing active medical issue. Patients with incidentally detected AAAs therefore may be at increased risk for surgery because of greater age or comorbidities or more anatomically complex AAAs than those whose AAA was detected through a screening program. The author thought to compare mortality rate within 30 days of elective surgery for AAA in men whose aneurysms were detected incidentally versus those that were detected from an invitation for an ultrasound screening. The data indicate that in men 65 years or older, the risk of death in a patient operated for an incidentally detected aneurysm is approximately 3 times that of a patient operated for a screen-detected AAA (Fig 2). The authors' data do not permit a drill down for reasons why patients operated for screened AAAs appear to have a lower mortality rate than those operated for incidentally detected

Study	30-day mortality		Weight (%)	Odds ratio	Odds ratio
	Screen-detected	Detected incidentally			
Chichester	0 of 39	0 of 21		Not estimable	
MASS	13 of 414	17 of 192	66·75	0·33 (0·16, 0·70)	
VIVA	0 of 75	1 of 11	7·64	0·05 (0·00, 1·21)	
Viborg	2 of 84	1 of 52	3·66	1·17 (0·10, 13·25)	
Western Australia	3 of 135	9 of 186	21·96	0·45 (0·12, 1·68)	
Total	18 of 747	28 of 459	100·00	0·37 (0·20, 0·68)	

Test for heterogeneity: $\chi^2 = 2·57$, 3 d.f., $P = 0·46$, $I^2 = 0\%$
Test for overall effect: $Z = 3·22$, $P = 0·001$

0·1 0·2 0·5 1 2 5 10
Favours treatment Favours control

FIGURE 2.—Meta-analysis of mortality within 30 days after elective repair of an abdominal aortic aneurysm detected by screening, or incidentally. Odds ratios are shown with 95 per cent confidence intervals. MASS, Multicentre Aneurysm Screening Study; VIVA, Viborg Vascular. (Reprinted from Lindholt JS, Norman PE. Meta-analysis of postoperative mortality after elective repair of abdominal aortic aneurysms detected by screening. *Br J Surg.* 2011;98:619-622, Copyright © 2011, British Journal of Surgery Society Ltd. Reproduced with permission. Permission is granted by John Wiley & Sons Ltd on behalf of the BJSS Ltd.)

AAAs. Reasons could include younger ages of screened patients, smaller aneurysm size, and/or less complex anatomy permitting a higher proportion of endovascular repairs. In addition, patients whose aneurysms were detected with screening may have fewer comorbidities than those whose aneurysms were operated in the workup of another illness. Overall, however, the authors' data provide another bit of evidence to encourage screening in patients at risk at for AAA.

G. L. Moneta, MD

Randomized clinical trial of mesh *versus* sutured wound closure after open abdominal aortic aneurysm surgery
Bevis PM, Windhaber RAJ, Lear PA, et al (Cheltenham General Hosp, UK; Univ of Bristol, UK; Southmead Hosp, Bristol, UK; et al)
Br J Surg 97:1497-1502, 2010

Background.—Incisional herniation is a common complication of abdominal aortic aneurysm (AAA) repair. This study investigated whether prophylactic mesh placement could reduce the rate of postoperative incisional hernia after open repair of AAA.

Methods.—This randomized clinical trial was undertaken in three hospitals. Patients undergoing elective open AAA repair were randomized to routine abdominal mass closure after AAA repair or to prophylactic placement of polypropylene mesh in the preperitoneal plane.

Results.—Eighty-five patients with a mean age of 73 (range 59—89) years were recruited, 77 (91 per cent) of whom were men. There were five perioperative deaths (6 per cent), two in the control group and three in the mesh group ($P = 0·663$), none related to the mesh. Sixteen patients in the control group and five in the mesh group developed a postoperative incisional hernia (hazard ratio 4·10, 95 per cent confidence interval 1·72 to 9·82; $P = 0·002$). Hernias developed between 170 and 585 days after surgery in the control group, and between 336 and 1122 days in the mesh group. Four patients in the control group and one in the mesh group underwent incisional hernia repair ($P = 0 \cdot 375$). No mesh became infected, but one was subsequently removed owing to seroma formation during laparotomy for small bowel obstruction.

Conclusion.—Mesh placement significantly reduced the rate of postoperative incisional hernia after open AAA repair without increasing the rate of complications. Registration number: ISRCTN28485581 (http://www.controlled-trials.com).

▶ Patients with abdominal aortic aneurysm are postulated to have a systemic connective tissue disorder that makes them more susceptible to developing abdominal hernia.[1] Rates of incisional hernia following abdominal aortic aneurysm repair may be as high as 38%.[2] There appears to be a significantly increased risk of incisional hernia in patients undergoing aortic surgery for an aneurysm compared with those undergoing aortic surgery for occlusive disease.[3] One study has suggested that prophylactic placement of prosthetic mesh in the peritoneal space during wound closure after open abdominal aortic aneurysm repair results in lower rates of incisional hernia.[4] There are significant concerns regarding placement of prophylactic polypropylene mesh. Certainly mesh has been associated with infection and adhesion to underlying bowel. Although these complications were not noted in this series, the number of patients is small. The study does confirm a high rate of hernia formation in patients undergoing midline incisions for abdominal aortic aneurysm repair. It also suggests that this rate of hernia formation can be reduced by prophylactic mesh replacement. The clinical significance of this is unclear, as the number of actual incisional hernia repairs was not statistically different in the patients undergoing routine mass closure versus those undergoing prophylactic mass closure, implying many of the hernias perhaps were small, asymptomatic, or did not trouble the patient.

G. L. Moneta, MD

References

1. Adey B, Luna G. Incidence of abdominal wall hernia in aortic surgery. *Am J Surg.* 1998;175:400-402.
2. Holland AJ, Castleden WM, Norman PE, Stacey MC. Incisional hernias are more common in aneurysmal arterial disease. *Eur J Vasc Endovasc Surg.* 1996;12:196-200.
3. Takagi H, Sugimoto M, Kato T, Matsuno Y, Umemoto T. Postoperative incision hernia in patients with abdominal aortic aneurysm and aortoiliac occlusive disease: a systematic review. *Eur J Vasc Endovasc Surg.* 2007;33:177-181.
4. O'Hare JL, Ward J, Earnshaw JJ. Late results of mesh wound closure after elective open aortic aneurysm repair. *Eur J Vasc Endovasc Surg.* 2007;33:412-413.

Rural Hospitals Face a Higher Burden of Ruptured Abdominal Aortic Aneurysm and Are More Likely to Transfer Patients for Emergent Repair

Maybury RS, Chang DC, Freischlag JA (Georgetown Univ Hosp, Washington, DC; Univ of California San Diego; The Johns Hopkins Med Institutions, Baltimore, MD)

J Am Coll Surg 212:1061-1067, 2011

Background.—The influence of rural hospital location on abdominal aortic aneurysm (AAA) outcomes is unknown. We undertook a study to determine the difference in the risk of ruptured AAA presentation and outcomes after ruptured AAA between rural and urban areas.

Study Design.—Patients in the Nationwide Inpatient Sample from 2001 to 2007, with intact AAA repair or ruptured AAA, were included. Patients transferred from another hospital, with unrecorded hospital ZIP code, or age less than 50 years were excluded. Health system variables were obtained from the Area Resource File. Vascular surgeon census was determined from the Society for Vascular Surgery online registry. Multivariable logistic regression was used to analyze outcomes in patients with AAA, adjusting for patient, hospital, and health system variables.

Results.—Rural hospital location was associated with higher risk of ruptured AAA presentation (odds ratio [OR] 2.46, 95% CI 1.90 to 3.19) and transfer to another hospital without ruptured AAA repair (9.3% vs 1.4%, p < 0.001). The adjusted risk of death was similar for patients with ruptured AAA admitted to rural and urban hospitals (OR 0.96, 95% CI 0.73 to 1.27). Hospital elective AAA repair volume less than 15 was a risk factor for death after ruptured AAA.

Conclusions.—Rural hospitals face a disproportionate burden of ruptured AAA and are more likely to transfer patients with ruptured AAA without performing repair, compared with urban hospitals. Solutions to rural disparity in ruptured AAA outcomes should focus on improving rural patients' access to vascular surgeons for elective and emergent AAA repair.

▶ Rural residence negatively affects surgical care. Patients needing solid-organ transplants are less likely to be registered on the wait-list if they reside in a rural area. Patients treated for breast cancer at rural hospitals are less likely to receive breast-conserving treatment, and obese patients in rural areas are less likely to undergo bariatric surgery. Vascular surgery expertise also tends to be concentrated in high-volume urban centers. In addition, abdominal aortic aneurysm (AAA) repair mortality and morbidity rates appear to be lower in high-volume centers. Therefore, there is reason to suspect that there may be a rural-urban discrepancy in outcomes of patients with ruptured AAA. The authors sought to determine the difference in risk of ruptured AAA presentation and outcome after ruptured AAAs between rural and urban areas. It is not surprising that the authors found patients in rural areas with ruptured AAA are more frequently transferred to larger-volume hospitals. Many small hospitals simply do not have local expertise to deal with this problem. It is, however, surprising that mortality rates were the same in rural and urban hospitals for ruptured AAAs. The authors suggest that this may be because of longer transport times in rural areas, selecting for patients who are more stable to undergo repair and who have a greater ability to survive hospitalization. In addition, more critically ill patients may actually be transferred to referring hospitals. It is really unrealistic to believe that outcomes will be the same in low-volume hospitals for emergent procedures as in high-volume hospitals. With decreasing experience of general surgical trainees in vascular surgery and concentration of vascular surgeons in urban areas, it seems likely that there will be, or perhaps already is, a significant discrepancy in outcomes of patients with ruptured AAAs in rural versus urban areas. It is doubtful that the solution will be increasing expertise in rural areas but rather improved screening of patients for AAA to facilitate treatment before my time.

G. L. Moneta, MD

The Ectatic Aorta: No Benefit in Surveillance
Gibbs DMR, Bown MJ, Hussey G, et al (Leicester Royal Infirmary, UK; Univ of Leicester, UK)
Ann Vasc Surg 24:908-911, 2010

Background.—To determine if patients presenting with an infrarenal aorta of 25-30 mm in diameter benefit from continued ultrasound surveillance, and if so to identify the frequency required.

Methods.—All patients in the Leicestershire abdominal aortic aneurysm (AAA) screening program with an initial AAA diameter of 25-30 mm and who had undergone two or more surveillance scans were identified (345 patients). The primary endpoint was death from AAA rupture, referral for elective repair, or presentation with rupture. This information together with the duration of surveillance was recorded.

Results.—A total of 345 patients were followed up for mean of 4.25 years (1-11). At 5 years surveillance, there was a 97% freedom from referral for repair or death from rupture.

Conclusion.—Patients presenting with an AAA diameter 25-30 mm may be safely deferred any further surveillance for a period of 5 years.

▶ The management of small abdominal aortic aneurysms (AAAs) has been largely clarified through recent large prospective studies. In addition, ultrasound screening of men aged 65 years and older appears effective in both reducing aneurysm-related mortality and cost.[1] There is, however, little consensus on follow-up of the so-called ectatic aorta. In this study, an ectatic aorta was defined as 25 to 30 mm in anteroposterior diameter. As many as one-third of patients presenting to a screening program for AAA will have an ectatic aorta.[2] Patients with aortas between 25 and 29 mm in diameter have unclear benefit of further screening. The authors therefore sought to determine if patients with aortic diameters between 25 and 30 mm should have continued surveillance or if they could be discharged from ultrasound screening follow-up. For screening of any medical condition to be both effective and cost-effective, there must be identification of appropriate subgroups of patients where a reasonable yield of the screening process is anticipated. One can certainly argue over what is a reasonable yield. However, it is difficult to argue that continued close surveillance of patients with AAas between 25 and 30 mm has any hope of being cost-effective. The information provided here, therefore, should be quite useful for those with an interest in designing and implementing aortic aneurysm screening programs in their community.

G. L. Moneta, MD

References

1. Ashton HA, Buxton MJ, Day NE, et al. The Multicentre Aneurysm Screening Study (MASS) into the effect of abdominal aortic aneurysm screening on mortality in men: a randomised controlled trial. *Lancet.* 2002;360:1531-1539.
2. Devaraj S, Dodds SR. Ultrasound surveillance of ectatic abdominal aortas. *Ann R Coll Surg Engl.* 2008;90:477-482.

Volume-Outcome Relationships and Abdominal Aortic Aneurysm Repair
Landon BE, O'Malley AJ, Giles K, et al (Harvard Med School, Boston, MA; Beth Israel Deaconess Med Ctr, Boston, MA; et al)
Circulation 122:1290-1297, 2010

Background.—There is a well-established literature relating procedure volume to outcomes, but incorporating such information into clinical decision making is problematic when there is >1 treatment option for a condition.

Methods and Results.—We used data from the Medicare program to investigate the relationship between institutional volume for open and endovascular abdominal aortic aneurysm (AAA) repair and outcomes, examine trends in volume, and explore the implications for physicians making referrals for AAA repair. Trends in institutional volume were measured for the time period 2001—2006, whereas outcomes were assessed with the use of a previously assembled propensity score-matched cohort covering the time period 2001—2004. Between 2001 and 2006, there were a total of 230 736 repairs of either an intact or ruptured AAA for traditional Medicare beneficiaries. During this time, the proportion of endovascular cases increased from ≈22% in 2001 to >50% of AAA repairs in 2006, but there was little shift in procedure volume to high-volume institutions. For endovascular repair, adjusted mortality by quintile showed a marked decrease between the first and second quintile, with continued smaller decreases over quintiles 3 to 5. For open repair, adjusted mortality showed a steady decrease across the quintiles of volume.

Conclusions.—We found a steady increase in survival with increasing volume of open repair but relatively little improvement after reaching a relatively low threshold for endovascular repair. Because hospital experience with one repair method does not translate into improved outcomes

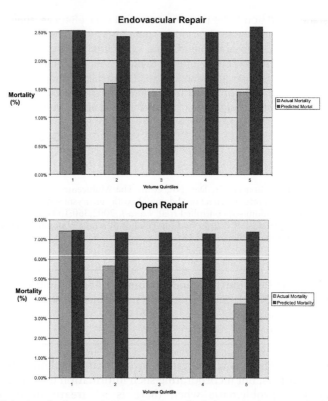

FIGURE 1.—Actual vs lowest-quintile predicted mortality by hospital volume (quintiles) for endovascular and open repair performed from 2001 to 2004. Predicted morality is calculated as if all cases were performed at a hospital in the lowest quintile of volume. All models control for baseline clinical and demographic characteristics. (Reprinted from Landon BE, O'Malley AJ, Giles K, et al. Volume-outcome relationships and abdominal aortic aneurysm repair. *Circulation.* 2010;122:1290-1297, with permission from American Heart Association, Inc.)

for the alternative method, referring clinicians must consider both treatment options when making referral decisions (Fig 1).

▶ For higher risk surgical procedures, it appears higher volume institutions and higher volume operators achieve better results. Infrarenal abdominal aortic aneurysm (AAA) may be repaired with either open or endovascular techniques. Surgeons who favor one approach over the other may have outcomes for the opposite approach that are not as good as their favored approach. Outcomes across procedures may not be related. The authors note that to date, there have been no studies examining volume-outcome relationship of AAA that take into consideration endovascular versus open AAA repair. The authors use Medicare data to investigate whether there was a relationship between institutional volume for endovascular and open AAA repair and outcome. Their data indicate that the number of hospitals with high volume of open AAA repair has declined dramatically. Almost 400 hospitals have stopped performing open AAA repair in the endovascular era! The data seem to justify this trend. For endovascular repair, repair mortality improvement occurs really only from lowest quintile to the second lowest quintile with little improvement beyond that for increasing volumes of endovascular repair. On the other hand, there appears to be a relatively constant relationship between increasing open repair volume and decreasing perioperative mortality (Fig 1). Given that referring physicians frequently do not know whether a patient will undergo open or endovascular AAA repair, the authors suggest that referral decisions should be made on the basis of open repair volume of a hospital rather than their total or endovascular repair volume. What is clear is that as endovascular repair increases, there are going to be fewer hospitals with adequate open repair volume to achieve optimal results with open AAA repair.

G. L. Moneta, MD

Activation of transglutaminase type 2 for aortic wall protection in a rat abdominal aortic aneurysm formation
Munezane T, Hasegawa T, Suritala, et al (Kobe Univ Graduate School of Medicine, Japan)
J Vasc Surg 52:967-974, 2010

Objective.—The altered structure and composition of the vascular extracellular matrix (ECM) influences the formation of abdominal aortic aneurysms (AAA). Transglutaminase type 2 (TG2), which is a Ca^{2+}-dependent cross-linking enzyme, has been proven the importance for ECM homeostasis, but there is no evidence of TG2 in AAA formation. The hypothesis was investigated that TG2 contributes to protect aortic walls during remodeling of the AAAs.

Methods.—In a rat abdominal aortic aneurysm model using a combination of intraluminal elastase infusion and extraluminal calcium chloride, TG2 expression and activity were evaluated at 1 and 8 weeks after the AAA preparation (n = 6 at each endpoint), compared with those of the non-prepared aorta (n = 6). Additionally, ex vivo experiments of isolated AAA tissue culture with recombinant human TG2, TG2 inhibitor cystamine, or tissue necrosis factor (TNF)-α were performed.

Results.—TG2 mRNA expression in the AAAs was significantly upregulated at both 1 and 8 weeks (22.4-fold and 5.4-fold increases of the non-prepared aorta, $P = .0022$ and $P = .0048$, respectively). TG2 protein expression and activity were also enhanced by fluorescent staining of the AAAs. Similar mRNA upregulation of TNF-α, interleukin-1β, matrix metalloproteinases (MMP)-2, MMP-9, and tissue inhibitors of metalloproteinases (TIMP)-1 and TIMP-2 was observed in the AAAs, and TG2 and TNF-α were colocalized in the aortic walls at 1 week. Ex vivo experiments showed that mRNA expressions of TNF-α, MMP-2, and MMP-9 in the cultured AAA tissue were decreased by exogenous TG2, whereas were increased by cystamine. TNF-α exposure to the AAA tissues was significantly upregulated TG2 mRNA expression ($P = .0333$).

Conclusion.—TG2 expression and activity in AAA formation were enhanced, possibly due to compensatory reaction. TG2 has a potential role of ECM protector in aortic walls during remodeling of the AAAs.

▶ In this study, the authors evaluate the function of transglutaminase type 2 (TG2), which is a Ca^{2+}-dependent cross-linking enzyme, and its biologic function is in extracellular matrix homeostasis interacting with a variety of intracellular and extracellular proteins, leading to effects on cell adhesion, wound healing, tissue fibrosis, extracellular matrix stability, inflammation, apoptosis, arterial calcification, and angiogenesis. However, TG2 has not been studied in abdominal aortic aneurysms (AAAs). The study demonstrated in a rat AAA model that the transcription product TG2 was significantly expressed compared with control normal aorta. In addition, the messenger RNA (mRNA) of tumor necrosis factor (TNF), matrix metalloproteinase (MMP)-2, MMP-9, interleukin 1, tissue inhibitors of metalloproteinase (TIMP)-1, and TIMP-2 were also elevated indicating the inflammatory molecules that are present in AAA formation, as well as inhibitors of MMPs. Another interesting finding of this study is that isolated AAA tissues were incubated with recombinant human TG2, TG2 inhibitor cystamine, or TNF. After 3-day incubation with exogenous TG2, mRNA expressions of TNF, MMP-2, and MMP-9 in the AAA tissues were decreased, compared with the control.

However, after 3-day incubation with cystamine, mRNA expressions of TNF, MMP-2, and MMP-9 in the AAA tissues were increased, compared with the control. Trinitroglycerin caused the expression of TG2, implicating its relation to TNF signaling in AAA. The importance of this study is that TG2 has an important function in the pathogenesis of AAA and may be useful as a marker of AAA formation and risk, AAA expansion, and it may potentially be useful as a therapeutic target for treatment. It would be interesting to determine if human aortic tissue expresses TG2 and if patients with AAA have overexpression of TG2. Further study will be required to answer these questions.

J. D. Raffetto, MD

Haptoglobin 2-1 phenotype predicts rapid growth of abdominal aortic aneurysms
Wiernicki I, Safranow K, Baranowska-Bosiacka I, et al (Pomeranian Med Univ, Szczecin, Poland)
J Vasc Surg 52:691-696, 2010

Background.—Haptoglobin (Hp) polymorphism is associated with the prevalence and clinical evolution of many inflammatory diseases and atherosclerosis. Circulating neutrophils and neutrophil-associated proteases are an important initial component of experimental abdominal aortic aneurysm (AAA) formation. Elastase and C-reactive protein (CRP) levels are elevated in patients with AAAs. This study assessed the relationship between AAA expansion and Hp phenotypes, neutrophil count, elastase, and CRP levels.

Methods.—Eighty-three consecutive AAA patients underwent annual ultrasound scans. Three major Hp phenotypes (1-1, 2-1, and 2-2) were determined, and the neutrophil count, serum elastase, and high-sensitivity (hs) CRP levels were measured at the initial examination. After initial screening, patients were rescanned at 6- to 12-month intervals up to a period of 2 to 7 years. The mean yearly growth of the AAA largest transverse diameter was estimated for each group of Hp patients. The results are presented as median (interquartile range).

Results.—Hp 2-1 patients had a significantly higher growth rate (3.69 [2.40] mm/y) of AAA compared with patients with Hp 2-2 (1.24 [0.79], $P < .00001$) and Hp 1-1 (1.45 [0.68], $P = .00004$). This association remained significant in the multivariate analysis. Elevated elastase serum activity was also evident in AAA patients with Hp 2-1 (0.119 [0.084] arbitrary units) in contrast to Hp 2-2 (0.064 [0.041], $P < .00001$) and Hp 1-1 (0.071 [0.040], $P = .0006$) patients. CRP serum levels (mg/L) were significantly higher in patients with Hp 2-1 (7.2 [7.1]) than in Hp 2-2 (3.4 [3.1], $P = .0058$) and Hp 1-1 (2.8 [4.1], $P = .044$). The neutrophil count was not significantly different among Hp groups.

Conclusions.—The Hp 2-1 phenotype showed a strong association with increased rates of the expansion of AAAs and may be a useful independent predictor of growth rate. Further large follow-up studies will be needed to investigate the pathomechanisms of association and the role of elastase and inflammation in the progression of AAA (Table 3).

▶ Haptoglobin has 3 genetic polymorphic phenotypes: 1-1, 2-1, and 2-2. This study evaluated if haptoglobin polymorphism was associated with an increase in abdominal aortic aneurysm (AAA) growth rate, neutrophil count, serum elastase, and C-reactive protein (CRP). The study found that patients with AAA

TABLE 3.—Comparison of Abdominal Aortic Aneurysm (AAA) Parameters, Serum Elastase Activity, and Inflammation Markers among Patients with Various Haptoglobin (Hp) Phenotypes

| Parameters | Hp phenotype, Median (IQR) | | | P Value[a] | | |
	1-1	2-1	2-2	2-1 vs 1-1	2-1 vs 2-2	2-2 vs 1-1
Age at initial examination, y	68 (10)	68 (14)	69 (11)	.89	.77	.91
AAA diameter, mm						
Initial	43 (15)	38 (6)	44 (12)	.023	.0081	.52
Final	56 (10)	52 (7)	51 (15)	.38	.79	.27
Increase[b]	8 (5)	15 (9)	8 (4)	.0074	.00007	.77
Follow-up, mon	66 (26)	45 (13)	62 (12)	.0028	<.00001	.81
Growth rate, mm/y	1.45 (0.68)	3.69 (2.40)	1.24 (0.79)	.00004	<.00001	.14
Elastase activity, AU[c]	0.071 (0.040)	0.119 (0.084)	0.064 (0.041)	.0006	<.00001	.65
CRP, mg/L	2.8 (4.1)	7.2 (7.1)	3.4 (3.1)	.044	.0058	.79
Neutrophil count, G/L	5.5 (2.0)	5.7 (2.5)	5.4 (1.8)	.55	.95	.57

CRP, C-reactive protein; IQR, interquartile range.
[a]Mann-Whitney test.
[b]Difference between final and initial AAA diameter.
[c]Arbitrary units based on absorbance change.

and haptoglobin 2-1 polymorphic phenotype had the greatest AAA growth rate, highest serum elastase activity, and highest CRP levels (Table III). On multivariate analysis, haptoglobin 2-1 phenotype was the only independent predictor of a higher AAA growth rate compared with haptoglobin 1-1 and 2-2 phenotypes. The clinical significance is that haptoglobin polymorphism potentially could be used as a genetic test to identify individuals with AAA who may be at increased risk for rapid aneurysm growth and rupture. As with many scientific studies, the results and conclusions usually always lead to more unanswered questions. Some questions worth considering from this study are the following: Were the ultrasound technicians blinded to the haptoglobin polymorphism status of the patients examined? Is ultrasound measurement the best test when evaluating millimeter differences of the abdominal aorta? Should patients with haptoglobin 2-1 have more aggressive surveillance than patients with haptoglobin 1-1 and 2-2 phenotypes? What is the pathomechanism of haptoglobin 2-1 leading to rapid aneurysm growth? Is haptoglobin polymorphism specific to AAA or also present in other aneurysms? Future studies will be required to answer these questions.

J. D. Raffetto, MD

Vascular smooth muscle cell peroxisome proliferator-activated receptor-γ deletion promotes abdominal aortic aneurysms
Hamblin M, Chang L, Zhang H, et al (Univ of Michigan Med Ctr, Ann Arbor)
J Vasc Surg 52:984-993, 2010

Objective.—Peroxisome proliferator-activated receptor-γ (PPARγ) plays an important role in the vasculature; however, the role of PPARγ in abdominal aortic aneurysms (AAA) is not well understood. We hypothesized that PPARγ in smooth muscle cells (SMCs) attenuates the development of AAA. We also investigated PPARγ-mediated signaling pathways that may prevent the development of AAA.

Methods.—We determined whether periaortic application of $CaCl_2$ renders vascular SMC-selective PPARγ knockout (SMPG KO) mice more susceptible to destruction of normal aortic wall architecture.

Results.—There is evidence of increased vessel dilatation in the abdominal aorta 6 weeks after 0.25 M periaortic $CaCl_2$ application in SMPG KO mice compared with littermate controls (1.4 ± 0.3 mm [n = 8] vs 1.1 ± 0.2 mm [n = 7]; $P =.000119$). Results from SMPG KO mice indicate medial layer elastin degradation was greater 6 weeks after abluminal application of $CaCl_2$ to the abdominal aorta ($P < .01$). Activated cathepsin S, a potent elastin-degrading enzyme, was increased in SMPG KO mice vs wild-type controls. To further identify a role of PPARγ signaling in reducing the development of AAA, we demonstrated that adenoviral-mediated PPARγ overexpression in cultured rat aortic SMCs decreases ($P =.022$) the messenger RNA levels of cathepsin S. In addition, a chromatin immunoprecipitation assay detected PPARγ bound to a peroxisome proliferator-activated receptor response element (PPRE) −141 to −159 bp upstream of the cathepsin S gene sequence in mouse aortic SMCs. Also, adenoviral-mediated PPARγ overexpression and knockdown in cultured rat aortic SMCs decreases ($P = .013$) and increases ($P = .018$) expression of activated cathepsin S. Finally, immunohistochemistry demonstrated a greater inflammatory infiltrate in SMPG KO mouse aortas, as evidenced by elevations in F4/80 and tumor necrosis factor-α expression.

Conclusion.—In this study, we identify PPARγ as an important contributor in attenuating the development of aortic aneurysms by demonstrating that loss of PPARγ in vascular SMCs promotes aortic dilatation and elastin degradation. Thus, PPARγ activation may be potentially promising medical therapy in reducing the risk of AAA progression and rupture.

▶ The study of aneurysm pathophysiology is complex and evolving as further studies are performed. This investigation focuses on the ligand-activated transcription factor peroxisome proliferator-activated receptor γ (PPARγ). PPAR is expressed in vascular smooth muscle cells (SMCs) and has a function in the vasculature through direct or indirect regulation of gene expression, important in blood pressure control, vascular smooth muscle restenosis, and atherosclerosis. Specifically to abdominal aortic aneurysms, PPAR reduces extracellular matrix proteases. PPAR facilitates the effects of angiotensin-receptor blocker (ARB) drugs that are used to treat hypertension. Recently it has been demonstrated that administering losartan or other ARBs may be effective in treating abdominal aortic aneurysm (AAA) in patients with Marfan syndrome. PPAR is the target of thiazolidinediones (TZDs), which are insulin-sensitizing compounds used for treating diabetes. Two recent studies provide evidence that rosiglitazone and pioglitazone, which are TZDs with high-affinity PPAR binding, are beneficial in experimentally reducing AAA. In this study, a mouse knockout for PPAR (SMC-selective PPARγ knockout [SMPG KO]) is used and compared with wild-type litter mates. In this mouse model, AAA is induced by the calcium chloride ($CaCl_2$) method with direct application to the infrarenal aorta for 15 minutes. The significant findings from this study are the following: (1) SMPG KO aorta at 6 weeks is significantly larger than wild type after $CaCl_2$ administration. (2) There was greater destruction of the elastic lamellae fiber network in SMPG KO mice compared with wild-type mice, indicating a potential role for PPAR in attenuating aortic aneurysmal development. (3) The overexpression of PPAR in vascular SMCs reduces cathepsin S, which has been shown to have elastin-degrading properties and is significantly increased in human AAA tissue, providing evidence that PPAR provides a vascular protective effect against destruction of the medial layer elastic network. (4) PPAR in attenuating $CaCl_2$-induced aortic dilatation and elastin degradation is not related to the regulation of matrix metalloproteinase (MMP) 2 or MMP-9 activity. (5) Activated cathepsin S protein expression is increased in SMPG KO mice compared with wild-type mice 1 week after $CaCl_2$ was administered. (6) PPAR overexpression in SMCs decreases active cathepsin S protein expression and activity. (7) PPAR inhibits cathepsin S expression at the genomic level through direct interaction with a putative PPAR response element in the cathepsin S promoter. (8) Vascular SMC PPAR is important in attenuating $CaCl_2$-induced increases in inflammatory cell recruitment and proinflammatory cytokine signaling in the medial layer of the aorta. For a basic scientist or translational scientist interested in the pathogenesis of AAA, this study offers a significant insight into the complex role of PPAR on AAA formation and should be read. However, for the clinician, the knowledge gained from such a study is to understand the importance of hypothesis-driven research, providing a better understanding on how disease pathology works and how to apply treatments and why. Future studies, as this article discusses, will involve the role of TZDs in PPAR knockout mouse model and determine if the treatment with TZD leads to attenuation of AAA formation and the histologic abnormalities identified during $CaCl_2$ administration in the mouse AAA model.

J. D. Raffetto, MD

A meta-analysis of clinical studies of statins for prevention of abdominal aortic aneurysm expansion
Takagi H, Matsui M, Umemoto T (Shizuoka Med Ctr, Japan)
J Vasc Surg 52:1675-1681, 2010

Background.—Despite the absence of a relationship between cholesterol and abdominal aortic aneurysm (AAA) expansion, there is evidence from a number of studies to suggest that statin therapy may influence AAA expansion, presumably through pleiotropic effects. To confirm whether statin therapy is associated with less AAA expansion, we performed a meta-analysis of clinical controlled studies of statin therapy for prevention of AAA expansion.

Methods.—To identify all clinical studies of statin therapy vs control (no statins) enrolling patients with small (≤ 55 mm) AAA, MEDLINE, EMBASE, and the Cochrane Central Register of Controlled Trials were searched. For each study, data regarding AAA expansion in both the statin and control groups were used to generate standardized mean differences (SMDs; <0 favoring statin therapy; >0 favoring control) and 95% confidence intervals (CIs). Study-specific estimates were combined using inverse variance-weighted averages of logarithmic SMDs in fixed-effects and random-effects models.

Results.—We identified five clinical controlled studies of statin therapy vs control enrolling patients with small AAA, including no randomized and five observational studies. Our meta-analysis included data on 697 patients with small AAA received statin therapy or no statins. Pooled analysis demonstrated that statin therapy was statistically significantly associated with less expansion rates (random-effects SMD, -0.50; 95% CI, -0.75 to -0.25; $P = .0001$). There was statistically significant trial heterogeneity of results ($P = .03$). Exclusion of any single trial from the analysis did not substantively alter the overall result of our analysis. There was no evidence of significant publication bias ($P = .81$).

Conclusion.—Statin therapy is associated with less expansion rates in patients with small AAA. To confirm our results and more accurately assess the effect of statins on AAA expansion, a large randomized trial is needed.

▶ As the circle of benefit for statin therapy seemingly widens, this meta-analysis suggests that statin therapy is associated with less expansion rates in patients with small abdominal aortic aneurysms (Aaas). As with any meta-analysis, it is important to note in the methods of this study that of 80 potentially relevant studies found via MEDLINE, only 5 clinical controlled studies met inclusion criteria and were used for collective data analysis. With the lack of randomized controlled trials, limitations with use of only observational studies is that treatment strategy was not based on randomized placebo-controlled assignment, subjecting the findings to selection bias and confounding variables. However, enough data are present here to suggest a possible relationship of statins and slowed AAA expansion to warrant further investigation with larger randomized clinical trials. Additional investigation should also evaluate whether the benefit of statins should also extend to prevention of AAA in higher-risk groups.

M. A. Passman, MD

Hyperglycemia limits experimental aortic aneurysm progression
Miyama N, Dua MM, Yeung JJ, et al (Stanford Univ School of Medicine, CA)
J Vasc Surg 52:975-983, 2010

Objective.—Diabetes mellitus (DM) is associated with reduced progression of abdominal aortic aneurysm (AAA) disease. Mechanisms responsible for this negative association remain unknown. We created AAAs in hyperglycemic mice to examine the influence of serum glucose concentration on experimental aneurysm progression.

Methods.—Aortic aneurysms were induced in hyperglycemic (DM) and normoglycemic models by using intra-aortic porcine pancreatic elastase (PPE) infusion in C57BL/6 mice or by systemic infusion of angiotensin II (ANG) in apolipoprotein E-deficient (ApoE$^{-/-}$) mice, respectively. In an additional DM cohort, insulin therapy was initiated after aneurysm induction. Aneurysmal aortic enlargement progression was monitored with serial transabdominal ultrasound measurements. At sacrifice, AAA cellularity and proteolytic activity were evaluated by immunohistochemistry and substrate zymography, respectively. Influences of serum glucose levels on macrophage migration were examined in separate models of thioglycollate-induced murine peritonitis.

Results.—At 14 days after PPE infusion, AAA enlargement in hyperglycemic mice (serum glucose ≥300 mg/dL) was less than that in euglycemic mice (PPE-DM: 54% ± 19% vs PPE: 84% ± 24%, $P < .0001$). PPE-DM mice also demonstrated reduced aortic mural macrophage infiltration (145 ± 87 vs 253 ± 119 cells/cross-sectional area, $P = .0325$), elastolysis (% residual elastin: 20% ± 7% vs 12% ± 6%, $P = .0209$), and neovascularization (12 ± 8 vs 20 ± 6 vessels/high powered field, $P = .0229$) compared with PPE mice. Hyperglycemia limited AAA enlargement after ANG infusion in ApoE$^{-/-}$ mice (ANG-DM: 38% ± 12% vs ANG: 61% ± 37% at day 28). Peritoneal macrophage production was reduced in response to thioglycollate stimulation in hyperglycemic mice, with limited augmentation noted in response to vascular endothelial growth factor administration. Insulin therapy reduced serum glucose levels and was associated with AAA enlargement rates intermediate between euglycemic and hyperglycemic mice (PPE: 1.21 ± 0.14 mm vs PPE-DM: 1.00 ± 0.04 mm vs PPE-DM + insulin: 1.14 ± 0.05 mm).

Conclusions.—Hyperglycemia reduces progression of experimental AAA disease; lowering of serum glucose levels with insulin treatment diminishes this protective effect. Identifying mechanisms of hyperglycemic aneurysm inhibition may accelerate development of novel clinical therapies for AAA disease.

▶ Based on clinical evidence that diabetes mellitus is associated with reduced progression of abdominal aortic aneurysm (AAA), this study examines the effect of serum glucose levels on AAA progression in a murine model. As an in vivo model, both AAA and hyperglycemia are induced using standardized techniques, and mice are sacrificed at 14 days with evaluation of AAA cellularity and proteolytic activities and influence of serum glucose levels on macrophage migration. Findings suggest that hyperglycemia is associated with attenuated mural neovascularization, macrophage infiltration, and medial elastolysis, all essential features of AAA disease in humans. While these findings are interesting, clinical extrapolation is difficult at this point given the murine model used, overlapping variables associated with induction of both AAA and hyperglycemia, and time frame studied. If this in vivo model for inhibition of AAA progression by hyperglycemia can translate to a human disease model and further clinical investigation is possible, potential therapeutic strategies directed at suppression of AAA progression may be a consideration in the future.

M. A. Passman, MD

The impact of body mass index on perioperative outcomes of open and endovascular abdominal aortic aneurysm repair from the National Surgical Quality Improvement Program, 2005-2007
Giles KA, Wyers MC, Pomposelli FB, et al (Beth Israel Deaconess Med Ctr, Boston, MA)
J Vasc Surg 52:1471-1477, 2010

Objectives.—Obesity and morbid obesity have been shown to increase wound infections and occasionally mortality after many surgical procedures. Little is known about the relative impact of body mass index (BMI) on these outcomes after open (OAR) and endovascular abdominal aortic aneurysm repair (EVAR).

Methods.—The 2005-2007 National Surgical Quality Improvement Program (NSQIP), a multi-institutional risk-adjusted database, was retrospectively queried to compare perioperative mortality (in-hospital or

30-day) and postoperative wound infections after OAR and EVAR. Patient demographics, comorbidities, and operative details were analyzed. Obesity was defined as a BMI >30 kg/m^2 and morbid obesity as a BMI >40 kg/m^2. Outcomes were compared with t test, Wilcoxon rank sum, χ^2, and multivariate logistic regression.

Results.—There were 2097 OARs and 3358 EVARs. Compared with EVAR, OAR patients were younger, more likely to be women (26% vs 17%, $P < .001$), and less obese (27% vs 32%, $P < .001$). Mortality was 3.7% after OAR vs 1.2% after EVAR (risk ratio, 3.1; $P < .001$), and overall morbidity was 28% vs 12%, respectively (relative risk, 2.3; $P < .001$). Morbidly obese patients had a higher mortality for both OAR (7.3%) and EVAR (2.4%) than obese patients (3.9% OAR; 1.5% EVAR) or nonobese patients (3.7% OAR; 1.1% EVAR). Obese patients had a higher rate of wound infection vs nonobese after OAR (6.3% vs 2.4%, $P < .001$) and EVAR (3.3% vs 1.5%, $P < .001$). Morbid obesity predicted death after OAR but not after EVAR, and obesity was an independent predictor of wound infection after OAR and EVAR.

Conclusions.—Morbid obesity confers a worse outcome for death after abdominal aortic aneurysm repair. Obesity is also a risk factor for infectious complications after OAR and EVAR. Obese patients and, particularly, morbidly obese patients should be treated with EVAR when anatomically feasible.

▶ With the US obesity epidemic, this study is part of a growing body of evidence that shows the effect of obesity on other diseases, which overall may translate to poorer outcomes. Using the National Surgical Quality Improvement Program data set and National Institutes of Health definitions for body mass index, comparison of obese versus nonobese patients undergoing abdominal aortic aneurysm (AAA) repair showed worse outcomes, including increased infection and wound complications after both open and endovascular repair and increased mortality after open repair, but no difference in mortality for endovascular repair. Although this study has some limitations related to data source validity, potential miscoding, and some missing details, this bias is likely evenly distributed throughout the data set. These findings reinforce concern for higher body mass index as an independent risk factor that should be considered when weighing benefit of AAA repair and may shift risk benefit toward endovascular approaches or surveillance in selected obese patients.

M. A. Passman, MD

Morphological and Mechanical Changes in Juxtarenal Aortic Segment and Aneurysm Before and After Open Surgical Repair of Abdominal Aortic Aneurysms
Majewski W, Stanišić M, Pawlaczyk K, et al (Poznań Univ of Med Sciences, Poland)
Eur J Vasc Endovasc Surg 40:202-208, 2010

Objective.—The aim of study was to assess how the ultrastructure of the wall of aortic aneurysms, sac and neck influences aortic wall distensibility and proximal dilatation 2 years after open repair.

Methods.—Biopsies for electron microscopy were taken from aneurysmal sac and neck of 30 patients. Patients were assessed by computed tomography (CT) and ultrasound for aneurysm diameter and distensibility (M-mode ultrasonography).

Results.—Postoperative CT of the aortic stump distinguished two groups. Group I ($n = 11$) with little enlargement, median 1 mm (1–3 mm) and group II ($n = 19$) with significant aortic enlargement, median 5.2 mm (4–12 mm). In group II, changes in elastic fibres in the aneurysm neck were comparable to, but as extreme as in the aneurysm sac. For group I, the distensibility of the aneurysmal sac was significantly lower than in the neck or at the renal arteries. For group II, the distensibility in both the neck and sac was significantly lower than at the juxtarenal segment ($p = 0.01$). The biopsies of group II patients showed the extensive degeneration of normal architecture, which was associated with altered wall distensibility in both the aneurysmal neck and sac.

Conclusions.—Disorganisation and destruction of normal aortic architecture at the ultrastructural level are associated with decreasing aortic distensibility. Low aortic neck distensibility is associated with proximal aortic dilatation at 2 years postoperatively.

▶ This study is a prospective observational cohort analysis of aortic neck morphology in patients undergoing open aneurysm repair. Thirty patients underwent ultrasound aortic distensibility measurements before surgical repair and during the follow-up period of 2 years. At the time of aneurysm repair, aortic pathology was obtained in the area of aneurysm as well as at the aortic neck. Pathology was correlated with preoperative aortic distensibility and continued aortic degeneration. Preoperative loss of aortic distensibility at the aortic neck correlated with elastic fiber degeneration and loss of collagen fibers, and it correlated with continued aortic diameter degeneration at 2 years of follow-up.

Gross aortic examination, CT, and MRI only estimate the beginning and end of aortic aneurysmal disease. Pathologic studies, like this one, have demonstrated aortic wall degeneration despite having a normal contour and diameter, which represents at-risk aorta for continued degeneration. This study correlates a dynamic ultrasound measurement, aortic distensibility, with occult aortic degeneration. While this study is not definitive, it does highlight our relatively poor understanding of the aortic neck and provides insight into late open and endovascular failures secondary to continued aortic degeneration.

Z. M. Arthurs, MD

8 Abdominal Aortic Endografting

Urgent Endovascular Treatment of Thoraco-abdominal Aneurysms Using a Sandwich Technique and Chimney Grafts — A Technical Description
Kolvenbach RR, Yoshida R, Pinter L, et al (Vascular Ctr Augusta Hosp and Catholic Clinics Duesseldorf, Germany; São Paulo State Univ, Botucatu, Brazil; et al)
Eur J Vasc Endovasc Surg 41:54-60, 2011

Introduction.—So far the only endovascular option to treat patients with thoraco abdominal aortic aneurysms is the deployment of branched grafts. We describe a technique consisting of the deployment of standard off-the- shelf grafts to treat urgent cases.

Material and Methods.—The sandwich technique consists of the deployment of ViaBahn chimney grafts in combination with standard thoracic and abdominal aortic stent grafts. The chimney grafts are deployed using a transbrachial and transaxillary access. These coaxial grafts are placed inside the thoracic tube graft. After deployment of the infrarenal bifurcated abdominal graft a bridging stent-a short tube graft is positioned inside the thoracic graft further stabilizing the chimney grafts.

Results.—5 patients with symptomatic thoraco abdominal aneurysms were treated. There was one Type I endoleak that resolved after 2 months. In all patients 3 stentgrafts had to be used When possible all visceral and renal branches were revascularized. A total number of 17 arteries were reconnected with covered branches. During follow up we lost one target vessel the right renal artery.

Conclusion.—The sandwich technique in combination with chimney grafts permits a total endovascular exclusion of thoraco abdominal aortic aneurysms. In all cases off-the shelf products and grafts could be used. The number of patients treated so far is still too small to draw further more robust conclusions with regard to long term performance and durability (Figs 2 and 3).

▶ Thoracoabdominal aortic aneurysm (TAA): as we sit and teeter on the brink between the past (extensive open operations with unacceptable rates of morbidity and mortality) and the future (minimally invasive endovascular procedures with off-the-shelf devices to suit a majority of complex aortic anatomy), we must keep our eyes and ears open for innovative endovascular

A   B

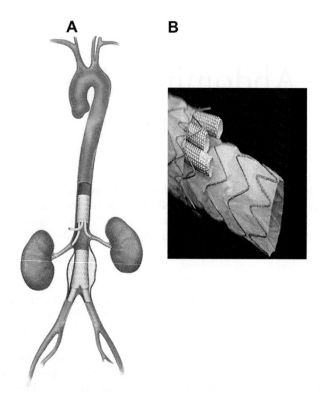

FIGURE 2.—A. Illustration of thoracic graft, chimney grafts and abdominal bifurcated graft. B. Relationship between stent graft and Via Bahn grafts. (Reprinted from Kolvenbach RR, Yoshida R, Pinter L, et al. Urgent Endovascular Treatment of Thoraco-abdominal Aneurysms Using a Sandwich Technique and Chimney Grafts − A Technical Description. *Eur J Vasc Endovasc Surg*. 2011;41:54-60. Copyright 2011, with permission from the European Society for Vascular Surgery.)

techniques that may potentially serve as a bridge to the future. I firmly believe that this report, based on a small experience with 5 patients, represents one of those bridges.

Kolvenbach et al report their early and impressive experience using what they refer to as the sandwich technique for the endovascular repair of TAA using chimney grafts. This technique, described in Figs 2 and 3, uses a stable chimney platform of Viabahn stent grafts (W.L. Gore, Flagstaff, AZ) sandwiched between conventional aortic stent grafts and reinforced with balloon-expandable stents.

The authors describe their results with 5 patients and 17 branch vessels. The rate of endoleak was small with only one type 1 and one type 2 endoleak after a mean follow-up of nearly 6 months. Eighty percent (4 patients) experienced sac regression of > 5 mm at 6 months. One branch vessel, a renal artery, was lost secondary to dissection intra-operatively. Fluoroscopy time was excessive at a mean of 135 minutes, but this will likely improve with increased experience.

At first glance, it is amazing that such a technique would actually work and obvious that longer-term follow-up on these types of patients and procedures is

A

B

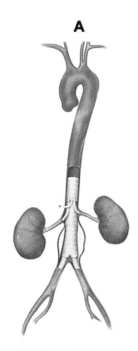

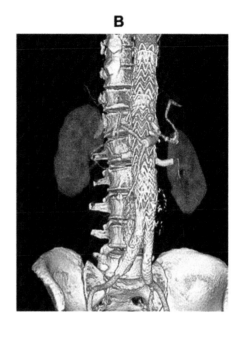

FIGURE 3.—A. Illustration of all grafts after complete deployment. B. Completion CT scans after TAAA exclusion. (Reprinted from Kolvenbach RR, Yoshida R, Pinter L, et al. Urgent Endovascular Treatment of Thoraco-abdominal Aneurysms Using a Sandwich Technique and Chimney Grafts — A Technical Description. *Eur J Vasc Endovasc Surg.* 2011;41:54-60. Copyright 2011, with permission from the European Society for Vascular Surgery.)

warranted. The authors appropriately credit Allaqaband et al for the initial description of this technique for branch vessel preservation in 2004.[1]

B. W. Starnes, MD

Reference

1. Allaqaband S, Kumar A, Bajwa T. A novel technique of aortomonoiliac AAA repair in patients with a single patent iliac artery: a "stent-graft sandwich". *J Endovasc Ther.* 2004;11:550-552.

Are intrasac pressure measurements useful after endovascular repair of abdominal aortic aneurysms?

Milner R, De Rango P, Verzini F, et al (Loyola Univ, Maywood, IL; Ospedale S. Maria della Misericordia, Perugia, Italy; et al)

J Vasc Surg 53:534-539, 2011

Few would argue with the need for long-term follow-up after endovascular repair of abdominal aortic aneurysms. A small risk of reintervention persists and the challenge remains to identify those patients that will require additional procedures to prevent subsequent complications. The ideal follow-up regimen remains elusive. Up until this point, most regimens have consisted of radiologic imaging, with either computed tomography (CT) scans or ultrasonography to identify continued aneurysm perfusion (endoleaks) and document sac dynamics, either shrinkage, growth, or stability. However, aneurysm sac growth or shrinkage serves only as a surrogate measurement for pressurization, and although it is uniformly believed that attachment site endoleaks require treatment, it remains controversial as to how to determine which type II endoleaks pressurize an aneurysm sufficiently to require therapy.

In response to these difficulties, several manufacturers have developed pressure sensors that can be implanted at the time of the initial repair. They have been shown capable of measuring intrasac pressures that have appropriately responded to reinterventions for endoleaks. However, are they the answer we are looking for? Are they ready for widespread use? Do they offer a reliable and consistent measure of intrasac pressure that can be trusted to determine the need, or lack of need, for further therapy? Our debaters will try to convince us one way or another.

▶ The development of endovascular repair of aortic aneurysms in the 1990s marked a revolution in alternative therapy for this deadly disease. Nearly 20 years later, however, we are still trying to understand the appropriate application of this technology. With the recent publication by Schanzer et al,[1] the topic of surveillance after endovascular aneurysm repair (EVAR) has become even more important. In this multicenter observational study, the authors reveal that compliance with EVAR device guidelines was low and post-EVAR aneurysm sac enlargement was high, raising concern for long-term risk of aneurysm rupture. The 5-year post-EVAR rate of abdominal aortic aneurysm (AAA) sac enlargement was 41%, and persistent endoleak after EVAR was an independent predictor of AAA sac enlargement.

The debate by Drs Milner and Cao highlights the use of intrasac pressure monitoring as one strategy to accomplish this monitoring without the continued use of CT scan and continued radiation exposure. This debate, however, highlights that despite being able to perform intrasac pressure monitoring, we still really don't know what to do with the information. Both authors in this debate highlight that the sensitivity/specificity of pressure measurements, including appropriate threshold pressures, is still unclear. Further work is needed to understand the clinical significance of type II endoleaks and the role of intrasac pressure measurements in following up with patients after endovascular aneurysm repair.

D. L. Gillespie, MD, RVT

Reference

1. Schanzer A, Greenberg RK, Hevelone N, et al. Predictors of abdominal aortic aneurysm sac enlargement after endovascular repair. *Circulation.* 2011;123: 2848-2855.

Endovascular aneurysm repair for ruptured abdominal aortic aneurysm: The Albany Vascular Group approach

Mehta M (The Ctr for Vascular Awareness, Inc, Albany, NY)
J Vasc Surg 52:1706-1712, 2010

Improvements in endovascular technology and techniques have allowed us to treat patients in ways we never thought possible. Today, endovascular treatment of ruptured abdominal aortic aneurysms is associated with markedly decreased morbidity and mortality compared with the open surgical approach, yet there are several fundamental obstacles in our ability to offer these endovascular techniques to most patients with ruptured aneurysms. This article will focus on the technical aspects of endovascular aneurysm repair for rupture, with particular attention to developing a standardized multidisciplinary approach that will help vascular surgeons deal with not just the technical aspects of these procedures but also address some of the challenges, including the availability of preoperative computed tomography, the choice of anesthesia, the percutaneous vs femoral cutdown approach, use of aortic occlusion balloons, need for bifurcated vs aortouniiliac stent grafts, need for adjunctive procedures, diagnosis and treatment of abdominal compartment syndrome, and conversion to open surgical repair.

▶ This is an excellent technique article that may help the individual practitioner develop their approach to using endovascular aneurysm repair for the treatment of ruptured abdominal aortic aneurysms (rAAAs). Dr Mehta details the Albany approach to setting up and accomplishing endovascular aneurysm repair (EVAR). The main components to address include having preoperative CT scans on all patients with rAAA, having dedicated operating room staff skilled in assisting with emergent EVAR at all times, having an inventory of off-the-shelf stent grafts, and last but not least making sure the surgeons have the experience and ability in managing unexpected endovascular issues during emergency repair. In addition, it is imperative that surgeons become facile with the use of intra-aortic balloon occlusion whether it be from a brachial or femoral approach.

As reported by Starnes et al,[1] implementation of a structured protocol for managing rAAA, has led to a relative risk reduction in 30-day mortality of 35% compared with the time before implementation of the protocol. In studies that used a structured protocol, the mortality rate after EVAR was 18% (95% confidence interval [CI], 10%-26%), whereas in those studies without such protocols, the mortality rate was 32% (95% CI, 20-44).

The implementation of a standardized protocol for the efficient evaluation and treatment of rAAAs is arguably at least as important as the introduction of EVAR for improvement in survival rates. Preparation is the hallmark of success to any emergency protocol!

D. L. Gillespie, MD, RVT

Reference

1. Starnes BW, Quiroga E, Hutter C, et al. Management of ruptured abdominal aortic aneurysm in the endovascular era. *J Vasc Surg.* 2010;51:9-18.

Endovascular chimney technique versus open repair of juxtarenal and suprarenal aneurysms

Bruen KJ, Feezor RJ, Daniels MJ, et al (Univ of Florida, Gainesville; et al)
J Vasc Surg 53:895-905, 2011

Objective.—To compare early outcomes of endovascular repair of juxtarenal and suprarenal aneurysms using the chimney technique with open repair in anatomically-matched patients.

Methods.—Between January 2008 and December 2009, 21 patients underwent endovascular repair of juxtarenal and suprarenal aortic aneurysms with chimney stenting (Ch-EVAR) of 1 or 2 renal and/or superior mesenteric artery (SMA) vessels. These were compared with 21 anatomically-matched patients that underwent open repair (OR) during the same time period. Primary end points were 30-day mortality, chimney stent patency, and type Ia endoleak. Secondary end points included early complications, renal function, blood loss, and length of stay (LOS).

Results.—Despite a higher proportion of women, oxygen-dependent pulmonary disease and lower baseline renal function, 30-day mortality was identical with one death (4.8%) in each group. Blood loss and total LOS were significantly less for Ch-EVAR. Six patients (29%) in the chimney group had acute kidney injury (AKI) compared with the open group, in which there were one (4.8%) AKI and four (19%) acute renal failures, of which two (9.5%) required chronic hemodialysis. Renal function at 12 months demonstrated similar declines in the overall estimated glomerular filtration rate (eGFR) in the Ch-EVAR and OR groups (11.1 ± 19.6 vs 10.4 ± 25.2, $P = $ NS, respectively). There was one asymptomatic SMA stent occlusion at 6 months and partial compression of a second SMA stent which underwent repeat balloon angioplasty. Primary patency at 6 and 12 months was 94% and 84%, respectively. There was one type Ia endoleak noted at 30 days which resolved by 6 months.

Conclusions.—Ch-EVAR may extend the anatomical eligibility of endovascular aneurysm repair using conventional devices. It appears to have similar mortality to open repair with less morbidity. Long-term durability and stent patency remain to be determined.

▶ The treatment of patients with juxtarenal aneurysms continues to be a challenge. Traditional open repair with renal artery bypass grafting or reimplantation has been the standard. This of course adds morbidity and mortality to these procedures. The use of fenestrated or branched grafts continues to be in development but still remains unavailable to most surgeons treating this disease. As such, innovating surgeons persist in finding alternative solutions to this problem. The technique of using covered stents to preserve flow to the renal arteries after inadvertently covering them has been a standard bailout procedure for years. The concept of using this technique to snorkel or protect a renal artery from encroachment on initial endovascular aneurysm repair implantation to treat patients with severely limited infrarenal aortic landing zone, however, is relatively new.

In this article, the authors report on their experience using off-the-shelf products to perform endovascular treatment of juxtarenal and pararenal aortic aneurysms. Furthermore, they compared their results with this technique to that obtained in 21 anatomically-matched patients who underwent open repair during the same period. This article shows that this technique is associated with good patency of the renal arteries as well as shorter length of stay. The incidence of acute and chronic renal failure was similar between groups as was the overall glomerular filtration rate after 1 year. Overall, 20 of 21 pts had their juxtarenal aneurysm successfully excluded using this technique.

Clearly the long-term durability of this technique remains to be proven with longer follow-up. Specifically, we will be following these patients to watch for the preservation of graft fixation, seal, and branch vessel patency. In addition, the controversial aspect of sacrificing 1 renal artery in cases of snorkeling the superior mesenteric artery needs further study. I think overall the article shows that using the snorkel technique is a viable option in patients determined to be too high risk for open repair.

D. L. Gillespie, MD, RVT

Predictors of Abdominal Aortic Aneurysm Sac Enlargement After Endovascular Repair

Schanzer A, Greenberg RK, Hevelone N, et al (Univ of Massachusetts Med School, Worcester; Cleveland Clinic Foundation, OH; Harvard School of Public Health, Boston, MA)
Circulation 123:2848-2855, 2011

Background.—The majority of infrarenal abdominal aortic aneurysm (AAA) repairs in the United States are performed with endovascular methods. Baseline aortoiliac arterial anatomic characteristics are fundamental criteria for appropriate patient selection for endovascular aortic repair (EVAR) and key determinants of long-term success. We evaluated compliance with anatomic guidelines for EVAR and the relationship between baseline aortoiliac arterial anatomy and post-EVAR AAA sac enlargement.

Methods and Results.—Patients with pre-EVAR and at least 1 post-EVAR computed tomography scan were identified from the M2S, Inc. imaging database (1999 to 2008). Preoperative baseline aortoiliac anatomic characteristics were reviewed for each patient. Data relating to the specific AAA endovascular device implanted were not available. Therefore, morphological measurements were compared with the most liberal and the most conservative published anatomic guidelines as stated in each manufacturer's instructions for use. The primary study outcome was post-EVAR AAA sac enlargement (>5-mm diameter increase). In 10 228 patients undergoing EVAR, 59% had a maximum AAA diameter below the 55-mm threshold at which intervention is recommended over surveillance. Only 42% of patients had anatomy that met the most conservative definition of device instructions for use; 69% met the most liberal definition of device instructions for use. The 5-year post-EVAR rate of AAA sac enlargement was 41%. Independent predictors of AAA sac enlargement included endoleak, age ≥80 years, aortic neck diameter ≥28 mm, aortic neck angle >60°, and common iliac artery diameter >20 mm.

Conclusion.—In this multicenter observational study, compliance with EVAR device guidelines was low and post-EVAR aneurysm sac enlargement was high, raising concern for long-term risk of aneurysm rupture (Fig 1).

▶ Companies marketing endovascular aortic repair (EVAR) devices measure technical factors, such as delivery accuracy, sealing ability, and fixation strength,

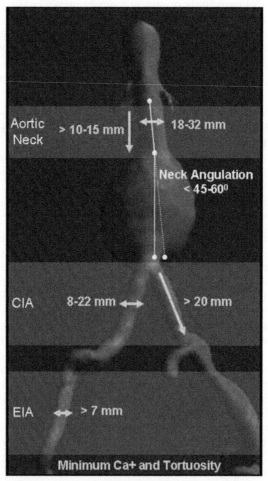

FIGURE 1.—The aortic and iliac arterial anatomy boundary conditions defined by the instructions for use that are packaged with each Food and Drug Administration—approved commercial endovascular aortic device. CIA, common iliac artery; EIA, external iliac artery. (Reprinted from Schanzer A, Greenberg RK, Hevelone N, et al. Predictors of abdominal aortic aneurysm sac enlargement after endovascular repair. *Circulation.* 2011;123:2848-2855, with permission from American Heart Association, Inc.)

in the laboratory. These measurements are used to generate instructions for use (IFU). IFUs are packaged with each EVAR device sold in the United States (Fig 1). The randomized trials comparing EVAR with open aneurysm repair used EVAR devices in accordance with IFUs; however, it is clear that many physicians perform EVAR in some cases without adherence to IFUs. It is unknown what proportion of patients have EVARs placed outside the IFU for the device used. Long-term and midterm results of EVAR performed outside IFUs are largely unknown. It is known, however, that a significant portion of late deaths after EVAR are a result of aneurysm rupture.[1,2] Late aneurysm rupture following EVAR has been linked with aneurysm sac enlargement. The authors sought to determine compliance with IFUs in EVAR placement over the past decade and to determine relationships between anatomic characteristics at baseline of aorta and iliac arteries and subsequent incidence of aortic aneurysm sac enlargement following EVAR. The data indicate that in many cases, those placing EVAR devices are acting in what may be considered an irresponsible fashion. In this study, most EVAR devices were placed in abdominal aortic aneurysms that were below the threshold for intervention justified by randomized trials. Even with the most liberal definition of IFUs, almost one-third of devices are placed outside the manufacturer's recommendations and more than 40% of aortas treated with EVAR have aneurysm sac enlargement at 5 years. These findings are quite disturbing. They raise significant questions about the ethics of aneurysm treatment and significant concerns about long-term risk of aneurysm rupture in patients treated with EVAR in the United States.

G. L. Moneta, MD

References

1. De Bruin JL, Baas AF, Buth J, et al. Long-term outcome of open or endovascular repair of abdominal aortic aneurysm. *N Engl J Med.* 2010;362:1881-1889.
2. Wyss TR, Brown LC, Powell JT, Greenhalgh RM. Rate and predictability of graft rupture after endovascular and open abdominal aortic aneurysm repair: data from the EVAR Trials. *Ann Surg.* 2010;252:805-812.

Rate and Predictability of Graft Rupture After Endovascular and Open Abdominal Aortic Aneurysm Repair: Data From the EVAR Trials
Wyss TR, Brown LC, Powell JT, et al (Imperial College, London, UK)
Ann Surg 252:805-812, 2010

Objective.—To assess the rate and factors associated with rupture after endovascular aneurysm repair (EVAR) or open repair (OR) of abdominal aortic aneurysm.

Background.—Graft rupture after EVAR has been reported, often preceded by graft-related complications. Graft rupture has also been reported after OR.

Methods.—By July 2009, a total of 848 elective EVARs and 594 elective ORs were performed in the United Kingdom EVAR trials 1 and 2. Patients were followed up for complications, reinterventions, and rupture. The incidence of rupture was explored in relation to baseline anatomy and subsequent complications in a Cox regression analysis.

Results.—There were no ruptures in the OR patients. A total of 27 ruptures occurred after EVAR during a mean follow-up of 4.8 years: crude rate $= 0.7$ [95% confidence interval (CI): $0.5-1.0$] ruptures per 100 person-years. Eighteen patients (67%) died within 30 days of rupture. Five ruptures occurred in the first 30 postoperative days and 22 after that: crude rates of rupture $= 7.2$ (95% CI: $3.0-17.4$) and 0.6 (95% CI: $0.4-0.9$) per 100 person-years, respectively. Previous complications (endoleak type 1, type 2 with sac expansion, type 3, migration or kinking) increased the risk of rupture, adjusted hazard ratio 8.83 (95% CI $3.76-20.76$), $P < 0.0001$.

Conclusions.—There were no ruptures after OR and a low rate after EVAR. Mortality after graft rupture is high and previous serious complications are significantly associated with the risk of rupture. Few ruptures after EVAR seem to be spontaneous without complications identified during optimal surveillance.

▶ Aneurysm rupture after endovascular aneurysm repair (EVAR) is a well-recognized complication of the procedure. Outcome of an endograft rupture has high mortality.[1] Graft-related complications after EVAR are frequent, and particular types of complications (endoleak types 1 and 3, stent graft disintegration and migration) increase the risk of an endograft rupture.[2] The United Kingdom EVAR trials have followed patients for up to 10 years, and final results have been published. The authors analyzed the patients in these trials to assess the rate and factors associated with rupture after EVAR or open repair of an abdominal aortic aneurysm (AAA). The data emphasized that EVAR is a form of management of AAA and not a cure for AAA. As such, patients must be continually followed for complications associated with potential rupture of an endograft-managed AAA. Patients with rupture fell into roughly 3 groups. Those that ruptured in the perioperative EVAR period likely reflect inadequate initial isolation of the aneurysm by the endograft. A small group of patients ruptured and had reasonable compliance with recommended surveillance. This group suggests that complications associated with EVAR that occur after a negative surveillance study may rapidly lead to rupture. Most ruptures, however, occurred in individuals who had an identified problem with their endovascular graft. Fifteen out of 17 in this group had documented sac expansion. Rupture after EVAR can be minimized by ensuring that prior to leaving the hospital, the patients have had technically satisfactory procedures and that sac expansion is evaluated, diagnosed, and aggressively treated.

G. L. Moneta, MD

References

1. Schlösser FJ, Gusberg RJ, Dardik A, et al. Aneurysm rupture after EVAR: can the ultimate failure be predicted? *Eur J Vasc Endovasc Surg.* 2009;37:15-22.
2. Fransen GA, Vallabhaneni SR Sr, van Marrewijk CJ, Laheij RJ, Harris PL, Buth J. Rupture of infra-renal aortic aneurysm after endovascular repair: a series from EUROSTAR registry. *Eur J Vasc Endovasc Surg.* 2003;26:487-493.

The effect of injectable biocompatible elastomer (PDMS) on the strength of the proximal fixation of endovascular aneurysm repair grafts: An in vitro study

Bosman W-MPF, van der Steenhoven TJ, Suárez DR, et al (Leiden Univ Med Ctr, The Netherlands; et al)

J Vasc Surg 52:152-158, 2010

Purpose.—One of the major concerns in the long-term success of endovascular aneurysm repair (EVAR) is stent graft migration, which can cause type I endoleak and even aneurysm rupture. Fixation depends on the mechanical forces between the graft and both the aortic neck and the blood flow. Therefore, there are anatomical restrictions for EVAR, such as short and angulated necks. To improve the fixation of EVAR grafts, elastomer (PDMS) can be injected in the aneurysm sac. The support given by the elastomer might prevent dislocation and migration of the graft. The aim of this study was to measure the influence of an injectable biocompatible elastomer on the fixation strength of different EVAR grafts in an in vitro model.

Methods.—The proximal part of three different stent grafts was inserted in a bovine artery with an attached latex aneurysm. The graft was connected to a tensile testing machine, applying force to the proximal fixation, while the artery with the aneurysm was fixated to the setup. The force to obtain graft dislodgement (DF) from the aorta was recorded in Newtons (N). Three different proximal seal lengths (5, 10, and 15 mm) were evaluated. The experiments were repeated after the space between the graft and the latex aneurysm was filled with the elastomer. Independent sample t tests were used for the comparison between the DF before and after elastomer treatment for each seal length.

Results.—The mean DF (mean ± SD) of all grafts without elastomer sac filling for a proximal seal length of 5, 10, and 15 mm were respectively, 4.4 ± 3.1 N, 12.2 ± 10.6 N, and 15.1 ± 6.9 N. After elastomer sac filling, the dislodgement forces increased significantly ($P < .001$) to 20.9 ± 3.8 N, 31.8 ± 9.8 N, and 36.0 ± 14.1 N, respectively.

Conclusions.—The present study shows that aneurysm sac filling may have a role as an adjuvant procedure to the present EVAR technique. The strength of the proximal fixation of three different stent grafts increases significantly in this in vitro setting. Further in vivo research must be done to see if this could facilitate the treatment of aneurysms with short infrarenal necks.

▶ The authors postulate that if the aneurysm sac following endovascular aneurysm repair was completely obliterated, then this would improve fixation of an endovascular graft. It is well known that short, angulated, and wide diameter proximal seal zones predispose to type 1 endoleak. The authors used an injectable biocompatible elastomer to fill the space between the aneurysm sac and the graft, theoretically providing increased support for the graft and increasing the forces required for proximal migration of the graft. The polymer used was polydimethylsiloxane. It sets up without exothermic heat and does not release byproducts into the circulation during the process of curing and cross-linking. The data clearly indicate an increase in dislodgment forces required for dislodgment of the graft with elastomer treatment compared with without elastomer treatment in the experimental model (Figs 2 and 4 in the original article).

This seems like a clever idea; however, there is clearly a large leap from the in vitro model using aortas from healthy young animals without calcification or thrombus to the in vivo situation where dislodgement forces are because of repetitive pulsations of blood flow. However, theoretically, adjunctive use of elastomer treatment at the time of endograft placement could reduce the possibility of both type 1 and type 2 endoleaks in follow-up.

G. L. Moneta, MD

Use of baseline factors to predict complications and reinterventions after endovascular repair of abdominal aortic aneurysm
Brown LC, on behalf of the EVAR Trial Participants (Imperial College London, UK; et al)
Br J Surg 97:1207-1217, 2010

Background.—It is uncertain which baseline factors are associated with graft-related complications and reinterventions after endovascular aneurysm repair (EVAR) in patients with a large abdominal aortic aneurysm.

Methods.—Patients randomized to elective EVAR in EVAR Trial 1 or 2 were followed for serious graft-related complications (type 2 endoleaks excluded) and reinterventions. Cox regression analysis was used to investigate whether any prespecified baseline factors were associated with time to first serious complication or reintervention.

Results.—A total of 756 patients who had elective EVAR were followed for a mean of 3·7 years, by which time there were 179 serious graft complications (rate 6·5 per 100 person years) and 114 reinterventions (rate 3·8 per 100 person years). The highest rate was during the first 6 months, with an apparent increase again after 2 years. Multivariable analysis indicated that graft-related complications increased significantly with larger initial aneurysm diameter ($P < 0·001$) and older age ($P = 0·040$). There was also evidence that patients with larger common iliac diameters experienced higher complication rates ($P = 0·011$).

Conclusion.—Graft-related complication and reintervention rates were common after EVAR in patients with a large aneurysm. Younger patients and those with aneurysms closer to the 5·5-cm threshold for intervention experienced lower rates (Figs 2 and 3).

▶ Use of endovascular aneurysm repair (EVAR) has escalated to the point that it is now used essentially in most patients who are anatomically suitable for an EVAR device. In the United Kingdom, the National Institute for Health and Clinical Excellence has concluded that EVAR should be offered to all patients who are suitable for both EVAR and open repair.[1]

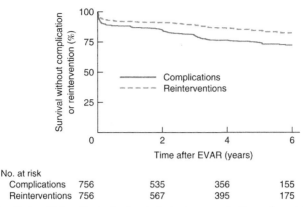

FIGURE 2.—Kaplan—Meier estimates for time to first serious complication or first reintervention for a serious complication after endovascular aneurysm repair (EVAR) for 756 patients in EVAR Trials 1 and 2. (Reprinted from Brown LC, on behalf of the EVAR Trial Participants. Use of baseline factors to predict complications and reinterventions after endovascular repair of abdominal aortic aneurysm. *Br J Surg.* 2010;97:1207-1217. Copyright © British Journal of Surgery Society Ltd. Reproduced with permission. Permission is granted by John Wiley & Sons Ltd on behalf of the BJSS Ltd.)

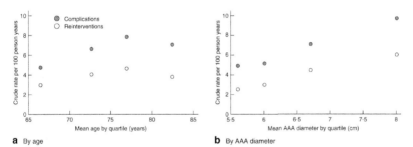

FIGURE 3.—Crude rates of serious complications and reinterventions across increasing quartile groups of **a** age and **b** abdominal aortic aneurysm (AAA) diameter. (Reprinted from Brown LC, on behalf of the EVAR Trial Participants. Use of baseline factors to predict complications and reinterventions after endovascular repair of abdominal aortic aneurysm. *Br J Surg.* 2010;97:1207-1217. Copyright © British Journal of Surgery Society Ltd. Reproduced with permission. Permission is granted by John Wiley & Sons Ltd on behalf of the BJSS Ltd.)

Clearly, however, defining anatomic suitability for EVAR can be complex and represents a balance between the patient under consideration and the characteristics of the individual devices. Surgeons also differ in their interpretation of anatomic suitability. The authors sought to determine baseline factors that were associated with graft-related complications and reinterventions after EVAR. The association of increasing aneurysm diameter with complication and reintervention rates stands out as the most telling finding in this study (Figs 2 and 3). The results, however, cannot be construed to justify EVAR in patients with small abdominal aortic aneurysms, as rupture rates in these patients are very low.[2,3] It is also important to note that patients in the EVAR 1 and 2 Trials had relatively strict criteria for inclusion. Relaxing anatomic selection criteria undoubtedly will result in higher complication and reintervention rates. Appropriate selection of anatomically suitable patients for EVAR remains crucial to the long-term success of the procedure.

G. L. Moneta, MD

References

1. National Institute for Health and Clinical Excellence (NICE) endovascular stent grafts for the treatment of abdominal aortic aneurysms, http://www.nice.org.uk/nicemedia/pdf/TA167Guidance.pdf. Accessed May 23, 2010.
2. Powell JT, Brown LC, Forbes JF, et al. Final 12-year follow-up of surgery versus surveillance in the UK Small Aneurysm Trial. *Br J Surg.* 2007;94:702-708.
3. Lederle FA, Wilson SE, Johnson GR, et al. Immediate repair compared with surveillance of small abdominal aortic aneurysms. *N Engl J Med.* 2002;346:1437-1444.

Evidence that Statins Protect Renal Function During Endovascular Repair of AAAS
Moulakakis KG, Matoussevitch V, Borgonio A, et al (Univ of Cologne, Germany)
Eur J Vasc Endovasc Surg 40:608-615, 2010

Objectives.—Several studies have documented a slight but significant deterioration of renal function after endovascular repair of abdominal aortic aneurysm (AAA) (EVAR). The aim of this retrospective study was therefore to investigate whether medication with statins may favourably affect perioperative renal function.

Material and Methods.—From January 2000 to January 2008, out of a total cohort of 287 elective patients receiving endovascular repair of their AAA or aortoiliac aneurysm, 127 patients were included in the present study, as their medication was reliably retrievable. Patients were divided according to whether their medication included statins (>3 months). Second, they were subdivided according to their supra- (SR) or infrarenal (IR) endo-graft fixation. Serum creatinine (SCr) and creatinine (CrCl) clearance were determined preoperatively, postoperatively, at 6 and 12 months. Patients with known pre-existing renal disease, with incorrect placement of the stent graft resulting in severe renal artery stenosis, and with occlusion or renal parenchymal infarction were excluded from the study.

Results.—Patients receiving an infrarenal fixation of their graft had no change in the renal function, regardless whether they were on statins or not. In patients with SR fixation not receiving statins, a deterioration in renal function was observed in the early postoperative period ((SCr) preoperative vs. SCr postoperative: 1.02 ± 0.2 vs. 1.11 ± 0.28, $p < 0.001$ and (Cr.Cl) preoperative vs. Cr.Cl postoperative: 74.1 ± 21.4 vs. 68.0 ± 21.4, $p < 0.001$), whereas patients on statins experienced no change in renal function (SCr preoperative vs. SCr postoperative: 0.99 ± 0.24 vs. 1.02 ± 0.20 n.s. and Cr.Cl preop vs. Cr.Clpostop.: 76.4 ± 19.1 vs. 74.28 ± 20.50, n.s.). During follow-up, a constant worsening of renal function at 6 and 12 months was observed, irrespective of the medication with statins.

Conclusions.—The present study suggests a slight immediate deterioration of the renal function using (SR) fixation, and this could be prevented by the use of statins. During follow-up, statins did not protect from further renal deterioration. Broader studies are needed to confirm a definitive relation between statin use and renal protection during the endovascular repair of AAA.

▶ The impact of endovascular aortic repair (EVAR) on long-term renal function has been conflicted with varied results. Renal artery embolization, iodinated contrast exposure, renal artery injury, and suprarenal fixation have all been implicated in worsening renal function. There are observational reports documenting statistically significant decrements in renal function over time (2-5 years), but it is rare for a patient to progress to renal failure and dialysis therapy. It is challenging to predict renal clearance and even more difficult to predict the impact of age, hypertension, and diabetes on long-term renal function. To date, no study has evaluated a randomized cohort of patients undergoing EVAR compared with a group of similar risk patients that did not undergo intervention. This study is plagued by the same limitations. They retrospectively evaluated a prospectively maintained database and found a statistical association between statin use and renal function following EVAR. They also found an association between suprarenal fixation and change in renal function. It is important to recognize the real clinical impact observed. Patients receiving statin therapy had a 0.1-mg/dL difference in creatinine compared with patients not taking statin therapy at 12 months following EVAR. The same magnitude of difference was observed in patients treated with suprarenal fixation. Does this really equate to clinical significance? Statin therapy may affect renal function following endograft therapy, but this study does not support statin therapy for that indication.

Z. M. Arthurs, MD

9 Visceral and Renal Artery Disease

Early Diagnosis of Intestinal Ischemia Using Urinary and Plasma Fatty Acid Binding Proteins
Thuijls G, van Wijck K, Grootjans J, et al (Maastricht Univ Med Ctr and NUTRIM School for Nutrition, The Netherlands)
Ann Surg 253:302-308, 2011

Objective.—This study aims at improving diagnosis of intestinal ischemia, by measuring plasma and urinary fatty acid binding protein (FABP) levels.

Methods.—Fifty consecutive patients suspected of intestinal ischemia were included and blood and urine were sampled at time of suspicion. Plasma and urinary concentrations of intestinal FABP (I-FABP), liver FABP (L-FABP) and ileal bile acid binding protein (I-BABP) were measured using enzyme linked immunosorbent assays.

Results.—Twenty-two patients suspected of intestinal ischemia were diagnosed with intestinal ischemia, 24 patients were diagnosed with other diseases, and 4 patients were excluded from further analysis fulfilling exclusion criteria. Median plasma concentrations of I-FABP and L-FABP and urinary concentrations of all 3 markers were significantly higher in patients with proven intestinal ischemia than in patients suspected of intestinal ischemia with other final diagnoses (plasma I-FABP; 653 pg/mL vs. 109 pg/mL, $P = 0.02$, plasma L-FABP; 117 ng/mL vs. 25 ng/mL, $P = 0.006$, urine I-FABP; 3377 pg/mL vs. 115 pg/mL, $P = 0.001$, urine L-FABP; 1,199 ng/mL vs. 37 ng/mL, $P = 0.004$, urine I-BABP; 48.6 ng/mL vs. 0.6 ng/mL, $P = 0.002$). Positive and negative likelihood ratios significantly increased positive posttest probability and decreased negative posttest probability on intestinal ischemia. In patients with intestinal ischemia a trend to higher plasma I-BABP levels was observed when the ileum was involved (18.4 ng/mL vs. 2.9 ng/mL, $P = 0.05$).

Conclusion.—Plasma and especially urinary I-FABP and L-FABP levels and urinary I-BABP levels can improve early diagnosis of intestinal ischemia. Furthermore, plasma I-BABP levels can help in localizing ileal ischemia (Figs 2 and 3).

▶ Diagnosis of intestinal ischemia is difficult. Clinical signs are nonspecific in the early phases, and in late phases the administration of sedative and analgesic

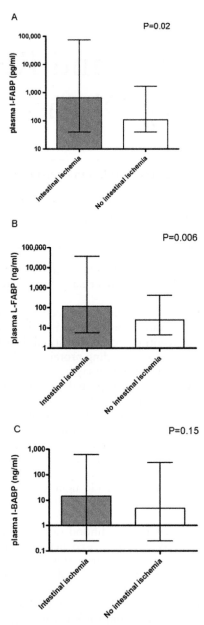

FIGURE 2.—A, Plasma I-FABP and B, L-FABP concentrations were significantly higher in patients with intestinal ischemia (n = 22) than in patients with other final diagnoses (n = 24). C, Plasma I-BABP levels did not differ between patients with intestinal ischemia (n = 22) and patients with other final diagnoses (n = 24). Data are reported as median and range. (Reprinted from Thuijls G, van Wijck K, Grootjans J, et al. Early diagnosis of intestinal ischemia using urinary and plasma fatty acid binding proteins. *Ann Surg.* 2011;253:302-308, with permission from Lippincott Williams & Wilkins.)

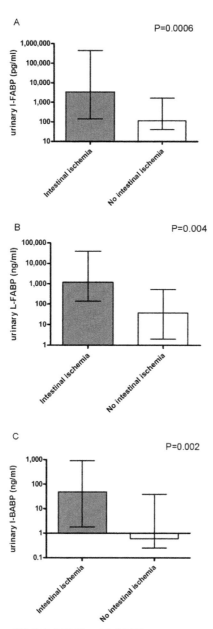

FIGURE 3.—A, Urinary I-FABP B, L-FABP and C, I-BABP concentrations were significantly higher in patients with intestinal ischemia (n = 10) than in patients with other final diagnoses (n = 9). Data are reported as median and range. (Reprinted from Thuijls G, van Wijck K, Grootjans J, et al. Early diagnosis of intestinal ischemia using urinary and plasma fatty acid binding proteins. *Ann Surg.* 2011;253:302-308, with permission from Lippincott Williams & Wilkins.)

agents may make clinical history taking and physical examination suspect. Early diagnosis of intestinal ischemia is crucial in that a diagnostic delay of 24 hours decreases survival rates by more than 20%.[1] Preliminary work suggests that fatty acid binding proteins (FABPs) may be a marker of intestinal ischemia. FABPs are small cytosolic proteins. They are released when enterocyte membrane integrity is lost. They are released into the circulation and cleared renally, allowing for an analysis of both plasma and urinary levels. Ileal FABP plasma and urine levels are increased in patients with intestinal ischemia compared with healthy controls.[2] The authors sought to answer the question of whether circulating urinary FABP levels can distinguish patients with intestinal ischemia from patients without intestinal ischemia where acute intestinal ischemia was initially suspected. The data suggest that plasma and urinary intestinal-FABP and liver-FABP levels and urinary ileal bile acid binding protein levels are increased at the time intestinal ischemia is suspected in patients who ultimately prove to have intestinal ischemia compared with patients with another final diagnosis. Overall, plasma FABP levels were only minimally increased. However, urinary FABP levels resulted in a markedly increased positive posttest probability of ischemia and a clearly decreased negative posttest probability of intestinal ischemia (Figs 2 and 3). The data suggest urinary levels of FABP may be the long-awaited laboratory diagnosis potentially providing confirmation of intestinal ischemia.

G. L. Moneta, MD

References

1. Oldenburg WA, Lau LL, Rodenberg TJ, Edmonds HJ, Burger CD. Acute mesenteric ischemia: a clinical review. *Arch Intern Med.* 2004;164:1054-1062.
2. Kanda T, Fujii H, Tani T, et al. Intestinal fatty acid-binding protein is a useful diagnostic marker for mesenteric infarction in humans. *Gastroenterology.* 1996;110: 339-343.

Efficacy of Revascularization For Renal Artery Stenosis Caused by Fibromuscular Dysplasia: A Systematic Review and Meta-Analysis
Trinquart L, Mounier-Vehier C, Sapoval M, et al (Institut National de la Santé et de la Recherche Médicale Centre d'Investigation Clinique et Epidémiologie Clinique 4, Paris, France; Université Lille 2, France; Université Paris Descartes, France; et al)
Hypertension 56:525-532, 2010

In patients with fibromuscular dysplasia and renal artery stenosis, renal artery revascularization has been used to cure hypertension or to improve blood pressure control. To provide an up-to-date assessment of the benefits and risks associated with revascularization in this condition, we performed a systematic review of studies in which hypertensive patients with fibromuscular dysplasia renal artery stenosis underwent percutaneous transluminal renal angioplasty or surgical reconstruction. We assessed how often periprocedural complications and hypertension cure and improvement occurred. We selected 47 angioplasty studies (1616 patients) and 23 surgery studies (1014 patients). Combined rates of hypertension cure, defined according to the criteria in each study, after angioplasty or surgery were estimated to be 46% (95% CI: 40% to 52%) and 58% (95% CI: 53% to 62%), respectively, with substantial variations across studies. The probability of being cured was negatively associated with patient age and time of publication. Cure rates using current definitions of hypertension cure (blood pressure <140/90 mm Hg without treatment) were only 36% and 54% after angioplasty and surgery, respectively. The combined risks of periprocedural complications were 12% and 17% after angioplasty and surgery, respectively, with less major complications after angioplasty than surgery (6% versus 15%). In conclusion, angioplasty or surgical revascularization yielded moderate benefits in patients with fibromuscular dysplasia renal artery stenosis, with substantial variation across studies. The blood pressure outcome was strongly influenced by patient age.

▶ Both surgery and percutaneous renal artery angioplasty are used to treat renal artery stenosis. Benefit for revascularization of atherosclerotic renal arteries stenosis is limited.[1-3] The limited benefit of revascularization of atherosclerotic renal artery stenosis is thought to reflect underlying renal parenchymal disease associated with age. However, patients with fibromuscular dysplasia (FMD) are younger, in their 30s and 40s, with normal kidney function. Patients with FMD are also primarily women. There have been no randomized control trials and no comprehensive systematic reviews assessing blood pressure outcome with revascularization for renal artery stenosis secondary to FMD. The primary objective of this systematic review was to assess the rate of hypertension cure after renal artery revascularization in patients with hypertension and FMD renal artery stenosis. Other objectives were to assess technical success rates of revascularization and risk of complication and to explore variation of outcomes across subgroups. This systematic review includes studies of both surgical and percutaneous revascularization of FMD renal artery stenosis. Overall this study found that the probability of cure for revascularization of renal artery stenosis secondary to FMD was negatively associated with age, known duration of hypertension, medial-type fibromuscular disease, time of publication, and a more strict definition of cure. This is the largest meta-analysis reported on this subject, and the authors utilized a replicable and transparent method to identify larger numbers of patients than previous reviews. The authors' identified factors associated with hypertension cure seem reasonable as increasing age and duration of hypertension are associated with renal parenchymal disease, other concurrent atherosclerotic disease, and alterations in aortic compliance. The authors note that future studies of revascularization for renal artery stenosis should include standardization of the definition of blood pressure cure using the recognized criteria of a blood pressure of less than 140/90 mm Hg without treatment as the definition of cure and that outcome assessment should occur at 6-month follow-up intervals for all patients. They also note that because only 1 patient in 3 has a normal blood pressure after percutaneous renal artery revascularization with a 12% risk of complications, a randomized trial comparing percutaneous renal artery angioplasty with medical treatment of FMD should be considered.

G. L. Moneta, MD

References

1. Nordmann AJ, Logan AG. Balloon angioplasty versus medical therapy for hypertensive patients with renal artery obstruction. *Cochrane Database Syst Rev.* 2003; (3). CD002944.
2. Balk E, Raman G, Chung M, et al. Effectiveness of management strategies for renal artery stenosis: a systematic review. *Ann Intern Med.* 2006;145:901-912.
3. ASTRAL Investigators, Wheatley K, Ives N, Gray R, et al. Revascularization versus medical therapy for renal-artery stenosis. *N Engl J Med.* 2009;361: 1953-1962.

Results of Single- and Two-Vessel Mesenteric Artery Stents for Chronic Mesenteric Ischemia
Malgor RD, Oderich GS, McKusick MA, et al (Mayo Clinic, Rochester, MN)
Ann Vasc Surg 24:1094-1101, 2010

Background.—To describe the outcomes of single- and two-vessel mesenteric artery stents in patients with chronic mesenteric ischemia (CMI).

Methods.—We reviewed 101 patients (41 men and 60 women; mean age, 73 ± 13 years) treated with mesenteric artery stents for atherosclerotic CMI between 1998 and 2008. Clinical data and outcomes were reviewed in patients treated with single superior mesenteric artery (SMA) stent (group A) or two-vessel celiac artery (CA) and SMA stent (group B). Isolated CA stenting was analyzed as a separate group (group C). End-points were taken as differences in morbidity and mortality and freedom from recurrent symptoms and reinterventions.

Results.—There were 61 patients in group A, 24 in group B, and 16 in group C. All three groups had similar demographics, cardiovascular risk factors, and clinical presentation. There were no differences in early mortality (2%, 4%, and 0%), morbidity (18%, 26%, and 12%), and symptom relief (95%, 78%, and 100%) between groups A, B, and C, respectively (p value was not significant). Mean follow-up was 41 ± 17 months. Freedom for reintervention at 1 and 3 years was similar among patients in groups A (86 ± 5% and 50 ± 9%), B (67 ± 11% and 67 ± 11%), and C (63 ± 13% and 63 ± 13%), respectively (p value was not significant). There were no significant differences in freedom from restenosis at 1 and 3 years among patients in groups A (54 ± 7% and 44 ± 9%), B (47 ± 12% and 39 ± 12%), and C (43 ± 13% and 34 ± 13%), respectively. Primary and secondary patency rates at 3 years were 57% and 96% for SMA and 61% and 87% for CA stents, respectively (p value was not significant). CA stent alone was associated with symptom recurrence in 6 of 16 patients (38%), as compared with the recurrence rate of 18% (11 of 61) in patients who underwent SMA stent placement ($p = 0.06$).

Conclusion.—Two-vessel CA and SMA stenting do not reduce the incidence of recurrent symptoms or reinterventions when compared with single-vessel SMA stents in patients with CMI. CA stent alone carries a high risk of recurrence.

▶ Mesenteric artery angioplasty and stenting is gaining wider acceptance in treatment of patients with chronic mesenteric ischemia (CMI). It relieves symptoms of mesenteric ischemia in 78% to 100% of patients and has lower morbidity and mortality compared with open surgical reconstruction. However, durability of mesenteric artery stenting remains in question. Primary patency has ranged from 30% to 82%, and 17% to 64% of patients have recurrent symptoms at 2 years of follow-up.[1,2] It is generally agreed that the superior mesenteric artery (SMA) is the primary target vessel for revascularization in patients with CMI. With regard to open surgical procedures, it is debated whether revascularization of the SMA alone is adequate treatment versus routine revascularization of both the celiac artery and SMA. In cases of endovascular therapy for CMI, it is also unclear whether stenting of the celiac artery in addition to the SMA adds to the durability of endovascular treatment of CMI. The purpose of this study was to describe the outcomes of single- versus 2-vessel mesenteric stent placement in patients with CMI secondary to atherosclerotic disease. The authors found no added benefit to 2-vessel stenting compared with single-vessel stenting for treatment of CMI. Long-term results are similar, with nearly identical rates of restenosis, reintervention, and recurrence of symptoms. However, 2-vessel stenting was associated with more complications compared with single-vessel stenting. The study is limited by its retrospective design, and it is possible that there was a bias toward placement of 2 stents in patients with more symptoms or when the anatomy of the SMA was suboptimal for stenting. Also, patients with poor collateralization between the celiac artery and SMA who have significant gastric ischemia may benefit from stenting of both arteries. Overall, however, the data did not support a policy of routine stenting of both the celiac artery and SMA for treatment of CMI.

G. L. Moneta, MD

References

1. Atkins MD, Kwolek CJ, LaMuraglia GM, et al. Surgical revascularization versus endovascular therapy for chronic mesenteric ischemia: a comparative experience. *J Vasc Surg.* 2007;45:1162-1171.
2. AbuRahma AF, Stone PA, Bates MC, Welch CA. Angioplasty/stenting of the superior mesenteric artery and celiac trunk: early and late outcomes. *J Endovasc Ther.* 2003;10:1046-1053.

Endovascular and open surgery for acute occlusion of the superior mesenteric artery

Block TA, Acosta S, Björck M (St Göran Hosp, Stockholm, Sweden; Malmö Univ Hosp, Sweden; Uppsala Univ, Sweden)
J Vasc Surg 52:959-966, 2010

Background.—Acute thromboembolic occlusion of the superior mesenteric artery (SMA) is associated with high mortality. Recent advances in diagnostics and surgical techniques may affect outcome.

Methods.—Through the Swedish Vascular Registry (Swedvasc), 121 open and 42 endovascular revascularizations of the SMA at 28 hospitals during 1999 to 2006 were identified. Patient medical records were retrieved, and survival was analyzed with multivariate Cox-regression analysis.

Results.—The number of revascularizations of the SMA increased over time with 41 operations in 2006, compared to 10 in 1999. Endovascular approach increased sixfold by 2006 as compared to 1999. The endovascular

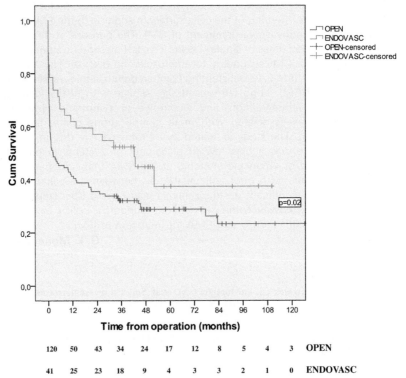

FIGURE 2.—Kaplan-Meier analysis of long-term survival in acute superior mesenteric artery occlusion comparing open and endovascular surgery (log-rank test; $P = .020$). Life tables show patients at risk for open and endovascular surgery at each respective time point. (Reprinted from Block TA, Acosta S, Björck M. Endovascular and open surgery for acute occlusion of the superior mesenteric artery. *J Vasc Surg*. 2010;52: 959-966. Copyright 2010, with permission from The Society for Vascular Surgery.)

group had thrombotic occlusion ($P < .001$) and history of abdominal angina ($P = .042$) more often, the open group had atrial fibrillation more frequently ($P = .031$). All the patients in the endovascular group, but only 34% after open surgery, underwent completion control of the vascular reconstruction ($P < .001$). Bowel resection ($P < .001$) and short bowel syndrome (SBS; $P = .009$) occurred more frequently in the open group. SBS (hazard ratio [HR], 2.6; 95% confidence interval [CI], 1.3-5.0) and age (HR, 1.03/year; 95% CI, 1.00-1.06) were independently associated with increased long-term mortality. Thirty-day and 1-year mortality rates were 42% vs 28% ($P = .03$) and 58% vs 39% ($P = .02$), for open and endovascular surgery, respectively. Long-term survival after endovascular treatment was better than after open surgery (log-rank, $P = .02$).

Conclusion.—The results after endovascular and open surgical revascularization of acute SMA occlusion were favorable, in particular among the endovascularly treated patients. Group differences need to be confirmed in a randomized trial (Fig 2, Table 1).

▶ This is an important study because it assesses a vascular problem not commonly treated. Using a highly validated vascular registry such as the

TABLE 1.—Clinical and Laboratory Data in Patients Undergoing Open vs Endovascular Surgery for Acute SMA Occlusion

	Open (n = 121)	Endovascular (n = 42)	*P* value
Gender (M/F)	55/66	18/24	.77
Age (IQR)	76 (66-81)	77 (59-82)	.50
Comorbidities	N (%)	N (%)	
IHD	51/118 (43)	21/41 (51)	.67
Atrial fibrillation	67/117 (57)	15/40 (38)	.031
History of abdominal angina	13/104 (12)	11/42 (26)	.042
Diabetes mellitus	15/121 (12)	5/42 (12)	.48
Smoking	25/121 (21)	10/42 (24)	.39
CVD	32/121 (26)	5/42 (12)	.053
Previous vascular surgery	24/121 (20)	15/42 (36)	.09
Symptoms			
Onset of symptoms			.61
Sudden	36/114 (32)	14/39 (36)	
Acute	55/114 (48)	12/39 (31)	
Insidious	23/114 (20)	13/39 (33)	
Vomiting	59/111 (53)	17/37 (46)	.59
Diarrhea	57/109 (52)	19/37 (51)	.93
Hematochezia	19/110 (17)	4/37 (11)	.57
Delay in hours	Median (IQR)	Median (IQR)	
Patient delay (n = 130)	6 (2-16)	8 (3-36)	.13
Doctor delay (n = 118)	12 (6-24)	24 (6-72)	.16
Total delay (n = 107)	24 (10-50)	36 (11-132)	.12
Laboratory tests			
CRP (mg/L; n = 102)	19 (5-133)	46 (14-148)	.29
WBC ($\times 10^9$/L; n = 88)	14.9 (11.5-21.0)	14.0 (11.1-18.2)	.76
Hb (g/L; n = 94)	143 (126-152)	134 (122-149)	.33
Creatinine (μmol/L; n = 98)	101 (78-131)	92 (79-120)	.49

CRP, C-reactive protein; *CVD*, cerebrovascular disease; *F*, female; *Hb*, hemoglobin; *IHD*, ischemic heart disease; *IQR*, interquartile range; *M*, male; *SMA*, superior mesenteric artery; *WBC*, white blood cell count.

Swedish Vascular Registry allows the examination of retrospectively reviewing vascular diseases of interest, in this study acute mesenteric ischemia with an intention to treat analysis. The interesting fact of this study is that there were 121 open and 42 endovascular revascularizations of the superior mesenteric artery at 28 hospitals during 1999 and 2006. Some important points to note in the treatment of acute mesenteric ischemia in this study are the following: (1) The number of total interventions increased from 10 in 1999 to 41 in 2006. (2) Endovascular treatment increased by over 6 times in 2006 compared with 1999. (3) Patients treated with open surgery had a higher frequency of embolic events versus thrombotic, higher frequency of bowel resection, second look operations, and short bowel syndrome. (4) Successful revascularization at the primary procedure occurred in 86% of open and 79% of endovascular patients ($P = .23$). (5) Thirty-day mortality was 42% for open and 24% for endovascular ($P = .034$). (6) The 1-year mortality was 59% for open and 38% for endovascular ($P = .021$). (7) On multivariate analysis, endovascular treatment was favorable with decreasing 30-day mortality (odds ratio, 3.7; 95% confidence interval, 1.2-11.6; $P = .025$). Although the 2 groups evaluated were relatively well matched (Table 1), one has to keep in mind that this is a retrospective study from a prospectively entered registry. However, as Fig 2 demonstrates, there is a clear advantage in long-term survival in patients who underwent endovascular revascularization for acute mesenteric ischemia. Obviously, a multicenter randomized controlled trial would be optimal to assess which treatment provides the most favorable outcomes. But given that this is not a common disease, registry data from this type of study provide valuable information for clinical decision making in the treatment of an uncommon but life-threatening vascular disease.

J. D. Raffetto, MD

Use of B-Type Natriuretic Peptide to Predict Blood Pressure Improvement after Percutaneous Revascularisation for Renal Artery Stenosis
Staub D, Zeller T, Trenk D, et al (Univ Hosp Basel, Switzerland; Herz-Zentrum Bad Krozingen, Germany)
Eur J Vasc Endovasc Surg 40:599-607, 2010

Objectives.—The purpose of this study was to evaluate the utility of B-type natriuretic peptide (BNP) to predict blood pressure (BP) response in patients with renal artery stenosis (RAS) after renal angioplasty and stenting (PTRA).

Methods.—In 120 patients with RAS and hypertension referred for PTRA, 24-h ambulatory BP recordings were obtained before and 6 months after intervention. BNP was measured before, 1 day and 6 months after PTRA.

Results.—BP improved in 54% of patients. Median BNP levels pre-intervention were 97 pg ml^{-1} (interquartile range (IQR) 35−250) and decreased significantly within 1 day of PTRA to 62 pg ml^{-1} (IQR 24−182) ($p < 0.001$), remaining at 75 pg ml^{-1} (IQR 31−190) at 6 months. The area under the receiver operating curve for pre-intervention BNP to predict BP improvement was 0.57 (95% confidence interval (CI) 0.46–0.67). Pre-intervention BNP >50 pg ml^{-1} was seen in 79% of patients with BP improvement compared with 56% in patients without improvement ($p = 0.01$). In a multivariate logistic regression analysis, BNP >50 pg ml^{-1} was significantly associated with BP improvement (odds ratio (OR) 4.0, 95% CI 1.2–13.2).

Conclusions.—BNP levels are elevated in patients with RAS and decrease after revascularisation. Although BNP does not seem useful as a continuous variable, pre-interventional BNP > 50 pg ml^{-1} may be helpful to identify patients in whom PTRA will improve BP.

▶ Renal artery stenosis has been associated with hypertension and chronic kidney disease, but treatment of this disease has failed to demonstrate a reliable response in either disease process. Most recently, the Angioplasty and Stenting for Renal Artery Lesions randomized 806 patients to either best medical therapy or percutaneous revascularization and best medical therapy.[1] There was no clear benefit to percutaneous revascularization. In addition, patients with bilateral disease, disease in a single functioning kidney, or with preocclusive lesions did not benefit from revascularization. Despite randomized data, there is still a search to identify patients who will benefit from treating renal artery stenosis.

In this study, the authors evaluate b-type natriuretic peptide (BNP) both before and after percutaneous revascularization in 127 consecutive patients. The authors point out that BNP is altered by several disease states, primarily congestive heart failure and renal failure. The main limitation of this study is lack of a medical treatment comparison group. The cutoff BNP level of > 50 pg/mL produced an area under the receiver operating curve of 0.57, which is marginal at best for identifying patients responding to therapy. It is likely that best medical therapy would have provided the same results in patients with an elevated BNP. This study, while intriguing, does not identify patients who should be treated with revascularization; I suspect that BNP identifies patients who should be aggressively treated with cardiac risk modification strategies.

Z. M. Arthurs, MD

Reference

1. ASTRAL Investigators, Wheatley K, Ives N, Gray R, et al. Revascularization versus medical therapy for renal-artery stenosis. *N Engl J Med.* 2009;361: 1953-1962.

10 Thoracic Aorta

Effectiveness of combination of losartan potassium and doxycycline versus single-drug treatments in the secondary prevention of thoracic aortic aneurysm in Marfan syndrome
Yang HHC, Kim JM, Chum E, et al (Univ of British Columbia, Vancouver, Canada)
J Thorac Cardiovasc Surg 140:305-312, 2010

Objective.—Losartan potassium (INN losartan), an antihypertensive drug, has been shown to prevent thoracic aortic aneurysm in Marfan syndrome through the inhibition of transforming growth factor β. Recently we reported that doxycycline, a nonspecific inhibitor of matrix metalloproteinases 2 and 9, normalized aortic vasomotor function and suppressed aneurysm growth. We hypothesized that a combination of losartan potassium and doxycycline would offer better secondary prevention treatment than would single-drug therapy to manage thoracic aortic aneurysm.

Methods.—A well-characterized mouse model of Marfan syndrome ($Fbn1^{C1039G/+}$) was used. At 4 months of age, when aneurysm had established, mice (n = 15/group) were given doxycycline alone (0.24 g/L), losartan potassium alone (0.6 g/L), or combined (0.12-g/L doxycycline and 0.3-g/L losartan potassium) in drinking water. Littermate $Fbn1^{+/+}$ mice served as control. Thoracic aortas at 6 and 9 months were studied.

Results.—At 9 months, aortic diameter in untreated group was increased by 40% relative to control. Losartan potassium or doxycycline reduced aortic diameter by 10% to 16% versus untreated aortas. Losartan potassium and doxycycline combined completely prevented thoracic aortic aneurysm and improved elastic fiber organization, also downregulating matrix metalloproteinases 2 and 9 and transforming growth factor β and normalizing aortic contractile and relaxation functions to control values.

Conclusions.—Neither losartan potassium nor doxycycline alone completely restored vascular integrity and cell function when given during delayed treatment, indicating the importance of timed pharmacologic intervention. Combined, however, they synergistically offered better aneurysm-suppressing effects than did single-drug medication in the secondary prevention of thoracic aortic aneurysm.

▶ In Marfan syndrome, 90% of mortality is from progressive thoracic aortic aneurysm enlargement, dissection, and rupture. Marfan syndrome is autosomal dominant. It results from mutations in the gene encoding fibrillin-1, the principal component of extracellular microfibrils. Microfibrils are crucial in organizing a scaffold for formation and maturation of aortic elastic fibers. Abnormal aortic elastic fibers result in altered load-bearing capacity of the aorta with degeneration, fibrosis, and microdissection. Progression of thoracic aortic aneurysm in Marfan syndrome is associated with upregulation of matrix metalloproteinases (MMPs): MMP-2 and MMP-9. Doxycycline can inhibit production of MMP-2 and MMP-9 and provides aneurysm-suppressing effects in a mouse model of Marfan syndrome.[1] It appears perturbations of transforming growth factor β (TGF-β) also contribute to clinical manifestations of Marfan syndrome. TGF-β can be antagonized with losartan potassium, an angiotensin II type 1 receptor antagonist. The authors hypothesize a combination of losartan potassium and doxycycline would therefore offer better treatment for inhibition of aortic degeneration in Marfan syndrome. The data suggest that combination drug treatment in a mouse model of Marfan syndrome appears to offer potentially extraordinary secondary prevention benefits. It is a long way from a mouse model to effective treatment in humans. While the model may not be representative of all cases of Marfan syndrome in humans, the mutation in this model does represent the most common mutation in classic Marfan syndrome. Both drugs used for secondary prevention in this study are readily available, and it seems a human study of combination therapy for prevention of aortic degeneration in patients with Marfan syndrome should not be long off.

G. L. Moneta, MD

Reference

1. Chung AW, Hsiang YN, Matzke LA, et al. Reduced expression of vascular endothelial growth factor paralleled with the increased angiostatin expression resulting from the upregulated activities of matrix metalloproteinase-2 and -9 in human type 2 diabetic arterial vasculature. *Circ Res.* 2006;99:140-148.

Endovascular Repair of Descending Thoracic Aneurysms: Results With "On-Label" Application in the Post Food and Drug Administration Approval Era

Hughes GC, Lee SM, Daneshmand MA, et al (Duke Univ Med Ctr, Durham, NC)

Ann Thorac Surg 90:83-89, 2010

Background.—Most studies of thoracic endovascular aortic repair (TEVAR) published since the technology gained US Food and Drug Administration (FDA) approval in March 2005 have included multiple applications including dissection, trauma, and "hybrid" approaches, all of which are currently "off-label." However, little post-approval data exist for the only FDA-approved application, namely descending thoracic aneurysm (DTA). The purpose of this study was to examine our experience with TEVAR for aneurysms limited to the descending thoracic aorta.

Methods.—Between March 23, 2005 (date of initial FDA approval) and April 6, 2009, 210 TEVAR procedures were performed at our institution.

Of these, 79 (38%) were for saccular (n = 31) or fusiform (n = 48) DTA and form the basis of this report. Patients requiring "hybrid" approaches other than carotid-subclavian bypass were excluded. Devices utilized were Gore TAG (W. L. Gore Associates, Flagstaff, AZ) (n = 67; 85%), Zenith TX2 (Cook Medical Incorporated, Bloomington, IN) (n = 10; 13%), and Medtronic Talent (Medtronic, Inc, Santa Rosa, CA) (n = 5; 6%); 3 (4%) patients received more than one type of device.

Results.—Median patient age was 73 ± 4 years; 35 (44%) were female. Mean aortic diameter was 5.8 ± 1.8 cm. Twenty-four (30%) procedures were urgent-emergent. Thirty-day in-hospital rates of death, stroke, and permanent paraplegia-paresis were 5.1% (n = 4; 1.9% elective mortality), 2.5% (n = 2), and 1.3% (n = 1), respectively. The median postoperative length of stay was 3.0 days (25th and 75th percentiles = 2 and 6, respectively). At a mean follow-up of 23 ± 17 months (range, 6 to 55), there were 2 (2.5%) late aortic deaths from graft infection (n = 1) and aneurysm rupture (n = 1). Overall actuarial midterm survival is 73% at 55 months, with an aorta-specific actuarial survival of 86% during this same time interval. Five patients (6.3%) required late (>30 days) secondary endovascular re-intervention for type I (n = 4) or type II (n = 1) endoleak; re-intervention was successful in 4 of 5.

Conclusions.—Despite the advanced age, comorbid conditions, and significant incidence of urgent-emergent status of patients presenting with DTA, on-label application of TEVAR yields excellent 30-day and midterm outcomes, especially when compared with historic rates of morbidity and mortality with open repair. However, "on-label" applications represent a minority of current TEVAR use, likely due to the relative scarcity of DTA. These data appear to support the increasing utilization of TEVAR as a treatment strategy for this pathology (Fig 1).

▶ In March of 2005, the Food and Drug Administration (FDA) approved the first endovascular device specifically designed for treatment of descending thoracic aortic aneurysms. Approval was based on highly selected trials of patients with descending thoracic aneurysms.[1,2] The authors point out that since the publication of these pivotal trials, most studies of thoracic endovascular aneurysm repair (TEVAR) document a mixture of indications, including dissection, trauma, and various hybrid approaches. All of these additional approaches to the treatment of thoracic aortic disease are off-label. The point of this article was to provide post-approval data on results of TEVAR when the device is used for an FDA-approved application (repair of descending thoracic aneurysm). This is the largest, post-FDA approval report of TEVAR for on-label application. The results compare very favorably with the pivotal trials of this technology (Fig 1). In the commentary accompanying the article, Dr Coselli points out that the results presented here are similar to the open results with descending thoracic aortic aneurysm in his series. However, in most surgeons' hands, in the older patient with degenerative thoracic aneurysm TEVAR is likely to produce better results than open surgery and should be considered the preferred technique. TEVAR when used in compliance with manufacturer instructions for use is effective treatment

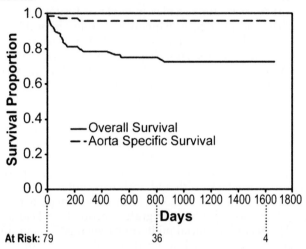

FIGURE 1.—Actuarial (Kaplan-Meier) overall (solid line) and aorta-specific (dashed line) survival at 55 months post-endovascular repair. (This article was published in The Annals of Thoracic Surgery, Hughes GC, Lee SM, Daneshmand MA, et al. Endovascular repair of descending thoracic aneurysms: results with "On-Label" application in the post food and drug administration approval era. *Ann Thorac Surg.* 2010;90:83-89. Copyright The Society of Thoracic Surgeons 2010.)

for on-label descending thoracic aortic aneurysm. The results provide validation of the FDA approval process.

G. L. Moneta, MD

References

1. Makaroun MS, Dillavou ED, Kee ST, et al. Endovascular treatment of thoracic aortic aneurysms: results of the phase II multicenter trial of the GORE TAG thoracic endoprosthesis. *J Vasc Surg.* 2005;41:1-9.
2. Bavaria JE, Appoo JJ, Makaroun MS, et al. Gore TAG Investigators. Endovascular stent grafting versus open surgical repair of descending thoracic aortic aneurysms in low-risk patients: a multicenter comparative trial. *J Thorac Cardiovasc Surg.* 2007;133:369-377.

Importance of Refractory Pain and Hypertension in Acute Type B Aortic Dissection: Insights From the International Registry of Acute Aortic Dissection (IRAD)

Trimarchi S, on behalf of the International Registry of Acute Aortic Dissection (IRAD) Investigators (Univ of Milano, Italy; et al)
Circulation 122:1283-1289, 2010

Background.—In patients with acute type B aortic dissection, presence of recurrent or refractory pain and/or refractory hypertension on medical therapy is sometimes used as an indication for invasive treatment. The International Registry of Acute Aortic Dissection (IRAD) was used to investigate the impact of refractory pain and/or refractory hypertension on the outcomes of acute type B aortic dissection.

Methods and Results.—Three hundred sixty-five patients affected by uncomplicated acute type B aortic dissection, enrolled in IRAD from 1996 to 2004, were categorized according to risk profile into 2 groups. Patients with recurrent and/or refractory pain or refractory hypertension (group I; n = 69) and patients without clinical complications at presentation (group II; n = 296) were compared. "High-risk" patients with classic complications were excluded from this analysis. The overall in-hospital mortality was 6.5% and was increased in group I compared with group II (17.4% versus 4.0%; $P = 0.0003$). The in-hospital mortality after medical management was significantly increased in group I compared with group II (35.6% versus 1.5%; $P = 0.0003$). Mortality rates after surgical (20% versus 28%; $P = 0.74$) or endovascular management (3.7% versus 9.1%; $P = 0.50$) did not differ significantly between group I and group II, respectively. A multivariable logistic regression model confirmed that recurrent and/or refractory pain or refractory hypertension was a predictor of in-hospital mortality (odds ratio, 3.31; 95% confidence interval, 1.04 to 10.45; $P = 0.041$).

Conclusions.—Recurrent pain and refractory hypertension appeared as clinical signs associated with increased in-hospital mortality, particularly when managed medically. These observations suggest that aortic intervention, such as via an endovascular approach, may be indicated in this intermediate-risk group.

▶ Complications of acute type B aortic dissection (ABAD) include organ malperfusion, shock, limb ischemia, periaortic bleeding, and rapidly expanding false lumen. Treatment of these complications with open surgery has mortality rates between 20% and 30%, and treatment with endovascular management has mortality rates between 10% and 20%. There are other, however, clinical conditions, such as refractory/recurrent pain or refractory hypertension, that may not result in hemodynamic instability or organ ischemia but may indicate a pending rupture or extending dissection. Currently, many have adopted repair with endovascular techniques for patients with ABAD and refractory hypertension or refractory pain. The authors used patients in the International Registry of Acute Aortic Dissection to investigate the impact of refractory hypertension and/or refractory pain on outcomes of ABAD. The data indicate that in uncomplicated patients with ABAD, medical therapy has excellent short-term outcome. However, in-hospital mortality is increased in patients with ABAD who have recurrent and/or refractory pain or refractory hypertension and are treated with medical management alone. These patients have outcomes that are worse than those with no complications of their type B aortic dissection, but their natural history appears to be better than those patients who have more adverse complications of aortic dissection such as limb ischemia or organ malperfusion. Given the mortality risk of the group with recurrent and/or refractory pain or refractory hypertension, endovascular management, when possible, seems appropriate.

G. L. Moneta, MD

Outcomes of Endovascular Repair of Ruptured Descending Thoracic Aortic Aneurysms

Jonker FHW, Verhagen HJM, Lin PH, et al (Yale Univ School of Medicine, New Haven, CT; Erasmus Univ Med Ctr, Rotterdam, the Netherlands; Baylor College of Medicine, Houston, TX; et al)
Circulation 121:2718-2723, 2010

Background.—Thoracic endovascular aortic repair offers a less invasive approach for the treatment of ruptured descending thoracic aortic aneurysms (rDTAA). Due to the low incidence of this life-threatening condition, little is known about the outcomes of endovascular repair of rDTAA and the factors that affect these outcomes.

Methods and Results.—We retrospectively investigated the outcomes of 87 patients who underwent thoracic endovascular aortic repair for rDTAA at 7 referral centers between 2002 and 2009. The mean age was 69.8 ± 12 years and 69.0% of the patients were men. Hypovolemic shock was present in 21.8% of patients, and 40.2% were hemodynamically unstable. The 30-day mortality rate was 18.4%, and hypovolemic shock (odds ratio 4.75; 95% confidence interval, 1.37 to 16.5; $P=0.014$) and hemothorax at admission (odds ratio 6.65; 95% confidence interval, 1.64 to 27.1; $P=0.008$) were associated with increased 30-day mortality after adjusting for age. Stroke and paraplegia occurred each in 8.0%, and endoleak was diagnosed in 18.4% of patients within the first 30 days after thoracic endovascular aortic repair. Four additional patients died as a result of procedure-related complications during a median follow-up of 13 months; the estimated aneurysm-related mortality at 4 years was 25.4%.

Conclusion.—Endovascular repair of rDTAA is associated with encouraging results. The endovascular approach was associated with considerable rates of neurological complications and procedure-related complications such as endoleak (Fig 3).

▶ Ruptured abdominal aortic aneurysms are the 13th leading cause of death in the United States. However, ruptured thoracic aortic aneurysms (TAAs) are relatively rare with reported incidence of only about 5 per 100 000. Mortality, however, is high and is thought to exceed 90%.[1] Because of the rarity of the condition, there is little information on endovascular treatment of ruptured TAAs. Ruptures of true degenerative TAAs are often lumped in other series combining traumatic aortic injuries, penetrating aortic ulcers, and complications of type B dissection. The authors therefore sought to accumulate a pure series of ruptured descending TAAs by identifying patients treated with endovascular repair for ruptured aneurysm of the descending thoracic aorta at 7 different centers in the United States and Europe between July 2002 and July 2009. Initial mortality rates of thoracic endovascular aortic repair (TEVAR) treatment of descending TAA rupture compare favorably with open repair of descending TAA rupture.[2] However, endovascular repair of a descending ruptured TAA appears to be associated with a high rate of neurologic and procedurally related complications, particularly type 1 endoleaks (Fig 3). The data make it

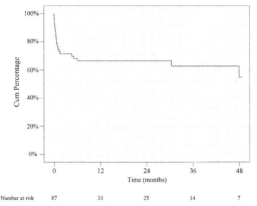

FIGURE 3.—Freedom from aneurysm-related death or thoracic aortic reintervention. Freedom from aneurysm-related death and aortic reintervention at 4 years was 54.9%. Thoracic aortic reintervention include all reinterventions that were required for complications related to the aneurysm and/or initial endovascular procedure such as endoleak, aneurysmal dilatation, and development of aortic fistulas. (Reprinted from Jonker FHW, Verhagen HJM, Lin PH, et al. Outcomes of endovascular repair of ruptured descending thoracic aortic aneurysms. *Circulation.* 2010;121:2718-2723, with permission from American Heart Association, Inc.)

reasonable to consider TEVAR for repair of a ruptured descending TAA, but morbidity and mortality are still significant.

G. L. Moneta, MD

References

1. Johannson G, Markström U, Swedenborg J. Ruptured thoracic aortic aneurysms: a study of incidence and mortality rates. *J Vasc Surg.* 1995;21:985-988.
2. Schermerhorn ML, Giles KA, Hamdan AD, Dalhberg SE, Hagberg R, Pomposelli F. Population-based outcomes of open descending thoracic aortic aneurysm repair. *J Vasc Surg.* 2008;48:821-827.

Pathogenesis of Acute Aortic Dissection: A Finite Element Stress Analysis
Nathan DP, Xu C, Gorman JH III, et al (Univ of Pennsylvania, Philadelphia; Univ of Iowa)
Ann Thorac Surg 91:458-464, 2011

Background.—Type A and type B aortic dissections typically result from intimal tears above the sinotubular junction and distal to the left subclavian artery (LSA) ostium, respectively. We hypothesized that this pathology results from elevated pressure-induced regional wall stress.

Methods.—We identified 47 individuals with normal thoracic aortas by electrocardiogram-gated computed tomography angiography. The thoracic aorta was segmented, reconstructed, and triangulated to create a geometric mesh. Finite element analysis using a systolic pressure load of 120 mm Hg was performed to predict regional thoracic aortic wall stress.

Results.—There were local maxima of wall stress above the sinotubular junction in the ascending aorta and distal to the ostia of the supraaortic vessels, including the LSA, in the aortic arch. No local maximum of wall stress was found in the descending thoracic aorta. Comparison of the mean peak wall stress above the sinotubular junction (0.43 ± 0.07 MPa), distal to the LSA (0.21 ± 0.07 MPa), and in the descending thoracic aorta (0.06 ± 0.01 MPa) showed a significant effect for wall stress by aortic region ($p < 0.001$).

Conclusions.—In the normal thoracic aorta, there are peaks in wall stress above the sinotubular junction and distal to the LSA ostium. This stress distribution may contribute to the pathogenesis of aortic dissections, given their colocalization. Future investigations to determine the utility of image-derived biomechanical calculations in predicting aortic dissection are warranted, and therapies designed to reduce the pressure load-induced wall stress in the thoracic aorta are rational (Figs 3 and 4).

▶ Approximately two-thirds of thoracic aortic dissections involve the ascending thoracic aorta (Stanford classification type A) with an overall incidence of thoracic aortic dissection of 3 to 4 per 100 000 person-years. In most cases, type A dissections and type B dissections originate with entry tears, respectively, above the sinotubular junction or distal to the left subclavian artery origin. Thoracic dissection is influenced by many components including aortic diameter, hypertension, and decreases in wall strength associated with Marfan syndrome or Ehlers-Danlos syndrome. However, the precise mechanistic rationale for

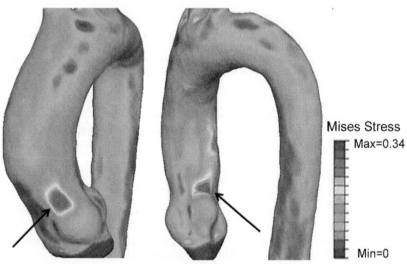

Mises Stress
Max=0.34

Min=0

FIGURE 3.—Three-dimensional wall stress distribution for the normal ascending aorta. Stress in mega-pascals (MPa) is mapped, with the highest stress in red and lowest stress in blue. The black arrows indicate maxima of stress on the (A) convex and (B) concave side of the ascending aorta. For interpretation of the references to color in this figure legend, the reader is referred to web version of this article. (This article was published in The Annals of Thoracic Surgery, Nathan DP, Xu C, Gorman JH III, et al. Pathogenesis of acute aortic dissection: a finite element stress analysis. *Ann Thorac Surg.* 2011;91:458-464. Copyright The Society of Thoracic Surgeons 2011.)

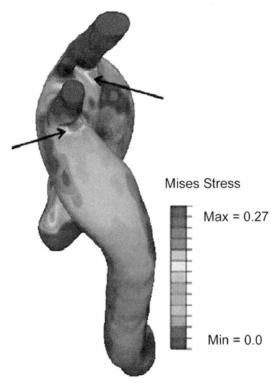

Mises Stress

Max = 0.27

Min = 0.0

FIGURE 4.—Three-dimensional wall stress distribution for the normal thoracic aorta. Stress in mega-pascals (MPa) is mapped, with the highest stress in red and the lowest stress in blue. The black arrows indicate maxima of stress distal to left subclavian and innominate arteries. For interpretation of the references to color in this figure legend, the reader is referred to web version of this article. (This article was published in The Annals of Thoracic Surgery, Nathan DP, Xu C, Gorman JH III, et al. Pathogenesis of acute aortic dissection: a finite element stress analysis. *Ann Thorac Surg.* 2011;91:458-464. Copyright The Society of Thoracic Surgeons 2011.)

origin of thoracic type A and type B dissections is not completely understood. The authors hypothesize that a biomechanical approach to predicting thoracic aortic wall stress may better define the risk of thoracic aortic dissection in individual patients. They therefore sought to map patterns of wall stress in the thoracic aorta in normal individuals, extrapolating wall stress patterns from normals to those with potential dissection. The data indicate that there are peaks in wall stress in the normal thoracic aorta above the sinotubular junction and just distal to the origin of the left subclavian artery (Figs 3 and 4). The implication that peaks in wall stress may contribute to aortic dissection is a bit of guilt by association. Preventing thoracic aortic dissection is likely to be a multifaceted task. Currently diameter, according to Laplace's law, is used as a noninvasive surrogate of aortic wall stress. Surgical intervention is timed to occur before wall stress exceeds maximal tensile strength of the aorta, estimated about 800 kPa. While the risk of acute aortic events is currently correlated roughly with size, even small aortas can have fatal dissections and ruptures. Improving wall strength of the aorta, decreasing expansion rates, and calculations of wall sheer stress will likely all be used in the future in the management of patients with both thoracic and abdominal aortic disease.

G. L. Moneta, MD

Rare Copy Number Variants Disrupt Genes Regulating Vascular Smooth Muscle Cell Adhesion and Contractility in Sporadic Thoracic Aortic Aneurysms and Dissections

Prakash SK, LeMaire SA, Guo D-C, et al (Baylor College of Medicine, Houston, TX; Univ of Texas Health Science Ctr at Houston)

Am J Hum Genet 87:743-756, 2010

Thoracic aortic aneurysms and dissections (TAAD) cause significant morbidity and mortality, but the genetic origins of TAAD remain largely unknown. In a genome-wide analysis of 418 sporadic TAAD cases, we identified 47 copy number variant (CNV) regions that were enriched in or unique to TAAD patients compared to population controls. Gene ontology, expression profiling, and network analysis showed that genes within TAAD CNVs regulate smooth muscle cell adhesion or contractility and interact with the smooth muscle-specific isoforms of α-actin and β-myosin, which are known to cause familial TAAD when altered. Enrichment of these gene functions in rare CNVs was replicated in independent cohorts with sporadic TAAD (STAAD, n = 387) and inherited TAAD (FTAAD, n = 88). The overall prevalence of rare CNVs (23%) was significantly increased in FTAAD compared with STAAD patients (Fisher's exact test, p = 0.03). Our findings suggest that rare CNVs disrupting smooth muscle adhesion or contraction contribute to both sporadic and familial disease.

▶ Twenty percent of patients with thoracic aortic aneurysms (TAAs) or dissections have a relative with a history of similar disease. The phenotype is generally inherited as autosomal dominant and is characterized by variable expression and incomplete penetrance.[1] Genes have been identified that contribute to familial TAA and dissection. These genes encode smooth muscle cell (SMC)-specific isoforms of actin and myosin, regulate expression of contractile proteins by vascular SMCs, or involve mutations of SMC adhesive or cytoskeletal proteins.[2,3] The authors hypothesize that there are variations in modifying genes that exert an influence on an individual's susceptibility to TAA or dissection. It is known that variation in copy numbers of genes, so-called copy number variations, can increase the risk for multifactorial diseases. This certainly appears to be the case with aneurysm disease, particularly thoracic aortic disease, in which both genetic and environmental factors are important. Gene products that relay environmental signals affecting genes that regulate SMC function would seem to be ideal candidates to modify the pathogenesis of aneurysm disease. The author's findings are consistent with a genetic model where copy number variant mutations contribute to aneurysm causation or predisposition. If such variants could be tested for clinically, patients with appropriate environmental factors that place them at risk for aneurysm disease could have their potential risk of aneurysm development identified with genetic testing. It is genetics that undoubtedly explains why some patients with similar environmental risk factors develop aneurysm disease and others develop occlusive disease of the aorta.

G. L. Moneta, MD

References

1. Milewicz DM, Chen H, Park ES, et al. Reduced penetrance and variable expressivity of familial thoracic aortic aneurysms/dissections. *Am J Cardiol.* 1998;82: 474-479.
2. Grainger DJ, Metcalfe JC, Grace AA, Mosedale DE. Transforming growth factor-beta dynamically regulates vascular smooth muscle differentiation in vivo. *J Cell Sci.* 1998;111:2977-2988.
3. Sheen VL, Jansen A, Chen MH, et al. Filamin A mutations cause periventricular heterotopia with Ehlers-Danlos syndrome. *Neurology.* 2005;64:254-262.

Superior nationwide outcomes of endovascular versus open repair for isolated descending thoracic aortic aneurysm in 11,669 patients
Gopaldas RR, Huh J, Dao TK, et al (Baylor College of Medicine, Houston, TX; Univ of Houston, TX)
J Thorac Cardiovasc Surg 140:1001-1010, 2010

Objectives.—Thoracic endovascular aneurysm repair (TEVAR) was introduced in 2005 to treat descending thoracic aortic aneurysms. Little is known about TEVAR's nationwide effect on patient outcomes. We evaluated nationwide data regarding the short-term outcomes of TEVAR and open aortic repair (OAR) procedures performed in the United States during a 2-year period.

Methods.—From the Nationwide Inpatient Sample data, we identified patients who had undergone surgery for an isolated descending thoracic aortic aneurysm from 2006 to 2007. Patients with aneurysm rupture, aortic dissection, vasculitis, connective tissue disorders, or concomitant aneurysms in other aortic segments were excluded. Of the remaining 11,669 patients, 9106 had undergone conventional OAR and 2563 had undergone TEVAR. Hierarchic regression analysis was used to assess the effect of TEVAR versus OAR after adjusting for confounding factors. The primary outcomes were mortality and the hospital length of stay (LOS). The secondary outcomes were the discharge status, morbidity, and hospital charges.

Results.—The patients who had undergone TEVAR were older (69.5 ± 12.7 vs 60.2 ± 14.2 years; $P < .001$) and had higher Deyo comorbidity scores (4.6 ± 1.8 vs 3.3 ± 1.8; $P < .001$). The unadjusted LOS was shorter for the TEVAR patients (7.7 ± 11 vs 8.8 ± 7.9 days), but the unadjusted mortality was similar (TEVAR 2.3% vs OAR 2.3%; $P = 1.0$). The proportion of nonelective interventions was similar between the 2 groups (TEVAR 15.9% vs OAR 15.8%; $P = .9$). The TEVAR and OAR techniques produced similar risk-adjusted mortality rates; however, the TEVAR patients had 60% fewer complications overall (odds ratio, 0.39; $P < .001$) and a shorter LOS (by 1.3 days). The TEVAR patients' hospital charges were greater by $6713 (95% confidence interval $1869 to $11,556; $P < .001$). However, the TEVAR patients were 4 times more likely to have a routine discharge to home.

Conclusions.—The nationwide data on TEVAR for descending thoracic aortic aneurysms have associated this procedure with better in-hospital outcomes than OAR, even though TEVAR was selectively performed in patients who were almost 1 decade older than the OAR patients. Compared with OAR, TEVAR was associated with a shorter hospital LOS and fewer complications but significantly greater hospital charges.

▶ Surgical procedures providing good outcomes and that are easy to perform will be adopted widely. More difficult procedures are likely to be restricted to high-volume centers. The results here show that adoption of thoracic endovascular aneurysm repair (TEVAR) is appropriate. Even though TEVAR was selectively performed in patients almost a decade older than patients having open aortic repair (OAR), outcomes were comparable, if not superior, for TEVAR versus OAR. TEVAR had significantly better risk-adjusted morbidity, stemming primarily from lower incidences of neurologic, respiratory, and pulmonary complications. Additional data are needed to determine whether TEVAR has volume-dependent outcomes or, as with endovascular abdominal aortic aneurysm repair, can be performed with relatively low morbidity in low-volume hospitals. Such data are needed to determine whether patients with thoracic aortic aneurysm should be treated in centers dedicated to treatment of aortic disease or if TEVAR will permit more widespread treatment of thoracic aortic pathology in community and smaller regional hospitals.

G. L. Moneta, MD

Left subclavian artery revascularization: Society for Vascular Surgery® Practice Guidelines
Matsumura JS, Rizvi AZ (Univ of Wisconsin School of Medicine and Public Health, Madison; Minneapolis Heart Inst at Abbott Northwestern Hosp)
J Vasc Surg 52:65S-70S, 2010

Background.—Management of the left subclavian artery (LSA) when coverage is needed for patients having thoracic endovascular aortic repair (TEVAR) varies from surgeon to surgeon. The Society for Vascular Surgery (SVS) noted complications of LSA coverage and offered recommendations and clinical practice guidelines.

Complications.—Stroke, spinal cord ischemia, and left upper extremity ischemia can complicate LSA coverage during TEVAR. Stroke incidence ranges from 3.8% to 6.3%, depending on patient and procedural variables. Over 60% of patients have a dominant left vertebral artery and an atretic or absent contralateral vertebral vessel. Covering the LSA artery with this anatomic variant can be risky. In comparison, LSA revascularization has lower rates of overall stroke (13% vs 2%) and posterior circulation stroke (5.5% vs 1.2%). Critical points in minimizing stroke include thorough understanding of arch and cerebral anatomy, routine LSA revascularization, and careful manipulation of wires, catheters, and device during stent graft deployment.

Spinal cord ischemia can result from periprocedural hypotension, embolization to the intercostal artery, intraspinal hematoma, or inadequate perfusion to the anterior spinal artery after collateral vessel coverage. A patent LSA reduces spinal cord ischemia risk.

Upper extremity ischemia is uncommon with LSA coverage (incidence 12% to 20%) and is usually tolerable, but severe symptoms are possible. An immediate threat is quite rare after TEVAR, so revascularization can be done less urgently.

Recommendations.—Coverage without revascularization is more likely to produce paraplegia, anterior circulation stroke, arm ischemia, and vertebrobasilar ischemia than preoperative LSA revascularization. Stroke and paraplegia represent clinically significant occurrences. Therefore for elective TEVAR where LSA coverage is needed to achieve adequate stent graft seal, the SVS recommends routine preoperative revascularization. When vessels in question perfuse vital organs, the SVS strongly recommends routine preoperative revascularization. In acute thoracic emergencies requiring urgent TEVAR with LSA coverage, revascularization is left to the individual surgeon, based on patient anatomy, urgency of the procedure, and availability of appropriate surgical expertise.

Clinical Practice Guidelines.—LSA revascularization has low morbidity and mortality. Subclavian-carotid transpositions have better patency rates than carotid-subclavian bypasses. Premade fenestrated stent grafts are seldom available in clinical settings, but percutaneous management of planned LSA coverage with stent grafts can be achieved with the double-barrel or chimney technique. A covered stent is positioned from a retrograde left brachial approach, deployed in a "kissing" fashion, and traverses the LSA origin when the thoracic stent graft is deployed. The thoracic stent graft forms a seal around the LSA stent and maintains anterograde flow. In situ fenestration for TEVAR involving the arch vessels can also be done. Such novel techniques maintain anterograde flow in the arch vessels and avoid surgical debranching procedures.

Conclusions.—Routine preoperative revascularization is suggested for LSA coverage during TEVAR and strongly recommended when collateral perfusion may be compromised. Emergency TEVAR and other circumstances that preclude preoperative LSA revascularization present exceptions to these recommendations. These approaches significantly reduce the risk of arm and vertebrobasilar ischemia.

► The Society for Vascular Surgery (SVS) Committee on Aortic Disease published these practice guidelines to provide recommendations regarding left subclavian artery (LSA) revascularization during thoracic endovascular aortic repair (TEVAR). This review provides a nice framework for recommendations regarding use of LSA revascularization with TEVAR when coverage of LSA is necessary for adequate stent graft seal prior to elective TEVAR (Grading of Recommendation Assessment, Development and Evaluation [GRADE] 2, level C), routinely prior to TEVAR when coverage of LSA would compromise perfusion to vital end organs (GRADE 1, level C), and selectively for emergent TEVAR based on patient anatomy, urgency of procedure, and availability of LSA revascularization expertise (GRADE 2, level C). While these practice guidelines for LSA revascularization for TEVAR seem reasonable, current evidence behind these is still weak (C level) with further clinical investigation needed in the future to better substantiate these clinical recommendations. Although publishing these SVS practice guidelines is helpful, it is important to note that these are made based on review of available data and group consensus of the SVS committee members with no specific structured methodology, which should be differentiated from the more rigorous process used in other formal consensus evidence-based guidelines.

M. A. Passman, MD

The Impact of Hypovolaemic Shock on the Aortic Diameter in a Porcine Model
Jonker FHW, Mojibian H, Schlösser FJV, et al (Yale Univ School of Medicine, New Haven, CT; et al)
Eur J Vasc Endovasc Surg 40:564-571, 2010

Objectives.—To investigate the impact of hypovolaemic shock on the aortic diameter in a porcine model, and to determine the implications for the endovascular management of hypovolaemic patients with traumatic thoracic aortic injury (TTAI).

Materials and Methods.—The circulating blood volume of seven Yorkshire pigs was gradually lowered in 10% increments. At 40% volume loss, an endograft was deployed in the descending thoracic aorta, followed by gradual fluid resuscitation. Potential changes in aortic diameter during the experiment were recorded using intravascular ultrasound (IVUS).

Results.—The aortic diameter decreased significantly at all evaluated levels during blood loss. The ascending aortic diameter decreased on average with 38% after 40% blood loss (range 24−62%, $p = 0.018$), the descending thoracic aorta with 32% (range 18−52%, $p = 0.018$) and the abdominal aorta with 28% (range 15−39%, $p = 0.018$). The aortic diameters regained their initial size during fluid resuscitation.

Conclusion.—The aortic diameter significantly decreases during blood loss in this porcine model. If these changes take place in hypovolaemic TTAI patients as well, it may have implications for thoracic endovascular aortic repair (TEVAR). Increased oversizing of the endograft, or additional computed tomography (CT) or IVUS imaging after fluid resuscitation for more adequate aortic measurements, may be needed in TTAI patients with considerable blood loss.

▶ This study is a porcine model for evaluating the impact of hypovolemia on aortic diameters. Using intravascular ultrasound for serial aortic measurements, controlled hypovolemia was induced at 10% blood volume increments. Aortic lumen diameters in the thoracic aorta decreased in a linear fashion with each increment of blood loss such that 20% blood loss equated to a 15% reduction in diameter and 40% blood loss equated to a 31% reduction in diameter. Blood pressure and heart rate also correlated with decreasing aortic diameters.

The authors are one of the first groups to investigate the impact of hypovolemic shock on the thoracic aorta. This study clearly demonstrates an impressive reduction in aortic diameter that could compromise a planned endograft repair. Determining the appropriate endograft size in a hypotensive patient remains a challenge. This study raises concern that the degree of oversizing should be increased in hypotensive patients or the procedures should be delayed until a true diameter measurement can be obtained. More importantly, using stent grafts designed for aneurysmal disease for this pathology is not ideal; devices designed for this disease process are needed.

Z. M. Arthurs, MD

11 Leg Ischemia

Arm vein conduit vs prosthetic graft in infrainguinal revascularization for critical leg ischemia

Arvela E, Söderström M, Albäck A, et al (Helsinki Univ Central Hosp, Finland)
J Vasc Surg 52:616-623, 2010

Background.—One-piece great saphenous vein (GSV) is the conduit of choice in infrainguinal revascularizations for critical limb ischemia (CLI). Unfortunately, adequate length of usable GSV is not always available. Despite inferior patency rates compared with GSV, prosthetic and arm vein conduits are generally considered usable. The purpose of this study was to compare the outcome of infrainguinal arm vein and prosthetic bypass.

Material and Methods.—We retrospectively reviewed 290 consecutive infrainguinal bypasses for CLI using arm vein conduit (n = 130) or prosthetic graft (n = 160) during January 2000 and December 2006 at our institution. The groups were compared for risk factors, indication for surgery, and runoff score. Survival, leg salvage, and patency rates were calculated with the Kaplan-Meier method.

Results.—Median surveillance time was 35 months (range 0-118 months). The age, gender, and usual risk factors were similar in arm vein and prosthetic groups, except cerebrovascular disease that was more common in the prosthetic group (P =.011). Indication for surgery was CLI. In the arm vein group, more than two-thirds (70.2%) of the procedures were for ischemic ulcer or gangrene, whereas in the prosthetic group the main indication was ischemic rest pain (51.3%). When the outcome of femoropopliteal bypasses was analyzed, the difference between groups was not statistically significant. However, in infrapopliteal revascularizations primary patency, assisted primary patency, and secondary patency rates at 3 years were significantly better in the arm vein group: 28.3% (SE ± 6.3%) vs 9.6% (SE ± 8.1%) (P =.031), 56.8% (SE ± 6.6%) vs 10.4% (SE ± 8.7%) (P =.000), and 57.4% (SE ± 6.6) vs 11.2% (SE ± 9.3%) (P =.000), respectively. Leg salvage and survival at 3 years were 75.0% (SE ± 4.9%) vs 57.1% (SE ± 8.8%) (P =.005) and 58.8% (SE ± 5.1%) vs 39.5% (SE ± 7.7%) (P =.007), respectively.

Conclusion.—Arm vein conduits, even when spliced, are superior to prosthetic grafts in terms of midterm assisted primary patency, secondary patency, and leg salvage in infrapopliteal bypasses for CLI (Figs 1 and 2).

▶ Greater saphenous veins in patients who are candidates for lower extremity bypass may be absent in 20% to 45% of cases. In such situations, above-knee

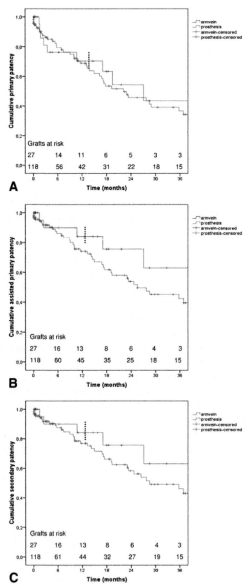

FIGURE 1.—In femoropopliteal bypasses. **A,** primary patency, **B,** assisted primary patency, and **C,** secondary patency were better in the arm vein group than in the prosthetic bypass group. The difference was not statistically significant ($P = .524$, $P = .128$, and $P = .451$, respectively). The standard error (SE) was <10% throughout the time interval, except in the arm vein group, where SE at 3 years was <10%. *Dashed line* cutting the curve at 12 months indicates that the number of grafts at risk thereafter is too small. (Reprinted from Arvela E, Söderström M, Albäck A, et al. Arm vein conduit vs prosthetic graft in infrainguinal revascularization for critical leg ischemia. *J Vasc Surg.* 2010;52:616-623. Copyright 2010, with permission from the Society for Vascular Surgery.)

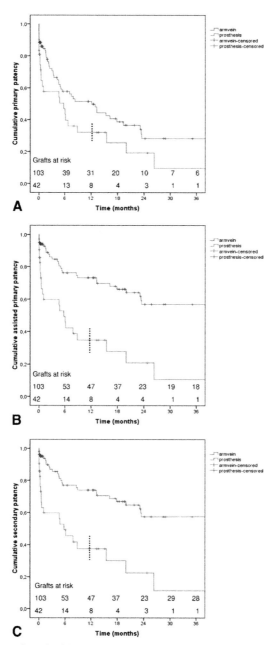

FIGURE 2.—In infrapopliteal bypasses. **A,** primary patency ($P = .031$), **B,** assisted primary patency ($P = .000$), and **C,** secondary patency ($P = .000$) were significantly better in the arm vein group. Standard error (SE) was <10% throughout the time interval. *Dashed line* cutting the curve at 12 months indicates that the number of grafts at risk thereafter is too small. (Reprinted from Arvela E, Söderström M, Albäck A, et al. Arm vein conduit vs prosthetic graft in infrainguinal revascularization for critical leg ischemia. *J Vasc Surg.* 2010;52:616-623. Copyright 2010, with permission from the Society for Vascular Surgery.)

femoral popliteal bypasses with synthetic conduits are reasonably well accepted. However, for infrapopliteal bypass, prosthetic conduits are more controversial and long-term patency of infrapopliteal prosthetic bypass appears, at best, moderate. Many surgeons prefer alternative vein conduits for patients requiring below-knee bypass who do not have a usable ipsilateral saphenous vein. In many cases, this may involve arm vein conduits and spliced veins. The relative effectiveness of an arm vein conduit versus a prosthetic graft for infrainguinal revascularization for critical limb ischemia is unknown. This article retrospectively reviewed 290 consecutive infrainguinal bypasses for critical limb ischemia using either arm vein (n = 130) or a prosthetic graft (n = 160) (Figs 1 and 2). The authors found that arm vein conduits, even when spliced, were superior to prosthetic grafts for infrapopliteal bypass in patients with critical limb ischemia. One could argue that the arm vein conduit patients and the prosthetic conduit patients were not all that well matched. The study was not randomized. However, despite this, the authors conclude an arm vein conduit, even if a spliced vein is required, is likely better than prosthetic for vascularization for critical limb ischemia. This conclusion is certainly in line with my personal experience in dealing with patients with critical limb ischemia who require bypass for limb salvage and have no usable greater saphenous vein.

G. L. Moneta, MD

Atheroembolic Disease—A Frequently Missed Diagnosis: Results of a 12-Year Matched-Pair Autopsy Study
Fries C, Roos M, Gaspert A, et al (Univ Hosp Zürich, Switzerland; Univ of Zürich, Switzerland; et al)
Medicine 89:126-132, 2010

Diagnosis of atheroembolic disease (AD) is challenging, because no specific test is available and AD often masquerades as other clinical conditions. We conducted the current study to investigate the relative frequency of autopsy-proven AD over time, to describe its clinical presentation, and to identify risk factors for AD. We screened 2066 autopsy reports from 1995 to 2006 for AD. For each AD case, a control patient without AD was matched for age, sex, and autopsy year. Diagnostic and therapeutic interventions (surgery, catheter interventions, and drug treatment) in the last 6 months before death, as well as clinical and laboratory parameters during the last hospitalization, were retrieved from electronic charts.

We identified 51 patients with AD. Among these only 6 (12%) had been diagnosed clinically. The organs most often affected were kidney (71%), spleen (37%), and lower gastrointestinal tract (22%). The relative AD frequency decreased over time from 3.5 to 0.5 per 100 autopsies, whereas the frequency of clinically suspected and biopsy-proven AD remained constant. Among clinical signs, skin lesions such as livedo reticularis and blue toe (33% vs. 14%; $p = 0.04$) were significantly increased in AD patients compared with the matched controls. We also observed a trend for higher incidence of eosinophilia and proteinuria in AD patients. Vascular

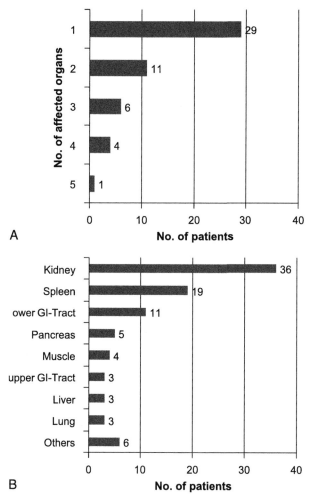

FIGURE 1.—Organ distribution of atheroemboli in autopsies. (A) Number of organs affected by AD. (B) Type of organs affected by AD. Multiple listings are possible. We divided the gastrointestinal tract (GI tract) into an upper tract including esophagus, stomach, and duodenum, and a lower tract including jejunum, ileum, and colon. (Reprinted from Fries C, Roos M, Gaspert A, et al. Atheroembolic disease—a frequently missed diagnosis: results of a 12-year matched-pair autopsy study. *Medicine.* 2010;89: 126-132, with permission from Lippincott Williams & Wilkins.)

interventions within 6 months before death were highly associated with AD (55% vs. 29%; p = 0.01), and in a multivariable analysis this remained the only significant risk factor for AD. Thus, the diagnosis of AD is frequently missed. Vascular interventions represent the most important risk factor for AD and should be performed restrictively in high-risk patients (Fig 1A, B).

▶ Atheroembolic disease is associated with a multitude of conditions. The most widely recognized are blue toe, livedo reticularis, and renal failure. However, atheroembolic disease has also been associated with pancreatitis, muscle pain, gastrointestinal bleeding, hypertension, peptic ulcer and inflammatory bowel disease, prostatitis, and hemorrhagic cystitis.[1,2] The present study indicates the widespread distribution of affected organs (Fig 1A, B) and that atheroembolic disease is missed premorbidly in more than 80% of the cases. Given the plethora of potential clinical manifestations of atheroembolic disease and that vascular interventions are the major risk factors for the disease, it is likely that the complication rate of vascular interventions is higher than suspected based on clinical criteria alone.

G. L. Moneta, MD

References

1. Moolenaar W, Kreuning J, Eulderink F, Lamers CB. Ischemic colitis and acalculous necrotizing cholecystitis as rare manifestations of cholesterol emboli in the same patient. *Am J Gastroenterol.* 1989;84:1421-1422.
2. Moolenaar W, Lamers CB. Cholesterol crystal embolization in the Netherlands. *Arch Intern Med.* 1996;156:653-657.

Infrapopliteal Percutaneous Transluminal Angioplasty Versus Bypass Surgery as First-Line Strategies in Critical Leg Ischemia: A Propensity Score Analysis
Söderström MI, Arvela EM, Korhonen M, et al (Helsinki Univ Central Hosp, Finland; et al)
Ann Surg 252:765-772, 2010

Introduction.—Recently, endovascular revascularization (percutaneous transluminal angioplasty [PTA]) has challenged surgery as a method for the salvage of critically ischemic legs (CLI). Comparison of surgical and endovascular techniques in randomized controlled trials is difficult because of differences in patient characteristics. To overcome this problem, we adjusted the differences by using propensity score analysis.

Materials and Methods.—The study cohort comprised 1023 patients treated for CLI with 262 endovascular and 761 surgical revascularization procedures to their crural or pedal arteries. A propensity score was used for adjustment in multivariable analysis, for stratification, and for one-to-one matching.

Results.—In the overall series, PTA and bypass surgery achieved similar 5-year leg salvage (75.3% vs 76.0%), survival (47.5% vs 43.3%), and amputation-free survival (37.7% vs 37.3%) rates and similar freedom from any further revascularization (77.3% vs 74.4%), whereas freedom from surgical revascularization was higher after bypass surgery (94.3% vs 86.2%, P < 0.001). In propensity-score-matched pairs, outcomes did not differ, except for freedom from surgical revascularization, which was significantly higher in the bypass surgery group (91.4% vs 85.3% at 5 years, P = 0.045). In a subgroup of patients who underwent isolated infrapopliteal revascularization, PTA was associated with better leg salvage (75.5% vs 68.0%, $P = 0.042$) and somewhat lower freedom from surgical revascularization (78.8% vs 85.2%, $P = 0.17$). This significant difference in the leg salvage rate was also observed after adjustment for propensity score ($P = 0.044$), but not in propensity-score-matched pairs ($P = 0.12$).

Conclusions.—When feasible, infrapopliteal PTA as a first-line strategy is expected to achieve similar long-term results to bypass surgery in CLI when redo surgery is actively utilized.

▶ Comparison of endovascular and open surgery for treatment of critically ischemic legs (CLI) in randomized controlled trials is almost impossible because of difficulties in forming comparable groups. Retrospective studies of patient characteristics in endovascular and surgical trials often differ significantly. Propensity score analysis can be used to adjust for important differences between treatment arms. The authors used propensity score analysis to compare outcomes in a consecutive series of patients who underwent percutaneous transluminal angioplasty and bypass surgery of infrapopliteal arteries. The propensity score analysis presented here is an interesting mathematical exercise. However, as pointed out by Dr JF Hamming in a discussion following the article, the authors are still comparing apples with oranges in that endovascular treatment was reserved for patients with shorter lesions and mostly stenosis and not occlusions. Therefore, we still have the underlying problem of trying to compare treatment modalities in patients with differing extent of disease. Because the authors have determined similar results in their endovascular and open surgical patients, what the article really demonstrates is that it is possible to be reasonably good at individualizing treatment in patients with CLI. The overall effectiveness of differing treatment modalities in patients with equal burdens of disease has not been answered by this study.

G. L. Moneta, MD

Randomized double-blind placebo-controlled crossover study of caffeine in patients with intermittent claudication
Momsen AH, Jensen MB, Norager CB, et al (Regional Hosp Herning, Denmark; Univ Hosp of Aarhus, Denmark; et al)
Br J Surg 97:1503-1510, 2010

Background.—Intermittent claudication is a disabling symptom of peripheral arterial disease for which few medical treatments are available. This study investigated the effect of caffeine on physical capacity in patients with intermittent claudication.

Methods.—This randomized double-blind placebo-controlled crossover study included 88 patients recruited by surgeons from outpatient clinics. The participants abstained from caffeine for 48 h before each test and then received either a placebo or oral caffeine (6 mg/kg). After 75 min, pain-free and maximal walking distance on a treadmill, perceived pain, reaction times, postural stability, maximal isometric knee extension strength, submaximal knee extension endurance and cognitive function were measured. The analysis was by intention to treat.

Results.—Caffeine increased the pain-free walking distance by 20·0 (95 per cent confidence interval 3·7 to 38·8) per cent ($P = 0·014$), maximal walking distance by 26·6 (12·1 to 43·0) per cent ($P < 0·001$), muscle strength by 9·8 (3·0 to 17·0) per cent ($P = 0·005$) and endurance by 21·4 (1·2 to 45·7) per cent ($P = 0·004$). However, postural stability was reduced significantly, by 22·1 (11·7 to 33·4) per cent with eyes open ($P < 0·001$) and by 21·8 (7·6 to 37·8) per cent with eyes closed ($P = 0·002$). Neither reaction time nor cognition was affected.

Conclusion.—In patients with moderate intermittent claudication, caffeine increased walking distance, maximal strength and endurance, but affected balance adversely. Registration number: NCT00388128 (http://www.clinicaltrials.gov).

▶ In patients with intermittent claudication, pharmacologic agents may modestly improve walking distance and statins may be the most effective drugs for this purpose.[1] The widely consumed central nervous system stimulant, caffeine, appears also to have potentially favorable effects on exercise and endurance. Caffeine increases endurance in young people when they exercise at 60% to 85% of maximum oxygen updtake.[2] Submaximal isometric contraction is also improved and rate of perceived exertion during exercise is decreased with caffeine.[3] In addition, caffeine has positive effects on cycling endurance and perceived exertion in healthy elderly people.[4] The authors therefore postulated that caffeine might be an effective drug to increase walking distance in patients with intermittent claudication. The effect of caffeine on intermittent claudication that was found in this study seems similar to that following administration of lipid-lowering agents and exceeds those reported in trials of various other agents, such as pentoxifylline. Recommendation of a drug to improve intermittent claudication, however, should not be based simply on increases in walking distance but rather on improvements in quality of life. Studies addressing caffeine consumption over time in conjunction with assessment by quality of life instruments are needed to judge the true potential impact of caffeine on quality of life in patients with intermittent claudication. In addition, the adverse effect of caffeine on balance is worrisome in an elderly population where falls are a significant source of morbidity and mortality. The study had multiple funding sources but Starbucks was not among the sponsors!

G. L. Moneta, MD

References

1. Momsen AH, Jensen MB, Norager CB, Madsen MR, Vestersgaard-Andersen T, Lindholt JS. Drug therapy for improving walking distance in intermittent claudication: a systematic review and meta-analysis of robust randomised controlled studies. *Eur J Vasc Endovasc Surg.* 2009;38:463-474.
2. Graham TE. Caffeine and exercise: metabolism, endurance and performance. *Sports Med.* 2001;31:785-807.

3. Falk B, Burstein R, Ashkenazi I, et al. The effect of caffeine ingestion on physical performance after prolonged exercise. *Eur J Appl Physiol Occup Physiol.* 1989;59: 168-173.
4. Norager CB, Jensen MB, Weimann A, Madsen MR. Metabolic effects of caffeine ingestion and physical work in 75-year old citizens. A randomized, double-blind, placebo-controlled, cross-over study. *Clin Endocrinol (Oxf).* 2006;65:223-228.

The impact of socioeconomic factors on outcome and hospital costs associated with femoropopliteal revascularization

Durham CA, Mohr MC, Parker FM, et al (East Carolina Univ, Greenville, NC)
J Vasc Surg 52:600-607, 2010

Introduction.—Within the context of healthcare system reform, the cost efficacy of lower extremity revascularization remains a timely topic. The impact of an individual patient's socioeconomic status represents an under-studied aspect of vascular care, especially with respect to longitudinal costs and outcomes. The purpose of this study is to examine the relationship between socioeconomic status and clinical outcomes as well as inpatient hospital costs.

Methods.—A retrospective femoropopliteal revascularization database, which included socioeconomic factors (household income, education level, and payor status), in addition to standard demographic, clinical, anatomical, and procedural variables were analyzed over a 3-year period. Patients were stratified by income level (low income [LI] <200% federal poverty level [$42,400 for a household of 4], and higher income [HI] >200% federal poverty level) and revascularization technique (open vs endovascular) and analyzed for the endpoints of primary assisted patency, amortized cost-per-day of patency, and limb salvage. Data were analyzed with univariate and multivariate techniques.

Results.—A total of 187 cases were identified with complete data for analysis, 146 in the LI and 41 in the HI cohorts. LI patients differed from HI patients by mean age (66.2 ± 1.0 vs 61.8 ± 1.5 years, $P = .04$), high school graduate rate (51.4% vs 85.4%, $P < .001$), presence of tissue loss (30.1% vs 14.6%, $P = .05$), female gender (43.7% vs 22.0%, $P = .01$) and preoperative statin use (45.8% vs 75.6%, $P < .001$). There were no differences with respect to other comorbidities including smoking status, presence of diabetes, renal insufficiency, anatomic factors or treatment modality (open vs endovascular). Ninety-seven patients underwent endovascular revascularization. The following outcomes were noted in the endovascular subset of LI and HI patients respectively: primary assisted patency (66% vs 71%, $P =$ NS) and 12-month cost-per-day of patency ($166.30 ± 77.40 vs $22.45 ± 12.45, $P = .05$). Ninety-eight patients underwent open revascularization, with the following outcomes in LI and HI patients respectively: primary assisted patency (78% vs 86%, $P =$ NS) and 12-month cost-per-day of patency ($319.43 ± 225.44 vs $40.47 ± 4.63, $P = .07$). Of the 77 patients with critical limb ischemia, 19 underwent eventual amputation. Multivariate analysis demonstrated that income above 100% of the federal poverty line was protective against limb loss (odds ratio 0.06, 95% confidence interval 0.01-0.51, $P < .001$).

Conclusion.—Income level correlates with advanced presentation, advanced age, and lack of statin use. Although primary assisted patency rate is not affected by income status, an increased cost-per-day of patency and inferior limb salvage is found in lower income patients.

▶ The article addresses an important issue: access to care and socioeconomic factors that influence quality of care. The multivariable analysis revealed that in patients with critical limb ischemia, an income > 100% of the federal poverty level was protective against limb loss after lower extremity revascularization. This is not surprising in that lower socioeconomic status has also been associated with poor overall health status. Lower socioeconomic status also appears to be associated with higher levels of vascular inflammatory markers.[1,2] Results of this study imply that removing barriers to care in low-income patients may lessen the gap between outcomes of patients with low incomes versus those who are more affluent. An additional potential benefit is a reduction in the financial burden of care of low-income patients on the health care system. Clearly, this study has many limitations. It is retrospective, and all the data were derived from a single institution. The socioeconomic data were not verified with tax returns. Education was not verified with school records, and all data were based primarily upon telephone survey. Nevertheless, there does appear to be a relationship between lower extremity revascularization success and income. The article demonstrates the financial and clinical burdens associated with caring for low-income patients.

G. L. Moneta, MD

References

1. Orszag PR, Ellis P. The challenge of rising health care costs—a view from the Congressional Budget Office. *N Engl J Med.* 2007;357:1793-1795.
2. Hong S, Nelesen RA, Krohn PL, Mills PJ, Dimsdale JE. The association of social status and blood pressure with markers of vascular inflammation. *Psychosom Med.* 2006;68:517-523.

12 Leg Ischemia and Aortoiliac Disease

Effect of fibroblast growth factor NV1FGF on amputation and death: a randomised placebo-controlled trial of gene therapy in critical limb ischaemia

Belch J, on behalf of the TAMARIS Committees and Investigators (Ninewells Hosp and Med School, Dundee, UK; et al)

Lancet 377:1929-1937, 2011

Background.—Patients with critical limb ischaemia have a high rate of amputation and mortality. We tested the hypothesis that non-viral 1 fibroblast growth factor (NV1FGF) would improve amputation-free survival.

Methods.—In this phase 3 trial (EFC6145/TAMARIS), 525 patients with critical limb ischaemia unsuitable for revascularisation were enrolled from 171 sites in 30 countries. All had ischaemic ulcer in legs or minor skin gangrene and met haemodynamic criteria (ankle pressure <70 mm Hg or a toe pressure <50 mm Hg, or both, or a transcutaneous oxygen pressure <30 mm Hg on the treated leg). Patients were randomly assigned to either NV1FGF at 0·2 mg/mL or matching placebo (visually identical) in a 1:1 ratio. Randomisation was done with a central interactive voice response system by block size 4 and was stratified by diabetes status and country. Investigators, patients, and study teams were masked to treatment. Patients received eight intramuscular injections of their assigned treatment in the index leg on days 1, 15, 29, and 43. The primary endpoint was time to major amputation or death at 1 year analysed by intention to treat with a log-rank test using a multivariate Cox proportional hazard model. This trial is registered with ClinicalTrials.gov, number NCT00566657.

Findings.—259 patients were assigned to NV1FGF and 266 to placebo. All 525 patients were analysed. The mean age was 70 years (range 50–92), 365 (70%) were men, 280 (53%) had diabetes, and 248 (47%) had a history of coronary artery disease. The primary endpoint or components of the primary did not differ between treatment groups, with major amputation or death in 86 patients (33%) in the placebo group, and 96 (36%) in the active group (hazard ratio 1·11, 95% CI 0·83–1·49; p=0·48). No significant safety issues were recorded.

Interpretation.—TAMARIS provided no evidence that NV1FGF is effective in reduction of amputation or death in patients with critical limb ischaemia. Thus, this group of patients remains a major therapeutic challenge for the clinician.

▶ Fibroblast growth factor type 1 (FGF1) enhances new blood vessel formation. It has been demonstrated to activate migration, proliferation, and differentiation of endothelial cells that result in sprouting of capillaries in preexisting vessels. A naked DNA plasmid including the gene encoding for human FGF1 when given intramuscularly in the calf or thigh leads to expression of human FGF1 protein. In an open label phase 1 trial of 51 patients, a single intramuscular administration of non-viral 1 fibroblast growth factor (NV1FGF) in patients with critical limb ischemia improved symptoms of pain and ulcer size as well as hemodynamic variables in the treated limb.[1] The TALISMAN trial was a phase 2 trial of administration of NV1FGF compared with placebo in patients with critical limb ischemia. This trial demonstrated a reduction of 63% in risk of major amputation and a 56% reduction of the risk of major amputation or death at 12 months compared with placebo even though there was no difference in the primary end point of ulcer healing.[2] These 2 previous trials provided the stimulus for the phase 3 trial reported here. A meta-analysis of trials that include both gene- and cell-based therapies in peripheral arterial disease concluded that such therapies had potential clinical benefit.[3] Unfortunately, this potential benefit has not been demonstrated as of yet to translate into actual clinical benefit in rigorously controlled phase 3 trials such as that

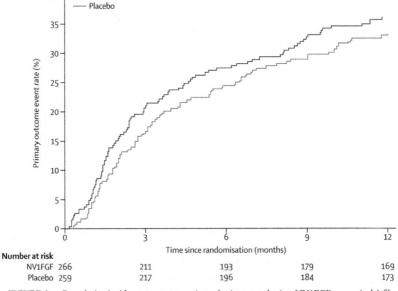

FIGURE 3.—Cumulative incidence curves over time of primary endpoint. NV1FGF=non-viral 1 fibroblast growth factor. (Reprinted from The Lancet, Belch J, on behalf of the TAMARIS Committees and Investigators. Effect of fibroblast growth factor NV1FGF on amputation and death: a randomised placebo-controlled trial of gene therapy in critical limb ischaemia. *Lancet.* 2011;377:1929-1937. Copyright 2011, with permission from Elsevier.)

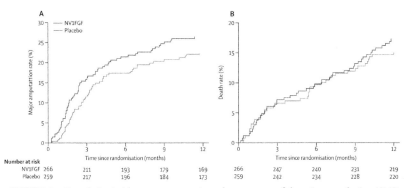

FIGURE 4.—Cumulative incidence curves over time of components of the primary endpoint. (A) First major amputation of the treated leg. (B) Death rate over time. NV1FGF=non-viral 1 fibroblast growth factor. (Reprinted from The Lancet, Belch J, on behalf of the TAMARIS Committees and Investigators. Effect of fibroblast growth factor NV1FGF on amputation and death: a randomised placebo-controlled trial of gene therapy in critical limb ischaemia. *Lancet.* 2011;377:1929-1937. Copyright 2011, with permission from Elsevier.)

presented here (Figs 3 and 4). One can perhaps question the concept that administration of a single gene where optimal dosage, routes of administration, duration of administration, and vectors of administration are unknown can result in clinical benefit. Gene therapy trials, as currently performed, can some-what pessimistically be described as shots in the dark and very expensive shots in the dark as well.

G. L. Moneta, MD

References

1. Comerota AJ, Throm RC, Miller KA, et al. Naked plasmid DNA encoding fibroblast growth factor type 1 for the treatment of end-stage unreconstructible lower extremity ischemia: preliminary results of a phase I trial. *J Vasc Surg.* 2002;35: 930-936.
2. Nikol S, Baumgartner I, Van Belle E, et al. Therapeutic angiogenesis with intramuscular NV1FGF improves amputation-free survival in patients with critical limb ischemia. *Mol Ther.* 2008;16:972-978.
3. De Haro J, Acin F, Lopez-Quintana A, Florez A, Martinez-Aguilar E, Varela C. Meta-analysis of randomized, controlled clinical trials in angiogenesis: gene and cell therapy in peripheral arterial disease. *Heart Vessels.* 2009;24:321-328.

Effectiveness of a Smoking Cessation Program for Peripheral Artery Disease Patients: A Randomized Controlled Trial

Hennrikus D, Joseph AM, Lando HA, et al (Univ of Minnesota, Minneapolis; et al)
J Am Coll Cardiol 56:2105-2112, 2010

Objectives.—This study tested the effectiveness of a smoking cessation program designed for patients with peripheral artery disease (PAD).

Background.—Tobacco use is the leading risk factor for PAD incidence and progression and for ischemic events. Tobacco cessation reduces PAD-related morbidity and mortality, yet few prospective clinical trials have evaluated smoking cessation interventions in PAD patients.

Methods.—We recruited outpatients with lower extremity PAD identified from medical records as cigarette smokers. Participants were randomly assigned to an intensive tailored PAD-specific counseling intervention or a minimal intervention. Participants completed surveys at baseline and at 3- and 6-month follow-up. Reported 7-day point prevalent smoking abstinence was confirmed by cotinine or carbon monoxide assessment.

Results.—In all, 687 outpatients were identified as probable smokers with lower extremity PAD; 232 met study eligibility requirements; and 124 (53% of eligible) enrolled. Participants were receptive to counselor contact: the median number of sessions was 8.5 (range 0 to 18). Participants randomly assigned to the intensive intervention group were significantly more likely to be confirmed abstinent at 6-month follow-up: 21.3% versus 6.8% in the minimal intervention group (chi-square = 5.21, $p = 0.023$).

Conclusions.—Many long-term smokers with PAD are willing to initiate a serious quit attempt and to engage in an intensive smoking cessation program. Intensive intervention for tobacco dependence is a more effective smoking cessation intervention than minimal care. Studies should be conducted to examine the long-term effectiveness of intensive smoking cessation programs in this population to examine the effect of this intervention on clinical outcomes related to PAD.

▶ The most important risk factor for development and progression of peripheral artery disease (PAD) is cigarette smoking. There is a 2.2-fold greater prevalence of symptomatic PAD in people who smoke compared with those who do not.[1] There has been only 1 randomized trial on the effectiveness of smoking cessation programs. This trial[2] evaluated the effectiveness of a nurse-conducted smoking cessation education program using nicotine gum. The study noted a difference between intervention and control groups' self-reported number of cigarettes smoked. However, biomarkers of tobacco use (urinary cotinine levels and expired carbon monoxide) provided conflicting results with the self-reported number of cigarettes smoked. The current study was designed to test the effectiveness of an intensive smoking cessation program in patients with PAD. This study shows many patients with PAD who are smokers are interested in quitting and receptive to a formal smoking cessation program. Those who chose to participate in the study almost universally indicate an understanding of the health risks of smoking. There was a demonstrated high desire to quit cigarette smoking as evidenced by the high level of engagement in the counseling sessions by those assigned to intensive intervention. One can conclude that the participants in this study were highly motivated to quit, yet only about one-fifth of the participants in the intensive intervention group were able to actually quit. The study confirms the powerful addictive nature of tobacco use and the importance of more intensive intervention in achieving abstinence from cigarette smoking. Perhaps most importantly, it points out the best we have to offer so far to achieve smoking cessation is still woefully inadequate even in the motivated patient.

G. L. Moneta, MD

References

1. Willigendael EM, Teijink JA, Bartelink ML, et al. Influence of smoking on incidence and prevalence of peripheral arterial disease. *J Vasc Surg.* 2004;40: 1158-1165.
2. Galvin K, Webb C, Hillier V. Assessing the impact of a nurse-led health education intervention for people with peripheral vascular disease who smoke: the use of physiological markers, nicotine dependence and withdrawal. *Int J Nurs Stud.* 2001;38:91-105.

Women With Peripheral Arterial Disease Experience Faster Functional Decline Than Men With Peripheral Arterial Disease

McDermott MM, Ferrucci L, Liu K, et al (Northwestern Univ, Chicago, IL; Natl Inst on Aging, Baltimore, MD; et al)
J Am Coll Cardiol 57:707-714, 2011

Objectives.—We hypothesized that women with lower extremity peripheral arterial disease (PAD) would have greater mobility loss and faster functional decline than men with PAD.

Background.—Whether rates of mobility loss or functional decline differ between men and women with PAD is currently unknown.

Methods.—Three hundred eighty men and women with PAD completed the 6-min walk, were assessed for mobility disability, and underwent measures of 4-m walking velocity at baseline and annually for up to 4 years. Computed tomography-assessed calf muscle characteristics were measured biannually. Outcomes included becoming unable to walk for 6 min continuously among participants who walked continuously for 6 min at baseline. Mobility loss was defined as becoming unable to walk for a quarter mile or to walk up and down 1 flight of stairs without assistance among those without baseline mobility disability. Results were adjusted for age, race, body mass index, physical activity, the ankle brachial index, comorbidities, and other confounders.

Results.—At 4 years of follow-up, women were more likely to become unable to walk for 6 min continuously (hazard ratio: 2.30, 95% confidence interval: 1.30 to 4.06, p = 0.004), more likely to develop mobility disability (hazard ratio: 1.79, 95% confidence interval: 1.30 to 3.03, p = 0.030), and had faster declines in walking velocity (p = 0.022) and the distance achieved in the 6-min walk (p = 0.041) compared with men. Sex differences in functional decline were attenuated after additional adjustment for baseline sex differences in calf muscle area.

Conclusions.—Women with PAD have faster functional decline and greater mobility loss than men with PAD. These sex differences may be attributable to smaller baseline calf muscle area among women with PAD.

▶ The prevalence of peripheral arterial disease (PAD) in older patients is at least the same in women as in men and may even be higher in women.[1] It has been previously demonstrated that women with PAD have decreased lower-extremity strength and greater functional impairment than men with PAD.[2] In this study, the authors determined whether there are sex differences in the rate of functional decline over time and whether there are differences in the rates of change of calf muscle characteristics over time between men and women with PAD.

This was a longitudinal observational study in which rates of mobility loss, decline in 6-minute walk performance, and decline in walking velocity between men and women with PAD were determined at baseline and at 4 years of follow-up. Baseline measurements of calf muscle characteristics and leg strength and changes in these muscle parameters between women and men with PAD were also determined at baseline and at 4 years of follow-up. In this study, women had smaller calf muscle area, lower calf muscle densities, and less knee extension strength at baseline compared with men. When these differences were adjusted for in the analysis, sex differences in functional decline in women versus men with PAD disappeared. This suggests that poor functional performance at baseline among women compared with men results in women being closer at baseline to thresholds for outcomes of mobility loss and physical dysfunction. It would be interesting to see if interventions to increase calf muscle area and improve lower-extremity strength among women with PAD would slow their functional decline.

G. L. Moneta, MD

References

1. Vavra AK, Kibbe MR. Women and peripheral arterial disease. *Womens Health (Lond Engl).* 2009;5:669-683.
2. McDermott MM, Greenland P, Liu K, et al. Sex differences in peripheral arterial disease: leg symptoms and physical functioning. *J Am Geriatr Soc.* 2003;51:222-228.

An elevated neutrophil-lymphocyte ratio independently predicts mortality in chronic critical limb ischemia
Spark JI, Sarveswaran J, Blest N, et al (Flinders Med Centre and Flinders Univ, Adelaide, South Australia; Leeds General Infirmary, UK)
J Vasc Surg 52:632-636, 2010

Background.—Atherogenesis represents an active inflammatory process with leucocytes playing a major role. An elevated white blood cell count has been shown to be predictive of death in coronary artery disease patients. The aim of this study was to examine the predictive ability of neutrophil count and neutrophil/lymphocyte ratio for predicting survival in patients with critical lower limb ischemia (CLI).

Methods.—All patients admitted to a single vascular unit with CCLI were identified prospectively over a 2-year period starting from January 2005. Patient demographics, clinical history, comorbidity, and risk factors for peripheral vascular disease were documented. The white blood count and differential cell count at admission was recorded. Overall, patient mortality was studied as the primary outcome.

Results.—One hundred forty-nine patients were identified, with a median age of 72 years (Interquartile range [IQR], 65.7-81). A neutrophil-lymphocyte ratio (NLR) of ≥5.25 was taken as the cutoff, based upon the receiver-operating-characteristic.The median follow up was 8.7 months (IQR, 3.1-16). During the follow-up period, there have been 62 deaths (43.4%). An elevated neutrophil/lymphocyte ratio and a high troponin level (>0.1) were found to be the only two factors independently associated with shorter survival on multivariate analysis using the Cox proportional hazards model.

Conclusions.—This study suggests that an elevated NLR can identify a poor-risk subset of patients among those being treated for critical limb

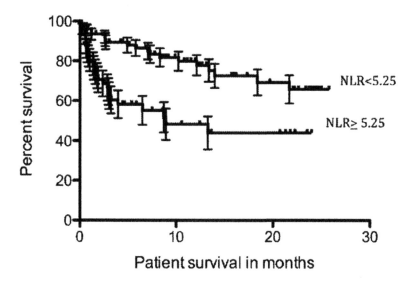

Patient survival in months

Patients at risk

NLR < 5.25	43	20	0
NLR ≥ 5.25	14	6	0

FIGURE 2.—Kaplan-Meier survival curve for neutrophil/lymphocyte ratio (*NLR*), with a cutoff of 5.25. (Reprinted from Spark JI, Sarveswaran J, Blest N, et al. An elevated neutrophil-lymphocyte ratio independently predicts mortality in chronic critical limb ischemia. *J Vasc Surg.* 2010;52:632-636. Copyright 2010, with permission from The Society for Vascular Surgery.)

TABLE 3.—Multivariate Analysis of Factors Affecting Mortality in Patients with Critical Limb Ischemia

	Hazard Ratio (95% Confidence Interval)	P Value
Elevated troponin	3.1 (1.6-5.6)	<.001
Neutrophil/lymphocyte ratio >5.25	2.3 (1.2-4.2)	.007
Diabetes mellitus	0.5 (0.2-1.1)	.1
Hypertension	1.4 (0.7-2.6)	.4
Previous myocardial infarction	1.2 (0.4-3.8)	.8
Renal failure	0.3 (0.05-3.7)	.3
Statin use	0.2 (0.06-0.7)	.013

ischemia. This simple, inexpensive test may, therefore, add to risk stratification of these high-risk patients (Fig 2, Table 3).

▶ The importance of the neutrophil-lymphocyte ratio (NLR) has been well characterized in the coronary literature. A high NLR has been associated with increased cardiac events and mortality. Because many patients presenting with critical limb ischemia (CLI) also have significant cardiac disease, the authors in this study assessed if NLR was associated with mortality in patients undergoing lower extremity revascularization for CLI. At a cutoff value of a NLR of 5.25, the study found that in patients with an elevated NLR (greater than 5.25), there were 38 deaths (all-cause mortality), and 24 mortalities occurred in the low NLR (less than or equal to 5.25) group (58.4% vs 28.6%, respectively; P less than .001; Fig 2). In fact, the multivariate analysis determined that both elevated troponin level and NLR were independent risk factors for all-cause mortality, while statin therapy was protective (Table 3). Several drawbacks from this study are worth mentioning. It is unclear when the blood work was analyzed (preoperative, postoperative) and at what time interval (days, weeks). It is unclear what a normal NLR is in subjects without peripheral vascular disease and the study lacked a control without disease. From the study, it is not clear which patients were on statins and from the multivariate analysis whether statin therapy favored protection from all-cause mortality. Having said this, it seems that such a simple blood test and ratio is as predictive of all-cause mortality in a complex biologic system as in patients with peripheral vascular diseases.

Prospective randomized controlled trials are needed to confirm these findings. More importantly, it would be necessary to identify therapeutic targets that would lead to normalization of the NLR, and one such consideration would be the use of statins.

J. D. Raffetto, MD

Four-year randomized prospective comparison of percutaneous ePTFE/nitinol self-expanding stent graft versus prosthetic femoral-popliteal bypass in the treatment of superficial femoral artery occlusive disease
McQuade K, Gable D, Pearl G, et al (Baylor Univ Med Ctr, Dallas, TX; et al)
J Vasc Surg 52:584-591, 2010

Background.—This is a randomized prospective study comparing the treatment of superficial femoral artery occlusive disease percutaneously with an expanded polytetrafluoroethylene (ePTFE)/nitinol self-expanding stent graft (stent graft) versus surgical femoral to above-knee popliteal artery bypass with synthetic graft material.

Methods.—One hundred limbs in 86 patients with superficial femoral artery occlusive disease were evaluated from March 2004 to May 2005. Patient symptoms included both claudication and limb threatening ischemia with or without tissue loss. Trans-Atlantic InterSociety Consensus (TASC II) A (n = 18), B (n = 56), C (n = 11), and D (n = 15) lesions were included. Patients were randomized prospectively into one of two treatment groups; a percutaneous treatment group (group A; n = 50) with angioplasty

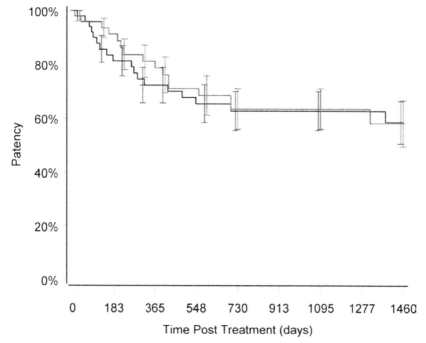

FIGURE 1.—Primary patency by treatment group. (Reprinted from McQuade K, Gable D, Pearl G, et al. Four-year randomized prospective comparison of percutaneous ePTFE/nitinol self-expanding stent graft versus prosthetic femoral-popliteal bypass in the treatment of superficial femoral artery occlusive disease. *J Vasc Surg*. 2010;52:584-591. Copyright 2010, with permission from the Society for Vascular Surgery.)

and placement of one or more stent grafts, or a surgical treatment group (group B; n = 50) with a femoral to above-knee popliteal artery bypass using synthetic conduit (Dacron or ePTFE). Patients were followed for 48 months. Follow-up evaluation included clinical assessment, physical examination, ankle-brachial indices, and color flow duplex sonography at 3, 6, 9, 12, 18, 24, 36, and 48 months.

Results.—Mean total lesion length of the treated arterial segment in the stent graft group was 25.6 cm (SD = 15 cm). The stent graft group demonstrated a primary patency of 72%, 63%, 63%, and 59% with a secondary patency of 83%, 74%, 74%, and 74% at 12, 24, 36, and 48 months, respectively. The surgical femoral-popliteal group demonstrated a primary patency of 76%, 63%, 63%, and 58% with a secondary patency of 86%, 76%, 76%, and 71% at 12, 24, 36, and 48 months, respectively. No statistical difference was found between the two groups with respect to primary ($P = .807$) or secondary ($P = .891$) patency.

Conclusion.—Management of superficial femoral artery occlusive disease with percutaneous stent grafts exhibits similar primary patency at 4-year (48 month) follow up when compared with conventional femoral-popliteal artery bypass grafting with synthetic conduit. This treatment

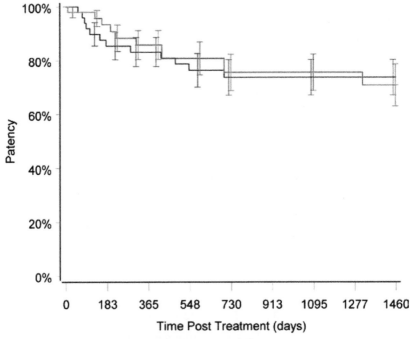

FIGURE 2.—Secondary patency by treatment group. (Reprinted from McQuade K, Gable D, Pearl G, et al. Four-year randomized prospective comparison of percutaneous ePTFE/nitinol self-expanding stent graft versus prosthetic femoral-popliteal bypass in the treatment of superficial femoral artery occlusive disease. *J Vasc Surg.* 2010;52:584-591. Copyright 2010, with permission from the Society for Vascular Surgery.)

method may offer an alternative to treatment of the superficial femoral artery segment for revascularization when prosthetic bypass is being considered or when autologous conduit is unavailable (Figs 1 and 2).

▶ This study is a continuation of a previously published study, with the difference of analyzing outcomes at 4 years. The study arms consist of open femoral-popliteal above-knee bypass with prosthetic graft versus percutaneous endovascular treatment with stent graft of the femoral-popliteal above-knee segment, well matched for demographics and risk factors, Trans-Atlantic InterSociety Consensus lesions, number of run-off vessels, and run-off score. The results were comparable in that initial technical success rates were the same in each arm, and primary and secondary patencies were similar (Figs 1 and 2). Additional information from the current or future studies that would be important in deciding which treatment a clinician would offer includes the following: (1) a cost analysis of the initial treatment, (2) a cost analysis of secondary interventions that were necessary for maintaining patency, and (3) most importantly, an analysis reporting quality of life for both general and disease-specific outcomes. Finally, this study used stent grafts and not bare metal stents. The mean lesion length was 25.6 cm. Although this study did not randomize stent grafts versus bare metal stents, the results with stent grafts that are comparable to bypass surgery would suggest that they may be more appropriate for longer segment lesion of the femoral-popliteal segment. The latter will require future trials.

J. D. Raffetto, MD

Histologic atherosclerotic plaque characteristics are associated with restenosis rates after endarterectomy of the common and superficial femoral arteries
Derksen WJM, de Vries J-PPM, Vink A, et al (Univ Med Ctr Utrecht, The Netherlands; St Antonius Hosp, Nieuwegein, The Netherlands; et al)
J Vasc Surg 52:592-599, 2010

Objectives.—This study assessed the predictive value of histologic plaque characteristics for the occurrence of restenosis after femoral artery endarterectomy.

Background.—It would be advantageous if patients at increased risk for restenosis after arterial endarterectomy could be identified by histologic characteristics of the dissected plaque. Differences in atherosclerotic plaque composition of the carotid artery have been associated with restenosis rates after surgical endarterectomy. However, whether atherosclerotic plaque characteristics are also predictive for restenosis in other vascular territories is unknown.

Methods.—Atherosclerotic plaques of 217 patients who underwent a common femoral artery endarterectomy (CFAE; n = 124) or remote superficial femoral artery endarterectomy (RSFAE; n = 93) were examined and scored microscopically for the presence of collagen, macrophages, smooth muscle cells, lipid core, intraplaque hemorrhage, and calcifications. The 12-month restenosis rate was assessed using duplex ultrasound imaging (peak systolic velocity [PSV] ratio ≥2.5).

Results.—The 1-year restenosis rate was 66% (61 of 93) after RSFAE compared to 21% (26 of 124) after CFAE. Plaque with characteristics of high collagen and smooth muscle cell content were positively associated with the occurrence of restenosis, with odds ratios (ORs) of 2.90 (95% confidence interval [CI], 1.82-4.68) and 2.20 (1.50-3.20) for superficial femoral artery (SFA) and common femoral artery (CFA), respectively. SFA plaques showed significantly heavier staining for collagen (69% vs 31% for CFA; $P < .001$) and smooth muscle cells (64% vs 36% for CFA; $P < .001$). After multivariate analysis, the operation type (CFAE or RSFAE), gender, and the presence of collagen were independent predictive variables for restenosis after endarterectomy of the CFA and SFA.

Conclusion.—Plaque composition of the CFA and SFA differs. Furthermore, the dissection of a fibrous collagen-rich plaque is an independent predictive variable for restenosis after endarterectomy of the CFA and SFA.

▶ Understanding the basic science of human arterial disease is paramount in developing improved strategies of identifying lesions at risk, improving treatments and outcomes. Atherosclerotic plaques are a principal disease affecting the vast majority of vascular diseases seen in clinical practice. A significant burden of arterial disease is seen in the common femoral and femoral artery. This study evaluated histological and biochemical characteristics of atherosclerotic plaques to determine if differences existed and affected restenosis rates after endarterectomy at 1 year. The study found that femoral artery plaques contained significantly more collagen and smooth muscle cells, and restenosis rates were more than 3 times greater in femoral plaques than in common femoral artery endarterectomized plaques (66% vs 21%, $P = .001$). Importantly, the presence of a fibrous collagen-rich atherosclerotic plaque is an independent predictive variable for restenosis after endarterectomy of the common femoral artery and femoral artery.

J. D. Raffetto, MD

Long-term outcomes of diabetic patients undergoing endovascular infrainguinal interventions
Abularrage CJ, Conrad MF, Hackney LA, et al (Massachusetts General Hosp and Harvard Med School, Boston)
J Vasc Surg 52:314-322, 2010

Objective.—Diabetes mellitus (DM) has traditionally predicted poor outcomes after lower extremity revascularization for peripheral vascular disease (PVD). This study assessed the influence of DM on long-term outcomes of percutaneous transluminal angioplasty, with or without stenting (PTA/stent), in patients with PVD.

Methods.—From January 2002 to December 2007, 920 patients underwent 1075 PTA/stent procedures. Patients were stratified into DM and non-DM cohorts. Study end points included primary patency (PP), assisted patency (AP), limb salvage, and survival and were evaluated using Kaplan-Meier and Cox regression analyses.

Results.—There were 533 DM and 542 non-DM limbs. Median follow-up was 34 months. Overall, the 5-year actuarial PP was 42% ± 2.4%, AP was 81% ± 2.0%, limb salvage was 89% ± 1.6%, and survival was 60% ± 2.4%. On univariate analysis, DM vs non-DM was associated with inferior 5-year PP (37% ± 3.4% vs 46% ± 3.3%; *P* =.009), limb salvage (84% ± 2.6% vs 93% ± 1.8%, *P* < .0001), and survival (52% ± 3.5% vs 68% ± 3.1%, *P* =.0001). AP did not differ between DM and non-DM patients (*P* =.18). In the entire cohort, DM (hazard ratio [HR], 1.25; 95% confidence interval [CI], 1.01-1.54; *P* =.04), single-vessel peroneal runoff (HR, 1.54; 95% CI, 1.16-2.08; *P* =.003), and dialysis (HR, 1.59; 95% CI, 1.10-2.33; *P* =.02) were associated with decreased PP on multivariate analysis. The only variables on multivariate analysis to predict limb loss and death were critical limb ischemia (HR, 9.09; 95% CI, 4.17-20.00; *P* < .0001; HR, 2.99; 95% CI, 2.01-4.44; *P* < .0001, respectively) and dialysis (HR, 2.94; 95% CI, 1.39-5.00; *P* =.003; HR, 4.24; 95% CI 2.80-6.45; *P* < .0001, respectively).

Conclusions.—DM is an independent predictor of decreased long-term primary patency after PTA/stent. Although acceptable assisted patency rates can be achieved with close surveillance and reintervention, long-term limb salvage remains inferior in diabetic patients compared with non-diabetic patients due to a more severe clinical presentation and poor runoff (Figs 1 and 2).

▶ The gold standard for treatment of patients with diabetes mellitus and critical limb ischemia is bypass surgery with the goal of restoring pulsatile blood flow to the foot. The advancement of endovascular techniques has challenged this dogma, and significant center experiences are appearing in the literature. This particular study, from a single center, evaluated patients with or without diabetes, assessing long-term outcomes of percutaneous transluminal angioplasty, with or without stenting, between 2002 and 2007. There are several results from this study that are worth mentioning: (1) 533 limbs with diabetes and 542 nondiabetic limbs were assessed. (2) The median follow-up was 34 months. (3) Diabetes versus nondiabetes treated limbs were associated with inferior 5-year primary patency (37% vs 46%, *P* = .009), limb salvage (84% vs 93%, *P* < .0001), and survival (52% vs 68%, *P* = .0001). There were no differences in assisted patency (reinterventions on stenosis or thrombosis). (4) In the entire cohort, diabetes (hazard ratio [HR] = 1.25; 95% confidence interval [CI], 1.01-1.54; *P* =.04), single-vessel peroneal runoff (HR, 1.54; 95% CI, 1.16-2.08; *P* = .003), and dialysis (HR, 1.59; 95% CI,1.10-2.33; *P* = .02) were associated with decreased primary patency on multivariate analysis. (5) The only variables on multivariate analysis to predict limb loss and death were critical limb ischemia (HR, 9.09; 95% CI, 4.17-20.00; *P* = .0001;

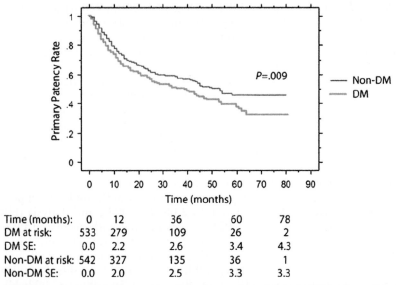

Time (months):	0	12	36	60	78
DM at risk:	533	279	109	26	2
DM SE:	0.0	2.2	2.6	3.4	4.3
Non-DM at risk:	542	327	135	36	1
Non-DM SE:	0.0	2.0	2.5	3.3	3.3

FIGURE 1.—Kaplan-Meier curves show the primary patency of diabetic (*DM*) and non-diabetic (*non-DM*) patients undergoing percutaneous transluminal angioplasty. (Reprinted from Abularrage CJ, Conrad MF, Hackney LA, et al. Long-term outcomes of diabetic patients undergoing endovascular infrainguinal interventions. *J Vasc Surg.* 2010;52:314-322. Copyright 2010, with permission from the Society for Vascular Surgery.)

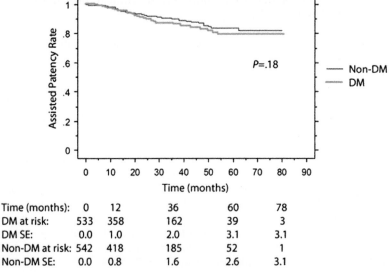

Time (months):	0	12	36	60	78
DM at risk:	533	358	162	39	3
DM SE:	0.0	1.0	2.0	3.1	3.1
Non-DM at risk:	542	418	185	52	1
Non-DM SE:	0.0	0.8	1.6	2.6	3.1

FIGURE 2.—Kaplan-Meier curves show the assisted patency of diabetic (*DM*) and non-diabetic (*non-DM*) patients undergoing percutaneous transluminal angioplasty. (Reprinted from Abularrage CJ, Conrad MF, Hackney LA, et al. Long-term outcomes of diabetic patients undergoing endovascular infrainguinal interventions. *J Vasc Surg.* 2010;52:314-322. Copyright 2010, with permission from the Society for Vascular Surgery.)

HR, 2.99; 95% CI, 2.01-4.44; $P = .0001$, respectively) and dialysis (HR, 2.94; 95% CI, 1.39-5.00; $P = .003$; HR, 4.24; 95% CI 2.80-6.45; $P = .0001$, respectively). Because of the study design consisting of a retrospective review of a prospectively entered database, clear guidelines cannot be established. However, the study does raise important questions and likely will require a controlled trial in patients with diabetes randomized to open revascularization or endovascular therapy. However, given the poor primary patency rates of 37% at 5 years in diabetic patients (Fig 1) and worse limb salvage in diabetic patients undergoing percutaneous endovascular interventions (Fig 2), it may be difficult to justify such a study, especially in diabetic patients with tissue loss and gangrene. Understanding how stents and angioplasty behave in patients with diabetes and improving endovascular treatments will be necessary before endovascular treatment can unequivocally become the standard of care in diabetic patients with severe limb-threatening disease.

J. D. Raffetto, MD

Prognostic values of C-reactive protein levels on clinical outcome after endovascular therapy in hemodialysis patients with peripheral artery disease

Ishii H, Kumada Y, Toriyama T, et al (Nagoya Univ Graduate School of Medicine, Japan; Nagoya Kyoritsu Hosp, Japan)
J Vasc Surg 52:854-859, 2010

Purpose.—Endovascular therapy (EVT) has been widely performed for peripheral artery disease. However, the high restenosis rate after EVT remains a major problem in patients on hemodialysis. Recent studies suggest that C-reactive protein (CRP) reflects vascular wall inflammation and can predict adverse events. We evaluated the possible prognostic values of CRP on outcomes in hemodialysis patients undergoing EVT.

Methods.—A total of 234 hemodialysis patients undergoing EVT for peripheral artery disease were enrolled and followed-up for up to 5 years. They were divided into tertiles according to serum CRP levels (lowest tertile, <1.4 mg/L; middle tertile, 1.4-6.0 mg/L; highest tertile, <6.0 mg/L). We analyzed the incidence of any reintervention or above-ankle amputation of the limb index (RAO) and any-cause death.

Results.—Kaplan-Meier analysis showed that the event-free rate from the composite end point of RAO and any-cause death for 5 years was 60.2% in the lowest tertile, 50.0% in the middle tertile, and 25.1% in the highest tertile ($P < .0001$). The survival rate from any-cause death for 5 years was 81.5% in the lowest tertile, 65.2% in the middle tertile, and 59.3% in the highest tertile ($P = .0078$). Even after adjusting for other risk factors at baseline, preprocedural CRP levels were a significant predictive factor for RAO and any-cause death after EVT in a multivariable Cox analysis.

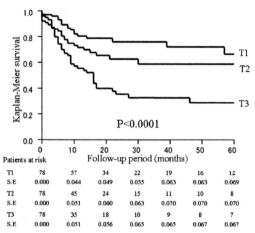

Patients at risk

T1	78	57	34	22	19	16	12
S.E	0.000	0.044	0.049	0.055	0.063	0.063	0.069
T2	78	45	24	15	11	10	8
S.E	0.000	0.051	0.060	0.063	0.070	0.070	0.070
T3	78	35	18	10	9	8	7
S.E	0.000	0.051	0.056	0.065	0.065	0.067	0.067

FIGURE 1.—Kaplan-Meier estimates show event-free survival, with the standard error (SE), from composite end points of any reintervention, defined as any repeat vascular procedure or above-ankle amputation of the limb index, in patients categorized by level of C-reactive protein into the lowest tertile (*T1*, <1.4 mg/L), middle tertile (*T2*, 1.4-6.0 mg/L), and highest tertile (*T3*, ≥6.0 mg/L). (Reprinted from Ishii H, Kumada Y, Toriyama T, et al. Prognostic values of C-reactive protein levels on clinical outcome after endovascular therapy in hemodialysis patients with peripheral artery disease. *J Vasc Surg.* 2010;52:854-859. Copyright 2010, with permission from The Society for Vascular Surgery.)

Conclusions.—Elevated preprocedural serum CRP levels were associated with RAO and any-cause death after EVT in hemodialysis patients with peripheral artery disease (Fig 1, Table 3).

▶ Patients who are on dialysis have significantly worse outcomes following revascularization, reflecting graft function, limb salvage, and mortality. Although medical therapy and dialysis help these patients with improving their quality of life, when a patient on dialysis is afflicted with limb-threatening ischemia and gangrene, the process can be prolonged with multiple hospital admissions, prolonged hospitalization, and significant morbidity. Having a prognostic test that can assess clinical outcomes would be of benefit especially in patients on dialysis and with severe peripheral vascular disease requiring interventions. In this study, which demonstrated patients undergoing endovascular treatment of iliofemoral and femoral-popliteal arterial disease, patients with C-reactive protein (CRP) levels in the highest tertile of greater than or equal to 6 mg/L had the greatest events rates of reinterventions, major limb amputation, and all-cause death reaching almost 75% at 5 years, while patients in the lowest tertile (CRP less than 1.4 mg/L) had the lowest rate (39.8%) of composite end points including death (Fig 1). Even after adjusting for other risk factors at baseline, preprocedural CRP levels (as well as the presence of ulcer or gangrene, and the TransAtlantic Inter-Society Consensus C and D lesions) were a significant independent predictive factor for reinterventions and limb amputation and any-cause death after endovascular treatment of peripheral arterial disease (Table 3). The interesting and somewhat puzzling aspect of this study is that in a series of 234 hemodialysis patients studied with significant

TABLE 3.—Predictive Value for RAO[a] by Cox Analysis

Variable	Univariate HR (95% CI)	P	Multivariate[b] HR (95% CI)	P
Serum CRP	1.01 (1.00-1.02)	.0059	1.01 (1.00-1.02)	.0046
Age	1.02 (0.99-1.04)	.14	...	...
Male, yes/no	1.23 (0.82-1.85)	.33	...	...
Diabetes, yes/no	1.06 (0.70-1.62)	.78	...	...
Hypertension, yes/no	1.10 (0.71-1.69)	.67	...	..
Dyslipidemia, yes/no	1.14 (0.72-1.78)	.57	...	...
Smoking, yes/no	1.05 (0.62-1.78)	.84	...	...
History of CAD, yes/no	1.17 (0.77-1.77)	.46	...	...
History of stroke, yes/no	1.53 (0.94-2.48)	.090	1.51 (0.85-2.67)	.16
Ulcer or gangrene, yes/no	2.14 (1.34-3.43)	.0015	2.20 (1.33-3.63)	.0021
Statins, yes/no	0.75 (0.44-1.27)	.28	...	...
Femoropopliteal lesion, yes/no	1.08 (0.69-1.68)	.74	...	...
TASC type C or D, yes/no	1.90 (1.15-3.14)	.012	2.15 (1.17-3.95)	.013
Stent use, yes/no	0.70 (0.47-1.04)	.084	0.76 (0.46-1.23)	.26

CAD, Coronary artery disease; CI, confidence interval; CRP, C-reactive protein; HR, hazard ratio; TASC, TransAtlantic Inter-Society Consensus.
[a]RAO: Any reintervention defined as any repeat vascular procedure or above-ankle amputation of the limb index, and any-cause death.
[b]Multivariate model includes variable with P < .10 by univariate analysis.

cardiovascular risk factors, only 12% to 15% of patients in each of the 3 CRP tertiles studied were on statins. Since CRP is a measure of the degree of inflammation in the arterial circulation, it would be interesting to see if the major primary outcomes studied would be affected if most hemodialysis patients were taking statins, especially in those with elevated preprocedural CRP levels. Other large studies (Heart Protection Study) have found a clear benefit in clinical outcomes in patients with peripheral vascular disease undergoing procedural interventions who were taking statins. Future studies will be required to determine if statin use has a clear and potential benefit (reinterventions, limb salvage, mortality) in patients on dialysis who present for endovascular treatment of critical limb ischemia.

J. D. Raffetto, MD

ACCF/AHA/ACR/SCAI/SIR/SVM/SVN/SVS 2010 performance measures for adults with peripheral artery disease. A Report of the American College of Cardiology Foundation/American Heart Association Task Force on Performance Measures, the American College of Radiology, the Society for Cardiac Angiography and Interventions, the Society for Interventional Radiology, the Society for Vascular Medicine, the Society for Vascular Nursing, and the Society for Vascular Surgery (Writing Committee to Develop Clinical Performance Measures for Peripheral Artery Disease). Developed in Collaboration With the American Association of Cardiovascular and Pulmonary Rehabilitation; the American Diabetes Association; the Society for Atherosclerosis Imaging and Prevention; the Society for Cardiovascular Magnetic Resonance; the Society of Cardiovascular Computed Tomography; and the PAD Coalition Endorsed by the American Academy of Podiatric Practice Management
American College of Cardiology Foundation, American Heart Association Task Force on Performance Measures, American College of Radiology, Society for Cardiac Angiography and Interventions, Society for Interventional Radiology, Society for Vascular Medicine, Society for Vascular Nursing, Society for Vascular Surgery, Olin JW (Society of Cardiovascular Computed Tomography Representative; et al)
J Vasc Surg 52:1616-1652, 2010

Background.—Recognition that care delivered often differs from care that ought to be delivered prompted the development of measures of quality of care and the use of such measures to improve quality and accountability in medical management. The American College of Cardiology Foundation (ACCF) and the American Heart Association (AHA) led in developing measures of quality of care for cardiovascular disease (CVD). The measures constructed could be used in prospective or retrospective environments, rely on readily documented clinical criteria, and, where appropriate, incorporate administrative data. They are linked to existing ACCF/AHA clinical data standards to promote uniform measurements of cardiovascular care. The initial measures focus on processes of medical care or actions taken by healthcare providers and are designed to improve quality, but they can be used for external review or public reporting of provider performance. The ACCF/AHA performance measure writing team commented on strengths and limitations of external reporting for specific CVDs or patient populations. The performance measures focus on peripheral artery disease (PAD) and address lower extremity and abdominal aortic disease in adults (age 18 years or older) in outpatient settings.

Definitions.—PAD includes several disorders marked by progressive stenosis or occlusion or aneurysmal dilation of the aorta and its noncoronary branch arteries. PAD is a marker of systemic atherosclerosis but has been underdiagnosed because it tends to present atypical symptoms or no ischemic symptoms related to the legs. Patients with PAD can manifest symptoms ranging from none to intermittent claudication, atypical leg pain, rest pain, ischemic ulcer, and gangrene. Studies indicate that more patients with PAD are asymptomatic or have atypical leg symptoms than have classic intermittent claudication. The two major consequences of PAD are decreased overall well-being and quality of life because of the claudication and leg pain and markedly increased cardiovascular morbidity and mortality. Both are the focus of treatment efforts. The PAD performance measures are directed at strategies designed to improve the diagnosis and treatment of patients, improve patients' walking distance and speed, give patients a better quality of life, and diminish the number of cardiovascular events related to PAD.

Performance Measures.—Criteria for selecting the performance measures include the specific evidence available, the ease or complexity of the measurement, and whether the measurement is included in previously published guidelines. Attribution and/or aggregation is included in each measure.

Most PAD patients require longitudinal follow-up by physicians from various specialties. All clinicians must effectively document in the patient's medical record complete clinical data for each PAD measure. This information must be shared among all the physicians caring for the patient on a regular basis.

All patients with PAD, regardless of symptom status, ankle-brachial artery index (ABI), or efficacy of revascularization, have a short-term risk of morbid or mortal ischemic events similar to that of patients with other CVDs, yet PAD patients are less consistently given treatments to address these issues. Both pharmacological and lifestyle interventions are commonly used to reduce risks in CVD patients, but physicians do not consistently recognize the cardiovascular risk associated with PAD and do not treat PAD patients as aggressively. Thus the use of risk-reduction interventions must be included as a PAD performance measure.

An ABI of 0.90 or less reliably and easily diagnoses PAD. This simple, inexpensive, noninvasive test is readily performed in most clinical settings and offers a sensitivity of 79% to 95% and a specificity of 95% to 100% for PAD. Abnormal ABI results are linked to significantly increased risk of coronary heart disease, stroke, and cardiovascular death. Thus the ABI should be measured in all patients at risk for PAD.

Antiplatelet therapy is recommended for the treatment of patients with PAD. In addition, PAD guidelines recommend supervised exercise to treat patients with PAD who have claudication. Such exercise has proven efficacious and safe. Patients with PAD should receive counseling concerning all their treatment options to encourage them to become fully engaged in the treatment process. Options include pharmacological management, supervised exercise, and/or various percutaneous or open surgical revascularization techniques.

Nonselected Test Measures.—Measures that were not included, although they were considered, include lower extremity endovascular revascularization surveillance, chronic critical limb ischemia and acute limb ischemia, renal and mesenteric artery disease, exercise treadmill testing, computed tomographic angiography and magnetic resonance angiography, management of hypertension and diabetes, screening for abdominal aortic aneurysm, and outcome measures. Usually these measures were rejected because they are difficult and time consuming to track and require resources for monitoring that may not be readily available or available at all.

▶ With the general trend in development of quality care measures, the American College of Cardiology Foundation/American Heart Association/American College of Radiology/Society for Cardiac Angiography and Interventions/Society for Interventional Radiology/Society for Vascular Medicine/Society for Vascular Nursing/Society for Vascular Surgery developed collective performance measures for peripheral artery disease (PAD) that are essentially an updated version from the American College of Cardiology/American Heart Association guidelines from 2005. With the inclusion of additional societies representing specialties beyond cardiology, including vascular surgery, vascular medicine, vascular nursing, and interventional radiology, the 2010 version offers a much more important consensus perspective. Although the specifics are beyond the scope of this review, the included appendices address recommendations for ankle brachial indices, cholesterol-lowering medications, smoking cessation, antiplatelet therapy, supervised exercise, lower extremity bypass graft surveillance, abdominal aortic aneurysm monitoring, vascular review of systems for lower extremity PAD, and pulse examination for identification of patients at risk for PAD. Also included is a sample prospective data collection flow sheet (Appendix E in the original article), which allows for standard recordings of these quality care performance measures. The source article should be required reading for any practitioner caring for patients with PAD and should help standardize quality care across all these specialties.

M. A. Passman, MD

Predictors of failure and success of tibial interventions for critical limb ischemia
Fernandez N, McEnaney R, Marone LK, et al (Univ of Pittsburgh Med Ctr, PA)
J Vasc Surg 52:834-842, 2010

Objective.—The efficacy of tibial artery endovascular intervention (TAEI) for critical limb ischemia (CLI) and particularly for wound healing is not fully defined. The purpose of this study is to determine predictors of failure and success for TAEI in the setting of CLI.

Methods.—All TAEI for tissue loss or rest pain (Rutherford classes 4, 5, and 6) from 2004 to 2008 were retrospectively reviewed. Clinical outcomes and patency rates were analyzed by multivariable Cox proportional hazards regression and life table analysis.

Results.—One hundred twenty-three limbs in 111 patients (62% male, mean age 74) were treated. Sixty-seven percent of patients were diabetics, 55% had renal insufficiency, and 21% required hemodialysis. One hundred two limbs (83%) exhibited tissue loss; all others had ischemic rest pain. All patients underwent tibial angioplasty (PTA). Tibial excimer laser atherectomy was performed in 14% of the patients. Interventions were performed on multiple tibial vessels in 20% of limbs. Isolated tibial procedures were performed on 50 limbs (41%), while 73 patients had concurrent ipsilateral superficial femoral artery or popliteal interventions. The mean distal popliteal and tibial runoff score improved from 11.8 ± 3.6 to 6.7 ± 1.6 ($P < .001$), and the mean ankle-brachial index increased from 0.61 ± 0.26 to 0.85 ± 0.22 ($P < .001$). Surgical bypass was required in seven patients (6%). The mean follow up was 6.8 ± 6.6 months, while the 1-year primary, primary-assisted, and secondary patency rates were 33%, 50%, and 56% respectively. Limb salvage rate at 1 year was 75%. Factors found to be associated with impaired limb salvage included renal insufficiency (hazard ratio [HR] = 5.7; $P = .03$) and the need for pedal intervention (HR = 13.75; $P = .04$). TAEI in an isolated peroneal artery (odds ratio = 7.80; $P = .01$) was associated with impaired wound healing, whereas multilevel intervention (HR = 2.1; $P = .009$) and tibial laser atherectomy (HR = 3.1; $P = .01$) were predictors of wound healing. In patients with tissue loss, 41% achieved complete closure (mean time to healing, 10.7 ± 7.4 months), and 39% exhibited partial wound healing (mean follow up, 4.4 ± 4.8 months) at last follow up. Diabetes, smoking, statin therapy, and revascularization of >1 tibial vessel had no impact on limb salvage or wound healing. Reintervention rate was 50% at 1 year.

Conclusions.—TAEI is an effective treatment for CLI with acceptable limb salvage and wound healing rates, but requires a high rate of reintervention. Patients with renal failure, pedal disease, or isolated peroneal runoff have poor outcomes with TAEI and should be considered for surgical bypass.

▶ While the authors conclude that tibial artery endovascular intervention (TAEI) is an effective treatment for critical limb ischemia (CLI), with acceptable limb salvage and wound healing rates, this conclusion is flawed. In this retrospective review of all TAEIs performed for patients with CLI, results may not be as promising as suggested by the authors. While an endovascular first approach is used, there are no further data on those patients who had failed attempts at TAEI because a lesion could not be crossed and may have required operative revascularization or amputation. On those who had what was considered a successful TAEI, 1-year primary patency, primary-assisted patency, and secondary patency were only 33%, 50%, and 56%, respectively, and 50% required re-intervention. While limb salvage is reported as 75% and subsequent operative bypass was required in only 6% at 1 year, the follow-up interval is rather short to declare a durable victory. If these surrogate outcomes are considered acceptable, one wonders what would be considered unacceptable. The problem in this study is that there is mixing of data sets: while all patients had tibial intervention, 50% required multilevel revascularization of a more proximal vessel; severity of occlusive disease is not stratified, and standard Trans Atlantic Inter-Societal Consensus document classification is not used; TAEIs include various combinations of angioplasty, stent, and atherectomy, each of which adds technical complexity to the case and potential negative confounding variables to the analysis. With a more stratified analysis of this data set, the routine endovascular first approach used should become more selective, which may impart improved and more durable outcomes for those selected for endovascular approach.

M. A. Passman, MD

Quality of life in patients with no-option critical limb ischemia underlines the need for new effective treatment

Sprengers RW, on behalf of the JUVENTAS and SMART study groups (Univ Med Ctr Utrecht, The Netherlands)
J Vasc Surg 52:843-849, 2010

Objective.—To provide a solid baseline reference for quality of life (QoL) in patients with no-option critical limb ischemia (CLI). CLI is associated with surgery, endovascular interventions, hospitalization, and a poor prognosis. An increasing number of clinical trials are, therefore, investigating new treatment strategies (eg, therapeutic neovascularization) in patients with CLI. QoL serves as an important secondary endpoint in many of these trials, but solid reference QoL data for patients with no-option CLI are lacking.

Methods.—The Medical Outcomes Study Short Form 36 (SF-36) and the EuroQol-5D (EQ-5D) questionnaires were used to obtain baseline QoL scores from 47 patients with no-option CLI participating in a therapeutic neovascularization trial. To allow for easy comparability, a norm-based scoring (NBS) method was used to report the results of the SF-36. Scores of patients with CLI were furthermore compared with scores of patients with milder forms of peripheral arterial disease (PAD) and with patients with cardiovascular risk factors only. Determinants of QoL in patients with PAD were identified using multiple linear regression methods.

Results.—Patients with no-option CLI reported QoL scores below the general population mean on every health dimension of the SF-36. Physical functioning, role physical functioning, and bodily pain were affected most intensively. These poor physical QoL scores were further underlined when compared with other patients with milder forms of PAD or patients with cardiovascular risk factors only. Patients with CLI scored poorly on the pain/discomfort and the usual activities domain of the EQ-5D. Diabetes, female gender, body mass index, and the ankle-brachial index at rest were significant determinants of the QoL in PAD on multivariate analysis.

Conclusion.—The QoL data of patients with no-option CLI using NBS methods for the SF-36 provide a baseline reference for ongoing clinical trials on new treatment strategies. Our data stress the need for new revascularization therapies in patients with no-option CLI.

▶ From a design standpoint, this study combines data sets from 2 ongoing clinical trails (JUVENTAS trial with 47 patients with critical limb ischemia [CLI] and no surgical or endovascular options for revascularization and Second Manifestations of ARTerial disease [SMART] cohort with 313 patients with mild peripheral arterial disease [PAD]; 1182 patients with cardiovascular risk factors but no manifestations of cardiovascular disease) to compare quality-of-life scoring from 36-Item Short Form Health Survey and EuroQol-5D questionnaires, using a norm-based scoring method to allow for comparability. Not surprisingly, patients with no-option CLI have poorer quality of life than those with mild or no PAD. There are significant design flaws in this study, including disparate sample size and distribution, combining data sets from the 2 completely different studies, and inability to identify other confounding variables that may have impacted quality-of-life parameters more than CLI or PAD. Predictably, this study does reinforce the notion that patients with end-stage PAD and no revascularization options tend to have worse prognosis on many levels and would be the group to have the highest potential benefit from future novel revascularization options currently under investigation.

M. A. Passman, MD

Safety and efficacy of patient specific intramuscular injection of HGF plasmid gene therapy on limb perfusion and wound healing in patients with ischemic lower extremity ulceration: Results of the HGF-0205 trial
Powell RJ, Goodney P, Mendelsohn FO, et al (Dartmouth Hitchcock Med Ctr, Lebanon, NH; Univ of Virginia Med School, Charlottesville)
J Vasc Surg 52:1525-1530, 2010

Objectives.—We have previously reported the results of a dose-finding phase II trial showing that HGF angiogenic gene therapy can increase TcPO2 compared with placebo in patients with critical limb ischemia (CLI). The purpose of this randomized placebo controlled multi-center trial was to further assess the safety and clinical efficacy of a modified HGF gene delivery technique in patients with CLI and no revascularization options.

Methods.—Patients with lower extremity ischemic tissue loss (Rutherford 5 and 6) received three sets of eight intramuscular injections every 2 weeks of HGF plasmid under duplex ultrasound guidance. Injection locations were individualized for each patient based on arteriographically defined vascular anatomy. Primary safety end point was incidence of adverse events (AE) or serious adverse events (SAE). Clinical end points included change from baseline in toe brachial index (TBI), rest pain assessment by a 10 cm visual analogue scale (VAS) as well as wound healing, amputation, and survival at 3 and 6 months.

Results.—Randomization ratio was 3:1 HGF (n = 21) vs placebo (n = 6). Mean age was 76 ± 2 years, with 56% male and 59% diabetic. There was no difference in demographics between groups. There was no difference in AEs or SAEs, which consisted mostly of transient injection site discomfort, worsening of CLI, and intercurrent illnesses. Change in TBI significantly improved from baseline at 6 months in the HGF-treated group compared with placebo (0.05 ± 0.05 vs −0.17 ± 0.04; $P = .047$). Change in VAS from baseline at 6 months was also significantly improved in the HGF-treated group compared with placebo (−1.9 ± 1.3 vs +0.06 ± 0.2; $P = .04$). Complete ulcer healing at 12 months occurred in 31% of the HGF group and 0% of the placebo ($P = .28$). There was no difference in major amputation of the treated limb (HGF 29% vs placebo 33%) or mortality at 12 months (HGF 19% vs placebo 17%) between groups.

Conclusion.—HGF gene therapy using a patient vascular anatomy specific delivery technique appears safe, maintained limb perfusion, and decreased rest pain in patients with CLI compared with placebo. A larger study to assess the efficacy of this therapy on more clinically relevant end points is warranted.

▶ There continues to be growing interest in therapeutic angiogenesis, and this clinical investigation evaluating the safety and efficacy of hepatocyte growth factor (HGF) gene therapy seems to have promising results of decreased rest pain, improved ulcer healing, and improved limb perfusion parameters when compared with placebo control in a prospective, 3:1 randomization, blinded design. Like other clinical investigations of therapeutic angiogenesis modalities, whether this translates to more clinically relevant efficacy is yet to be determined. However, the most interesting part of this study is the use of a novel directed HGF delivery based on patient-specific vascular anatomy. Using preinjection arteriography, MR angiography, or CT angiography, this directed technique used ultrasound-guided injection into the muscle bed distribution of occluded tibial vessels. By delivering gene therapy into the anatomic region of most severe vascular disease, there is theoretical advantage of focusing the angiogenesis effect on the area that would most benefit from these novel therapies. Further validation would be important to determine whether there is added benefit of optimal directed delivery of therapeutic angiogenesis agents over the more common nonspecific approaches used in other studies.

M. A. Passman, MD

Inframalleolar Bypass Grafts for Limb Salvage
Brochado Neto FC, Cury MVM, Costa VS, et al (Hospital do Servidor Publico Estadual Sao Paulo (HSPE)-Dept of Vascular Surgery, Brazil)
Eur J Vasc Endovasc Surg 40:747-753, 2010

Objective.—To report our experience of long-term results of inframalleolar bypass.

Design.—Retrospective analysis.

Materials and Methods.—We analysed 122 inframalleolar bypasses performed between January 1991 and June 2005 in 116 patients. Most patients were treated for critical ischaemia (97%). The indication for the use of podalic arteries was a lack of tibial arteries with run-off to the foot. The dorsalis pedis was predominantly used for distal anastomoses (62.3%) and the greater saphenous vein (84.4%) as the conduit. The follow-up periods ranged from 1 to 60 months. The endpoints analysed were graft patency, limb salvage, preservation of deambulation and survival rate.

Results.—The cumulative patency was 58.2% at 3 years and 53.4% at 5 years. The best results were achieved with the devalvulated greater saphenous veins. Limb salvage was 70.0% at 3 years and 50.4% at 5 years, with preserved deambulation rates of 57.3% and 47.1%, respectively. There were 36 major and 45 minor amputations. At 3 years, the survival rate was 50.2% and the surgical mortality 13%. Female sex was associated with worse results for cumulative patency and limb salvage (*P* < 0.01).

Conclusions.—In the long term, inframalleolar bypass is a satisfactory option for limb salvage.

▶ This retrospective study of inframalleolar bypass grafts for limb salvage from a single institution reveals the continued utility of this procedure in patients with critical limb ischemia. The authors describe their experience with 116 patients (122 inframalleolar bypasses). The cumulative patency was 58.2% at 3 years and 53.4% at 5 years, and limb salvage was 70% at 3 years and 50.4% at 5 years.

As would be expected in this population, most patients were male (67%) with diabetes mellitus (84%), and tissue loss and infection (total of 91.7%) were the indications for the procedure. The most common outflow artery was the dorsalis pedis (62.3%), which has been demonstrated historically to be a durable vessel for limb salvage in diabetic patients. The most common procedure was a below-knee popliteal artery to dorsalis pedis artery bypass, which was classified as a short bypass (short bypass below the knee origin total, 57.3%; long bypass above the knee origin, 52.6%). Interestingly, there was no statistical difference in the patency of the long and short bypasses as has been demonstrated in other series. A total of 21 bypass procedures were performed to the vicariate branches of pedal arteries (medial plantar artery in 13, lateral plantar in 3, and lateral tarsal in 5). The authors found no statistical difference in diabetic and nondiabetic patients in regard to cumulative patency and limb salvage, which is likely a reflection of the fewer nondiabetic patients (16%) in the study.

This study again demonstrates that limb salvage is attainable in this patient population, and avoidance of a major amputation (36 total major amputations) can be achieved with a careful approach to distal bypass procedures. Again the authors reinforce what other trials such as the Bypass Versus Angioplasty in Severe Ischaemia of the Leg (BASIL) trial have revealed that in patients with TransAtlantic InterSociety Consensus (TASC) C and D lesions who can undergo a bypass procedure, it is the better choice.

N. Singh, MD

Quality of Life Among Lower Extremity Peripheral Arterial Disease Patients who have Undergone Endovascular or Surgical Revascularization: A Case-control Study

Remes L, Isoaho R, Vahlberg T, et al (Univ of Turku, Finland; et al)
Eur J Vasc Endovasc Surg 40:618-625, 2010

Objectives.—To assess the quality of life (QoL) of peripheral arterial disease (PAD) patients who have undergone either percutaneous transluminal angioplasty (PTA) only and/or one or more surgical revascularizations.

Design.—A postal questionnaire study in which a case-control methodology was applied.

Materials and methods.—131 patients with PTAs (mean age 70.7, SD 10.4 yrs; range 39—89, 58% men) and 100 with surgical revascularizations (mean age 67.8, SD 10.4 yrs; range 43—91, 62% men), in 1998—2003, and their age- and gender-matched controls were studied. The mean time since the last revascularization for PTA was 2.7, SD 1.3 yrs and for operated patients 3.5, SD 1.8 yrs. Ankle—brachial pressure index (ABI) and Mini-Mental-State Examination (MMSE) score were obtained from 70% of the patients.

QoL was assessed using 15D Health-related QoL instrument, Rand-36 Physical Functioning subscale, 6-item Brief Social Support Questionnaire, Geriatric Depression Scale (GDS), Self-reported Life Satisfaction (LS) score, and one 'perceived state of health' question.

Results.—Patients after endovascular and/or surgical revascularization (most with ABIs 0.5—0.89 and without cognitive impairment), had similarly lower QoL, GDS and LS indicated more depression than their controls.

Conclusion.—Poor QoL and depression should be thoroughly considered, alongside proper follow-up and ABI-measurements.

▶ A case-control model was undertaken in this study of peripheral arterial disease (PAD) patients who had undergone either endovascular or surgical revascularization in regard to the quality of life (QoL) and depression. The control group was age-matched and gender-matched from the same community, and postal questionnaires were used. Numerous standardized scales were used to assess not only health-related QoL but also social support, physical functioning status, as well as the Geriatric Depression Scale and Life Satisfaction score. A Mini-Mental State Examination (MMSE) and ankle-brachial index were also performed.

Other than cognitive impairment based on the MMSE, the PAD patients fared worse in every category. Thirty-nine percent of PAD patients had the expected findings of a lot of limitations in walking 500 m versus only 10% of the controls. For the Geriatric Depression Scale, 53% of PAD patients had scores of 5 to > 10 versus 23% of the controls, and 41% had Life Satisfaction scores of 12 to 20 versus 12% of the control group. Both these indicate a lower perceived QoL in this patient population.

The authors mention that the strength of the study is that all of original patients with revascularizations from the same district were covered and compared with similar controls from the district. It would be interesting to see if there was a difference within the PAD group (ie, those with claudication vs those who have critical limb ischemia). Nevertheless, the authors are to be commended for bringing the concept of depression to light in these patients we often follow for PAD symptoms only.

N. Singh, MD

Results of Catheter-Directed Endovascular Thrombolytic Treatment of Acute Ischaemia of the Leg
Løkse Nilssen GA, Svendsen D, Singh K, et al (Univ Hosp of North Norway and Univ of Tromsø, Norway; Univ Hosp of North Norway, Tromsø, Norway; et al)
Eur J Vasc Endovasc Surg 41:91-96, 2011

Objectives.—To observe immediate and late results of catheter-directed endovascular thrombolytic treatment of acute ischaemia of the leg.
Design, Material and Methods.—A total of 212 patients treated with Actilyse® at the University Hospital of North Norway because of acute arterial ischaemia of the leg during the period 01 January 2000—30 June 2006 were analysed retrospectively.
Results.—The radiologic outcome was judged to be successful in 101 (48%), adequate in 80 (38%) and failed in 31 (14%). At 1-year follow-up, 158 (75%) were alive without amputation, 14 (7%) were alive with amputation, 20 (9%) were dead without amputation and 20 (9%) were dead with amputation. Altogether, 34 (16%) were amputated and 40 (19%) were dead after 1 year. After an average observation period of 3.25 years, 111 (52%) were alive without amputation, 16 (8%) were alive with amputation, 60 (28%) were dead without amputation and 25 (12%) were dead with amputation. A total of 41 (19%) were amputated and 85 (40%) were dead. Fifty complications were registered; 30 (14%) patients had a compartment syndrome, eight (4%) had cerebral stroke and 12 (6%) had a myocardial infarction.
Conclusions.—The results are at least as good as historic controls and similar to international series. Especially, it appears as though the long-term results are somewhat better. The complication rate and morbidity are less than in surgery alone.

▶ This retrospective study of catheter-directed thrombolysis reviews the outcome of this therapy in conjunction with endovascular or open revascularization in patients presenting with acute ischemia. The authors describe their experience with Actilyse, a human plasminogen activator, and immediate and late results. Immediate results were classified as successful from the interventionist if there was contrast in all 3 leg arteries, adequate if some increase of contrast in the leg arteries was noted, and failed if no contrast in the leg arteries was apparent. Late results were defined as being alive or dead with and without an amputation.

In brief 48% were found to be immediately successful and 38% adequate. One-year follow-up revealed that 75% of patients were alive without an amputation and this dropped to 52% at 3.25 years. Interestingly, at 3.25 years in those patients who were alive without an amputation, thrombosis was the cause of acute ischemia in 41% versus 33% who had embolism as a cause and 26% with combination of thrombosis and embolism, while in patients who were dead without an amputation, thrombosis was the cause in 38%, embolism in 52%, and a combination of thrombosis and embolism in 10% demonstrating the confinement of chronic disease to the extremity and the likely lethal effects of embolic events.

The results are better than other series in regard to 1-year findings, however; even with these superior results, the overall mortality in this group of patients continues to be extremely high (40% at 3.25 years), underscoring the global issues in this patient population.

N. Singh, MD

13 Upper Extremity and Dialysis Access

Preoperative thrombolysis and venoplasty affords no benefit in patency following first rib resection and scalenectomy for subacute and chronic subclavian vein thrombosis

Guzzo JL, Chang K, Demos J, et al (The Johns Hopkins Hosp, Baltimore, MD)

J Vasc Surg 52:658-663, 2010

Background.—Axillosubclavian vein thrombosis, also known as Paget-Schroetter syndrome, is a rare presentation of thoracic outlet syndrome (TOS) representing approximately 5% of all cases. Conventional management consists of routine anticoagulation, operative decompression via first rib resection and scalenectomy (FRRS), and, recently, thrombolysis. The purpose of our study was to retrospectively review our experience with this condition and compare the effectiveness of preoperative endovascular intervention with thrombolysis and venoplasty to anticoagulation alone in those undergoing FRRS to preserve subclavian vein patency.

Methods.—A retrospective review was conducted for all venous TOS patients from July 2003 to May 2009 from a prospectively maintained database. Preoperative clinic notes were reviewed to allow stratification into two groups. One group consisted of patients undergoing preoperative endovascular intervention with thrombolysis and venoplasty, while the other group consisted of patients managed medically with anticoagulation alone prior to FRSS. Operative notes, postoperative venograms, and postoperative duplex imaging results were reviewed for presence of recanalization, chronic nonocclusive thrombus, or continued occlusion.

Results.—One hundred three patients had 110 FRRS for subclavian vein thrombosis (53 men, 50 women), seven of which had contralateral FRRS for thrombosis. The cohort averaged 31 years of age (range, 16-54 years) with an overall, mean follow-up time of 16 months (range, 1-52 months). Of the 110 veins evaluated, 45 underwent endovascular intervention (thombolysis, with or without venoplasty) prior to FRRS, and at 1 year, 41 (91%) were patent with improvement of symptoms. In the 65 veins on anticoagulation alone, 59 (91%) ultimately were patent, with symptomatic improvement in all. Overall, 91% (100/110) of subclavian veins were patent in patients completing follow-up, were asymptomatic, and back to their previous active lifestyle.

Conclusions.—Preoperative endovascular intervention offered no benefit over simple anticoagulation prior to FRRS, since the use of thrombolysis prior to FRRS, regardless of need for postoperative venoplasty, had little impact on overall rates of patency. The optimal treatment algorithm may merely be routine anticoagulation for all effort thrombosis patients prior to FRRS followed by venography with venoplasty if needed. The role of thrombolysis for Paget-Schroetter syndrome should be further investigated in randomized trials.

▶ One has to wonder whether this article is a step forward or backward in the assessment and treatment of patients with venous thoracic outlet syndrome. Perhaps it is a step forward in that it suggests that expensive and time-intensive preoperative thrombolysis is not necessary in patients who undergo first rib resection and scalenectomy for treatment of venous thoracic outlet syndrome. On the other hand, it may be a step backward in that many of us have seen patients with venous thoracic outlet syndrome obtain short-term dramatic relief of congestive symptoms with thrombolytic therapy. Making someone feel better, even in the short term, may not be a bad thing. Perhaps one could also argue that thrombolytic therapy followed by anticoagulation itself is adequate therapy for the large majority of patients with venous thoracic outlet syndrome? If it is really possible to operate on these patients and achieve reasonable results several months down the road, why not adopt a policy of thrombolytic therapy followed by anticoagulation and then select the first rib resection for those patients who have inadequate symptom relief?

G. L. Moneta, MD

Primary balloon angioplasty plus balloon angioplasty maturation to upgrade small-caliber veins (<3 mm) for arteriovenous fistulas
De Marco Garcia LP, Davila-Santini LR, Feng Q, et al (North Shore-Long Island Jewish Health System, Manhasset, NY)
J Vasc Surg 52:139-144, 2010

Objective.—Small-diameter veins are often a limiting factor for the successful creation of arteriovenous fistulas (AVFs). This study evaluated the use of intraoperative primary balloon angioplasty (PBA) as a technique to upgrade small-diameter veins during AVF creation. Sequential balloon angioplasty maturation (BAM) was evaluated as a technique to salvage failed fistulas, expedite maturation, and improve the patency of AVFs after PBA.

Methods.—Sixty-two PBAs were performed in 55 patients with an intent-to-treat using an all-autologous policy. PBAs of veins were performed just before AVF creation using 2.5- to 4-mm angioplasty balloons (1- to 1.5-mm larger than the nominal vein diameter). PBAs were performed through the spatulated end of the vein for a length of up to 8 cm using hydrophilic guidewires and hand inflations without fluoroscopy.

BAM was performed in 53 of the 62 PBAs at 2, 4, and 6 weeks after the PBA. Successful outcome was determined as the functional ability to use the fistula for hemodialysis without surgical revision.

Results.—Of the 62 PBAs, 53 (85.4%), comprising 47 of the original AVFs and 6 new site AVFs created at other sites, remained patent and subsequently underwent BAM with a resulting functional AVF. Fifteen of the 47 original AVFs: 14 due to occlusion; one AVF with a steal was ligated. Seven of the 14 fistulas that occluded were salvaged using recanalization techniques during sequential BAMs. Two of the seven fistulas that were not salvaged required AVGs (3%), and five patients underwent redo AVFs using alternative veins. These five cases were also performed using PBAs and BAMs technique. One patient with a functioning fistula underwent intentional ligation for steal syndrome and also underwent an alternative site AVF, PBA, and BAM. At 3 months, 53 AVFs were functional and successfully used for dialysis. Overall, a working AVF was obtained at the initial site in 47 of 55 patients (85.4%), and 53 (96.3%) received working AVFs that were functioning for dialysis access.

Conclusions.—Small or suboptimal veins can undergo PBA and then be matured to create functioning AVFs <2 months. Overall, >90% autogenous AVF rates can be achieved using PBA and BAM. BAM can be successfully used to mature AVFs created from small veins and salvage thrombosed AVFs in many cases. The use of these techniques may decrease the number of patients requiring AVGs and indwelling catheters.

▶ This is an extension of the authors' previous work where they have advocated repetitive balloon angioplasties post fistula placement (so-called balloon-assisted maturation) to aid in maturation of arteriovenous fistulas placed for dialysis access using smaller-caliber veins. Veins were measured preoperatively using ultrasound and with a tourniquet. Those ≤3 mm were treated with the authors' technique (Table 1 and Figs 1 and 2 in the original article). The authors feel their technique has advantages over intraoperative dilatation of the veins with vasodilating agents and rigid dilators. They feel balloon angioplasty techniques provide greater disruption of fibrotic areas within the smaller veins. We have tried this on a couple of occasions in our practice and anecdotally found that while the veins could be dilated, the amount of additional work following the initial procedure both in terms of additional imaging studies and follow-up angioplasties seemed excessive if an alternative site for construction of an arteriovenous fistula was available.

G. L. Moneta, MD

Achieving the Goal of the Fistula First Breakthrough Initiative for Prevalent Maintenance Hemodialysis Patients

Lynch JR, Wasse H, Armistead NC, et al (Mid-Atlantic Renal Coalition, Midlothian, VA; Emory Univ School of Medicine, Atlanta, GA)
Am J Kidney Dis 57:78-89, 2011

Background.—The Centers for Medicare & Medicaid Services (CMS) established a national goal of 66% arteriovenous fistula (AVF) use in prevalent hemodialysis (HD) patients for the current Fistula First Breakthrough Initiative. The feasibility of achieving the goal has been debated. We examined contemporary patterns of AVF use in prevalent patients to assess the potential for attaining the goal by dialysis facilities and their associated End-Stage Renal Disease Networks in the United States.

Study Design.—Observational study.

Setting & Participants.—US dialysis facilities with a mean HD patient census of 10 or more during the 40-month study period, January 2007-April 2010.

Outcomes & Measurements.—Mean changes in facility-level AVF use and percentage of facilities achieving the 66% prevalent AVF goal within the United States and each network.

Results.—Mean prevalent AVF use within dialysis facilities increased from 45.3% to 55.5% ($P < 0.001$) in the United States, but varied substantially across regions. The percentage of facilities achieving the 66% AVF use goal increased from 6.4% to 19.0% ($P < 0.001$). During the 40 months, 35.9% of facilities achieved the CMS goal for at least 1 month. On average, these facilities sustained mean use ≥66% for 12.9 ± 11.7 (SD) months. Case-mix and other facility characteristics explained 20% of the variation in proportion of facility patients using an AVF in the last measured month, leaving substantial unexplained variability.

Limitations.—This analysis is limited by the absence of facility case-mix data over time, and the national scope of the initiative precludes use of a comparison group.

Conclusions.—Achieving the CMS goal of 66% prevalent AVF use is feasible for individual dialysis facilities. There is a need to decrease regional variation before the CMS goal can be fully realized for US HD facilities (Fig 2).

▶ National Kidney Foundation Kidney Disease Outcome Quality Initiative guidelines recommend the use of arteriovenous fistula at the onset of renal replacement therapy.[1] Following these guidelines, the Centers for Medicare & Medicaid Services (CMS) developed the Fistula First Breakthrough Initiative (FFBI). The purpose was to disseminate information to improve arteriovenous fistula (AVF) use in the United States and to collect and analyze data on fistula use. The initial FFBI goal was 40% prevalence of AVF use. Once this was achieved, CMS then established a new national quality goal of 66% AVF use by June of 2009 in patients currently undergoing hemodialysis. The target of

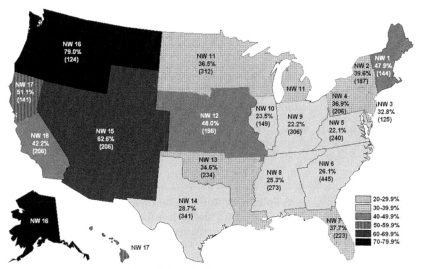

FIGURE 2.—Percentage of hemodialysis facilities (with ≥10 patients and 40 months of data) achieving the Centers for Medicare & Medicaid Services goal of 66% for prevalent arteriovenous fistula use at least once between January 2007 and April 2010. Source: Centers for Medicare & Medicaid Services, Vascular Access Data Set as delivered by the Network Information Technology Support contractor to Fistula First Breakthrough Initiative contractor, January 2007-April 2010. (Reprinted from Lynch JR, Wasse H, Armistead NC, et al. Achieving the goal of the Fistula First Breakthrough Initiative for prevalent maintenance hemodialysis patients. *Am J Kidney Dis.* 2011;57:78-89, with permission from the National Kidney Foundation, Inc.)

66% was based on observations that AVF use for hemodialysis in Asia and Europe generally exceeds 60% and can be as high as 90%.[2] However, some question that the end-stage renal disease (ESRD) population in Asia and Europe may not be similar to that of the United States. In addition, AVF use in the United States is measured for the entire ESRD population. International estimates, however, may be based on treatment facility samples that do not fully capture the entire ESRD population. This has led some to question the appropriateness of the CMS goal of 66% AVF fistula use in the US hemodialysis population. The data suggest the CMS goal of achieving 66% prevalent hemodialysis use is obtainable but not easily obtainable. It is not clear why some facilities are able to obtain this goal and others do not do as well. There can be vastly different performances in geographically contiguous networks (Fig 2). It was noted that facilities with higher percentages of white and Hispanic patients, patients with diabetes as a primary cause of ESRD, patients with glomerulonephritis as the primary cause of ESRD, and patients beginning long-term hemodialysis therapy tended to have a higher prevalence of AVF use. AVF use was lower in facilities with higher percentages of women, in patients starting long-term hemodialysis who also had peripheral vascular disease, and in facilities with older populations. However, case mix explains only a proportion of the variation of facility AVF use, and much work needs to be done to fully understand regional variability. Finally, it needs to be emphasized that the slogan "Fistula first," does not mean all patients should receive an

AVF. Patients with poor likelihood of maturation of a fistula or a shorter life expectancy may be better candidates for a graft rather than a fistula.

G. L. Moneta, MD

References

1. National Kidney Foundation: KDOQI. Clinical practice guidelines and clinical practice recommendations for vascular access 2006. *Am J Kidney Dis.* 2006;48: S176-S322.
2. Ethier J, Mendelssohn DC, Elder SJ, et al. Vascular access use and outcomes: an international perspective from the Dialysis Outcomes and Practice Patterns Study. *Nephrol Dial Transplant.* 2008;23:3219-3226.

Infectious Complications Following Conversion to Buttonhole Cannulation of Native Arteriovenous Fistulas: A Quality Improvement Report
Labriola L, Crott R, Desmet C, et al (Université Catholique de Louvain, Brussels, Belgium)
Am J Kidney Dis 57:442-448, 2011

Background.—Constant-site or buttonhole cannulation of native arteriovenous fistulas (AVFs) has gained in popularity compared with rope-ladder cannulation. However, cannulating nonhealed skin might increase the risk of (AVF-related) infectious events, as suggested by small reports.
Study Design.—Quality improvement report.
Setting & Participants.—All patients on in-center hemodialysis therapy using a native AVF from January 1, 2001, to June 30, 2010.
Quality Improvement Plan.—Shift to buttonhole cannulation between August 2004 and January 2005. Because the infectious event rate increased after the shift, educational workshops were held in May 2008 for all nurses, with review of every step of buttonhole protocol.
Outcomes.—Infectious events (unexplained bacteremia caused by skin bacteria and/or local AVF infection) and complicated infectious events (resulting in metastatic infection, death, or AVF surgery) were ascertained during 4 periods: (1) rope-ladder technique in all, (2) switch to buttonhole, (3) buttonhole in all before workshops, and (4) buttonhole in all after workshops.
Results.—177 patients (aged 70.4 ± 11.5 years) with 193 AVFs were analyzed, including 186,481 AVF-days. 57 infectious events occurred (0.31 events/1,000 AVF-days). The incidence of infectious events increased after the switch to the buttonhole method (0.17 [95% CI, 0.086-0.31], 0.11 [95% CI, 0.0014-0.63], and 0.43 [95% CI, 0.29-0.61] events/ 1,000 AVF-days in periods 1, 2, and 3, respectively; $P = 0.003$). This reached significance during only the second full year of buttonhole cannulation. During period 4, the incidence tended to decrease (0.34 events/ 1,000 AVF-days). Complicated infectious events (n = 12) were virtually restricted to period 3 (n = 11; 0.153 [95% CI, 0.076-0.273] events/ 1,000 AVF-days), with a significant decrease in period 4 (n = 1; 0.024

[95% CI, 0.001-0.118] events/1,000 AVF-days; RR for period 3 vs period 4, 6.37 [95% CI, 1.09-138.4]; $P = 0.04$).
Limitations.—Observational partly retrospective design.
Conclusion.—Intensive staff education regarding strict protocol for the buttonhole procedure was associated with a decrease in infectious events.

▶ Twardowski[1] reported the use of buttonhole cannulation of native arteriovenous fistulas (AVFs) with blunt needles in 1977. This technique has recently gained popularity and differs from the traditional rope-ladder method of access cannulation. In the buttonhole technique, the AVF is repeatedly accessed at the same site with blunt needles. A tunnel can be created from the skin to the vessel using a constant site over 6 hemodialysis sessions. In theory, in subsequent cannulation, this tunnel guides the blunt needle to the access vessel. Careful disinfection and withdrawing of the scab formed at the cannulation site are critical to success of the buttonhole technique. Proponents of the technique argue that it provides for easier cannulation, fewer missed sticks, less pain, and faster hemostasis after needle removal, as well as fewer hematomas and aneurysms. Because the buttonhole technique essentially requires cannulation through nonhealed skin, it is also possible that the technique may lead to an increased risk of infectious events associated with arteriovenous fistulas. The authors conducted an observational study to determine whether patients with AVFs who switched to buttonhole cannulation had an increase in rates of infectious

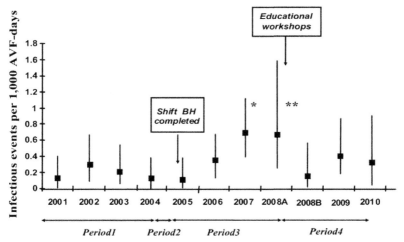

FIGURE 1.—Annual incidence of infectious events. Lines around the squares indicate 95% confidence intervals; *$P < 0.05$ (compared with 2001, 2002, 2003, 2004, 2005, 2006, and 2008B); **$P < 0.05$ (compared with 2001, 2003, 2004, 2005, and 2008B). Period 1 (January 1, 2001, to August 3, 2004): all patients using rope-ladder technique with sharp needles; period 2 (August 4, 2004, to January 31, 2005): progressive switch to buttonhole (BH) method using blunt needles; period 3 (February 1, 2005, to May 19, 2008): all patients using BH method, before educational workshops; and period 4 (May 20, 2008, to June 30, 2010): all patients using BH method, after educational workshops. Abbreviation: AVF, arteriovenous fistula. (Reprinted from Labriola L, Crott R, Desmet C, et al. Infectious complications following conversion to buttonhole cannulation of native arteriovenous fistulas: a quality improvement report. *Am J Kidney Dis.* 2011;57:442-448. Reprinted from American Journal of Kidney Diseases, copyright 2011 with permission from the National Kidney Foundation.)

events. There are not many infections of native AVFs, but this article documented an increase in infections and complications associated with the switch to buttonhole cannulations. The increase did not reach statistical significance until after the third year of the switch to the buttonhole technique. The authors' suspicion is that technicians accessing the fistulas became complacent with the hygiene protocol of the buttonhole technique. The suspicion is somewhat supported by a subsequent decrease in infectious complications after institution of an educational program emphasizing proper hygiene in accessing of the AVFs with the buttonhole technique (Fig 1). The data are consistent with the recent emphasis on meticulous hygiene with access of any type of indwelling intravenous line or permanent vascular access device.

G. L. Moneta, MD

Reference

1. Twardowski Z. The "buttonhole" method of needle insertion takes center stage in the attempt to revive daily home hemodialysis. *Contemp Dial Nephrol.* 1977;18: 18-19.

14 Carotid and Cerebrovascular Disease

10-year stroke prevention after successful carotid endarterectomy for asymptomatic stenosis (ACST-1): a multicentre randomised trial
Halliday A, on behalf of the Asymptomatic Carotid Surgery Trial (ACST) Collaborative Group (John Radcliffe Hosp, Oxford, UK; et al)
Lancet 376:1074-1084, 2010

Background.—If carotid artery narrowing remains asymptomatic (ie, has caused no recent stroke or other neurological symptoms), successful carotid endarterectomy (CEA) reduces stroke incidence for some years. We assessed the long-term effects of successful CEA.

Methods.—Between 1993 and 2003, 3120 asymptomatic patients from 126 centres in 30 countries were allocated equally, by blinded minimised randomisation, to immediate CEA (median delay 1 month, IQR $0\cdot3-2\cdot5$) or to indefinite deferral of any carotid procedure, and were followed up until death or for a median among survivors of 9 years (IQR 6−11). The primary outcomes were perioperative mortality and morbidity (death or stroke within 30 days) and non-perioperative stroke. Kaplan-Meier percentages and logrank p values are from intention-to-treat analyses. This study is registered, number ISRCTN26156392.

Findings.—1560 patients were allocated immediate CEA versus 1560 allocated deferral of any carotid procedure. The proportions operated on while still asymptomatic were $89\cdot7\%$ versus $4\cdot8\%$ at 1 year (and $92\cdot1\%$ *vs* $16\cdot5\%$ at 5 years). Perioperative risk of stroke or death within 30 days was $3\cdot0\%$ (95% CI $2\cdot4-3\cdot9$; 26 non-disabling strokes plus 34 disabling or fatal perioperative events in 1979 CEAs). Excluding perioperative events and non-stroke mortality, stroke risks (immediate *vs* deferred CEA) were $4\cdot1\%$ versus $10\cdot0\%$ at 5 years (gain $5\cdot9\%$, 95% CI $4\cdot0-7\cdot8$) and $10\cdot8\%$ versus $16\cdot9\%$ at 10 years (gain $6\cdot1\%$, $2\cdot7-9\cdot4$); ratio of stroke incidence rates $0\cdot54$, 95% CI $0\cdot43-0\cdot68$, p<$0\cdot0001$. 62 versus 104 had a disabling or fatal stroke, and 37 versus 84 others had a non-disabling stroke. Combining perioperative events and strokes, net risks were $6\cdot9\%$ versus $10\cdot9\%$ at 5 years (gain $4\cdot1\%$, $2\cdot0-6\cdot2$) and $13\cdot4\%$ versus $17\cdot9\%$ at 10 years (gain $4\cdot6\%$, $1\cdot2-7\cdot9$). Medication was similar

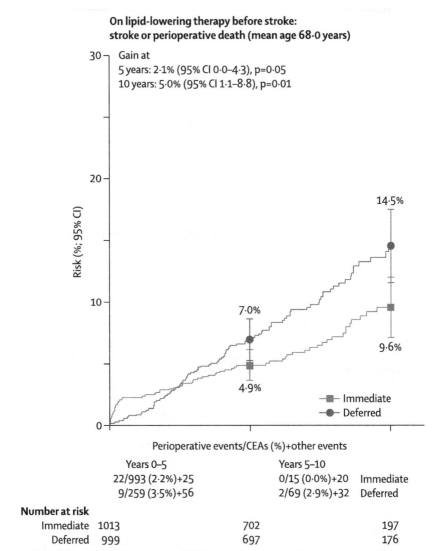

On lipid-lowering therapy before stroke:
stroke or perioperative death (mean age 68·0 years)

Gain at
5 years: 2·1% (95% CI 0·0–4·3), p=0·05
10 years: 5·0% (95% CI 1·1–8·8), p=0·01

14·5%

7·0%

9·6%

4·9%

Immediate
Deferred

Perioperative events/CEAs (%)+other events

Years 0–5	Years 5–10	
22/993 (2·2%)+25	0/15 (0·0%)+20	Immediate
9/259 (3·5%)+56	2/69 (2·9%)+32	Deferred

Number at risk

Immediate	1013	702	197
Deferred	999	697	176

FIGURE 5.—10-year risks, by current lipid-lowering therapy (at or after randomisation). CEA=carotid endarterectomy. py=per year. (Reprinted from The Lancet, Halliday A, on behalf of the Asymptomatic Carotid Surgery Trial (ACST) Collaborative Group. 10-year stroke prevention after successful carotid endarterectomy for asymptomatic stenosis (ACST-1): a multicentre randomised trial. *Lancet.* 2010;376:1074-1084. Copyright 2010, with permission from Elsevier.)

in both groups; throughout the study, most were on antithrombotic and antihypertensive therapy. Net benefits were significant both for those on lipid-lowering therapy and for those not, and both for men and for women up to 75 years of age at entry (although not for older patients).

Interpretation.—Successful CEA for asymptomatic patients younger than 75 years of age reduces 10-year stroke risks. Half this reduction is in disabling or fatal strokes. Net benefit in future patients will depend on their risks from unoperated carotid lesions (which will be reduced by medication), on future surgical risks (which might differ from those in trials), and on whether life expectancy exceeds 10 years (Fig 5).

▶ From 1993 to 2003, the Asymptomatic Carotid Surgery Trial (ACST-1) randomly assigned patients to immediate carotid endarterectomy (CEA) or deferral of a carotid procedure until a more definitive indication arose. Patients were followed up until 2006-2008. Median-term results of this trial were reported in 2004.[1] In this article, the authors described 10-year results of the ACST trial and delineated benefits by participants' medical treatment and characteristics. The study provides long-term evidence of the effectiveness of CEA for stroke prevention in patients with initially asymptomatic high-grade carotid stenosis. The authors point out that their data suggest that potential long-term benefits of CEA are limited in those who have < 10 years of life expectancy. Fig 5 suggests compliant patients with effective antithrombotic lipid lowering and antihypertensive therapy and little likelihood of death from other causes within 10 years would have a predicted absolute 10-year stroke reduction of about 5%, suggesting about 20 endarterectomies will be required to avoid 1 stroke at 10 years. Cost-effectiveness versus medical effectiveness with such an approach will, of course, be debated. Overall, the trial suggests that for otherwise healthy males and females < 75 years of age, there is a net modest benefit in stroke reduction for prophylactic CEA in patients with asymptomatic high-grade internal carotid artery stenosis.

G. L. Moneta, MD

Reference

1. Halliday A, Mansfield A, Marro J, et al. Prevention of disabling and fatal strokes by successful carotid endarterectomy in patients without recent neurological symptoms: randomised controlled trial. *Lancet.* 2004;363:1491-1502.

A Cost-Effectiveness Analysis of Carotid Artery Stenting Compared With Endarterectomy
Young KC, Holloway RG, Burgin WS, et al (Univ of Rochester Med Ctr, NY)
J Stroke Cerebrovasc Dis 19:404-409, 2010

Endarterectomy and angioplasty with stenting have emerged as 2 alternative treatments for carotid artery stenosis. This study's objective was to determine the cost-effectiveness of carotid artery stenting (CAS) compared with carotid endarterectomy (CEA) in symptomatic subjects who are suitable for either intervention. A Markov analysis of these 2 revascularization procedures was conducted using direct Medicare costs (2007 US$) and characteristics of a symptomatic 70-year-old cohort over a lifetime. In the base case analysis, CAS produced 8.97 quality-adjusted life-years, compared with 9.64 quality-adjusted life-years for CEA. The incremental cost of stenting was $17,700, and thus CAS was dominated by CEA. Sensitivity analyses show that the long-term probabilities of major stroke or mortality influenced the results. In the base case analysis, CEA for patients with symptomatic stenosis has a greater benefit than CAS, with lower direct costs. With 59% probability, CEA will be the optimal intervention when all of the model assumptions are varied simultaneously.

▶ In this analysis, carotid endarterectomy (CEA) was the most cost-effective option for the treatment of symptomatic carotid stenosis in a hypothetical cohort suitable for either carotid artery stenting (CAS) or CEA. Of the 2 options, CEA or CAS, CEA maximizes health benefits and cost savings. The authors' analysis incorporated weighted averages (by trial size) for stroke or death beyond 30 days. These weighted averages, from the randomized trials available at the time the article was prepared, show a higher long-term risk of stroke following CAS. Additional analyses indicated that assumptions with respect to long-term stroke risk and mortality further influence the finding that CEA is the most cost-effective option for treatment of symptomatic carotid stenosis. With lower thresholds for cost-effectiveness, the probability that CEA is the treatment of choice increases further from 59% to 68%. The authors' conclusion, "Given the uncertainty about the effectiveness and cost-effectiveness of CAS compared with CEA, CAS should remain limited to randomized trials or select populations of patients with carotid stenosis," seems very reasonable.

G. L. Moneta, MD

Anatomical and Technical Factors Associated With Stroke or Death During Carotid Angioplasty and Stenting: Results From the Endarterectomy Versus Angioplasty in Patients With Symptomatic Severe Carotid Stenosis (EVA-3S) Trial and Systematic Review
Naggara O, for the EVA-3S Investigators (Université Paris Descartes, France; et al)
Stroke 42:380-388, 2011

Background and Purpose.—The purposes of this study were to assess the relationships between anatomic and technical factors and the 30-day risk of stroke or death after carotid angioplasty and stenting in the Endarterectomy versus Stenting in Patients with Symptomatic Severe Carotid Stenosis (EVA-3S) trial and to perform a systematic review of the literature.

Methods.—We included patients from EVA-3S in whom carotid stenting was attempted irrespective of allocated treatment. Two radiologists blinded to clinical data independently assessed the aortic arch and carotid arteries on procedural angiograms. In addition, we performed a systematic review of studies that reported 30-day risk of stroke or death in relation with arterial anatomy and technique. Outcomes were stroke or death and stroke occurring within 30 days of the carotid angioplasty and stenting procedure.

Results.—Two hundred sixty-two patients from EVA-3S fulfilled the inclusion criteria (including 1 initially allocated to surgery and 13 in whom stent insertion failed). Within 30 days after the procedure, 25 (9.5%) patients had a stroke or had died. The risk of stroke or death was higher in patients with internal carotid artery—common carotid artery angulation ≥60° (relative risk, 4.96; 2.29 to 10.74) and lower in those treated with cerebral protection devices (relative risk [RR], 0.38; 0.17 to 0.85). In the systematic review (56 studies; 34 398 patients), the risk of stroke or death was higher in patients with left-sided carotid angioplasty and stenting (RR, 1.29; 1.05 to 1.58), increased internal carotid artery-common carotid artery angulation (RR, 3.41; 1.52 to 7.63), and when the target internal carotid artery stenosis was >10 mm (RR, 2.36; 1.28 to 3.38). There was no significant increase in risk of stroke or death in patients with Type III aortic arch, aortic arch calcification, or with ostial involvement, calcification, ulceration or degree of stenosis of the target internal carotid artery stenosis. The use of a cerebral protection device was associated with a lower risk of stroke or death (RR, 0.55; 0.41 to 0.73). Risk was not related with stent or cerebral protection device type.

Conclusions.—Our results strongly suggest that some technical and anatomic factors, especially extreme angulation of the carotid artery, have an impact on the risks of carotid angioplasty and stenting (Figs 3 and 4).

▶ There are some widely recognized anatomic factors that may influence the risk of stroke following carotid angioplasty and stenting (CAS). It seems quite clear at this point that large randomized clinical trials of 30-day stroke and death rates favor carotid endarterectomy (CEA) over CAS. However, once the perioperative period has passed, both CAS and CEA appear effective in preventing midterm stroke. The implication is that decreasing periprocedural rates of CAS would make the procedure more attractive, as long-term stroke prevention following CAS or CEA is more equivalent. The authors therefore sought to assess relationships

	N Studies	N Patients	Pooled RR (95% IC) for Stroke or death	RR (95% CI)	I^2	P (Het)	P (Sig)
Anatomical factors							
Type III aortic arch	2	488		1.82 (0.97-3.41)	0	0.81	0.06
Left vs right side	5	9384		1.29 (1.05-1.58)	26.55	0.24	0.02
Increased ICA-CCA angulation	2	406		3.41 (1.52-7.63)	45.13	0.18	<0.001
Aortic arch calcification	2	341		1.80 (0.74-4.37)	22.00	0.26	0.19
Contralateral ICA occlusion	8	4050		0.83 (0.48-1.44)	0	0.88	0.50
Target stenosis							
Lesion length > 10mm	3	634		2.36 (1.28-3.38)	14.36	0.31	0.01
Calcification	5	1334		1.62 (0.99-2.64)	0	0.67	0.05
Ostial location	2	781		1.75 (0.99-3.11)	0	0.54	0.06
Stenosis≥90% (NASCET)	5	4547		1.29 (0.64-2.58)	70.87	0.01	0.88
Ulceration	3	906		1.73 (0.64-4.69)	53.81	0.11	0.15
Technical factors							
Cerebral protection	23	15702		0.55 (0.41-0.73)	40.67	0.02	<0.001
Closed vs open cells stent	4	4830		0.80 (0.47-1.37)	55.66	0.08	0.15
Filter vs balloon	3	3987		0.88 (0.45-1.71)	0	0.84	0.71
Eccentric vs concentric filter	3	3253		1.64 (0.71-3.76)	0	0.45	0.25

0 0.5 1.0 1.5 2.0 2.5 3.0 3.5 4.0

FIGURE 3.—Pooled risks of 30-day stroke or death according to different subgroups. (Reprinted from Naggara O, for the EVA-3S Investigators. Anatomical and technical factors associated with stroke or death during carotid angioplasty and stenting: results from the endarterectomy versus angioplasty in patients with symptomatic severe carotid stenosis (EVA-3S) trial and systematic review. *Stroke.* 2011;42:380-388, with permission from American Heart Association, Inc.)

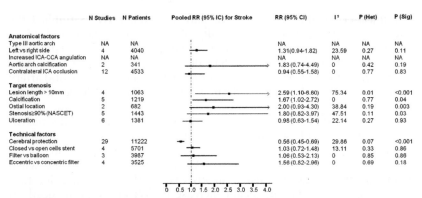

	N Studies	N Patients	Pooled RR (95% IC) for Stroke	RR (95% CI)	I²	P (Het)	P (Sig)
Anatomical factors							
Type III aortic arch	NA	NA		NA	NA	NA	NA
Left vs right side	4	4040		1.31(0.94-1.82)	23.59	0.27	0.11
Increased ICA-CCA angulation	NA	NA		NA	NA	NA	NA
Aortic arch calcification	2	341		1.83 (0.74-4.49)	0	0.42	0.19
Contralateral ICA occlusion	12	4533		0.94 (0.55-1.58)	0	0.77	0.83
Target stenosis							
Lesion length > 10mm	4	1063		2.59 (1.10-6.60)	75.34	0.01	<0.001
Calcification	5	1219		1.67 (1.02-2.72)	0	0.77	0.04
Ostial location	2	682		2.00 (0.93-4.30)	38.84	0.19	0.003
Stenosis≥90% (NASCET)	5	1443		1.80 (0.82-3.97)	47.51	0.11	0.03
Ulceration	6	1381		0.98 (0.63-1.54)	22.14	0.27	0.93
Technical factors							
Cerebral protection	29	11222		0.56 (0.45-0.69)	29.86	0.07	<0.001
Closed vs open cells stent	4	5701		1.03 (0.72-1.48)	13.11	0.33	0.86
Filter vs balloon	3	3987		1.06 (0.53-2.13)	0	0.85	0.86
Eccentric vs concentric filter	4	3525		1.56 (0.82-2.96)	0	0.69	0.18

0 0.5 1.0 1.5 2.0 2.5 3.0 3.5 4.0

FIGURE 4.—Pooled risks of 30-day stroke according to different subgroups. ICA indicates internal carotid artery; NASCET, North American Symptomatic Carotid Endarterectomy Trial; p(het), probability value associated to Cochran χ^2 statistical test for heterogeneity; I², percentage of the variability in effect estimates that is due to heterogeneity rather than sampling error (chance); NA, not assessable. In the forest plots, boxes correspond to RRs and their 95% CI. (Reprinted from Naggara O, for the EVA-3S Investigators. Anatomical and technical factors associated with stroke or death during carotid angioplasty and stenting: results from the endarterectomy versus angioplasty in patients with symptomatic severe carotid stenosis (EVA-3S) trial and systematic review. *Stroke.* 2011;42:380-388, with permission from American Heart Association, Inc.)

between anatomic and technical factors and 30-day risk of stroke and death following CAS. By improving patient selection for CAS, overall efficacy of CAS may be improved by decreasing periprocedural complications. There is in fact no procedure in which the risk of the procedure cannot be diminished by improved patient selection. In that regard, this article by the Endarterectomy versus Stenting in Patients with Symptomatic Severe Carotid Stenosis (EVA-3S) investigators is an important contribution to the CAS literature. Both CEA and CAS are potentially important modalities in decreasing the risk of stroke in patients with internal carotid artery stenosis (Figs 3 and 4). Unfortunately, many of the anatomic risk factors identified for CAS will be discovered only during the course of the angiogram accompanying the procedure. Perhaps the incidence of 30-day stroke or death associated with CAS could be decreased if the operators were willing to back out of the procedure when an anatomic risk factor for an adverse outcome is identified during their preliminary angiogram?

G. L. Moneta, MD

Carotid Artery Stenting vs Carotid Endarterectomy: Meta-analysis and Diversity-Adjusted Trial Sequential Analysis of Randomized Trials

Bangalore S, Kumar S, Wetterslev J, et al (New York Univ School of Medicine; Univ of Nebraska Med Ctr, Omaha; Copenhagen Univ Hosp, Denmark; et al)
Arch Neurol 68:172-184, 2011

Background.—The role of carotid artery stenting (CAS) when compared with carotid endarterectomy (CEA) is controversial, with recent trials showing an increased risk of harm with CAS.

Objective.—To evaluate the periprocedural and intermediate to long-term benefits and harms of CAS compared with CEA.

Data Sources and Study Selection.—PubMed, EMBASE, and Cochrane Central Register of Controlled Trials searches for randomized clinical trials until June 2010 of CAS compared with CEA for carotid artery disease. Periprocedural (≤30-day) outcomes (death, myocardial infarction [MI], or stroke; death or any stroke; any stroke; and MI) and intermediate to long-term outcomes (outcomes as in the Stenting and Angioplasty With Protection in Patients at High Risk for Endarterectomy [SAPPHIRE] trial: composite of periprocedural death, MI, or stroke plus ipsilateral stroke or death thereafter; periprocedural death or stroke plus ipsilateral stroke thereafter; death or any stroke; and any stroke) were evaluated.

Data Extraction.—Two of us independently extracted data in duplicate. Baseline characteristics, inclusion and exclusion criteria, use of an embolic protection device, US vs non-US study, and the earlier-mentioned outcomes of interest were extracted from each trial.

Data Synthesis.—We identified 13 randomized clinical trials randomizing 7477 participants. Carotid artery stenting was associated with an increased risk of periprocedural outcomes of death, MI, or stroke (odds ratio = 1.31; 95% confidence interval, 1.08-1.59), 65% and 67% increases in death or stroke and any stroke, respectively, but with 55% and 85% reductions in the risk of MI and cranial nerve injury, respectively, when compared with CEA. The trial sequential monitoring boundary was crossed by the cumulative z curve, suggesting firm evidence for at least a 20% relative risk increase of periprocedural death or stroke and any stroke and at least a 15% reduction in MI with CAS compared with CEA. Similarly, CAS was associated with 19%, 38%, 24%, and 48% increases in the intermediate to long-term outcomes of SAPPHIRE-like outcome, periprocedural death or stroke and ipsilateral stroke thereafter, death or any stroke, and any stroke, respectively. The trial sequential monitoring boundary was crossed by the cumulative z curve, suggesting firm evidence for at least a 20% relative risk increase of any stroke.

Conclusions.—In this largest and most comprehensive meta-analysis to date using outcomes that are standard in contemporary studies, CAS was associated with an increased risk of both periprocedural and intermediate to long-term outcomes, but with a reduction in periprocedural MI and cranial nerve injury. Strategies are urgently needed to identify patients who are best served by CAS vs CEA.

▶ Prior to this meta-analysis, the most recent meta-analysis of the results of carotid endarterectomy (CEA) versus carotid artery stenting (CAS) was performed by Meier et al.[1] The authors felt a new meta-analysis was appropriate given that since the Meier et al publication, the Carotid Revascularization Endarterectomy Versus Stent Trial (CREST) was published as well as the long-term results of the Carotid and Vertebral Artery Transluminal Angioplasty Study (CAVATAS) and Stent-supported Percutaneous Angioplasty of the Carotid Artery Versus Endarterectomy (SPACE). The purpose of this new meta-analysis was therefore to provide a comprehensive approach incorporating both short- and long-term comparisons between CEA and CAS using all available data from published randomized trials. The results suggest the frequently reported advantages of CEA over CAS in preventing short-term risk of stroke (Fig 1 in the original article) are continued in the long term (Fig 2 in the original article). There are, of course, still many questions regarding the use of CEA or CAS. We do not know whether one or the other intervention is better in patients with acute stroke nor do we know which is associated with less long-term restenosis. Overall, in younger patients, CEA and CAS may be roughly equivalent with regard to neurologic outcome. However, in older patients, if the goal is to prevent stroke, CEA is more effective in preventing stroke than CAS.

G. L. Moneta, MD

Reference

1. Meier P, Knapp G, Tamhane U, Chaturvedi S, Gurm HS. Short term and interme- diate term comparison of endarterectomy versus stenting for carotid artery stenosis: systematic review and meta-analysis of randomised controlled clinical trials. *BMJ.* 2010;340:c467.

Carotid Bruits and Cerebrovascular Disease Risk: A Meta-Analysis
Pickett CA, Jackson JL, Hemann BA, et al (Keller Army Hosp, West Point, NY; Zablocki VA Med Ctr, Milwaukee, WI; Walter Reed Army Med Ctr, Washington, DC)
Stroke 41:2295-2302, 2010

Background and Purpose.—Current guidelines recommend against routine auscultation of carotid arteries, believing that carotid bruits are poor predictors of either underlying carotid stenosis or stroke risk in asymptomatic patients. We investigated whether the presence of a carotid bruit is associated with increased risk for transient ischemic attack, stroke, or death by stroke (stroke death).

Methods.—We searched Medline (1966 to December 2009) and EMBASE (1974 to December 2009) with the terms "carotid" and "bruit." Bibliographies of all retrieved articles were also searched. Articles were included if they prospectively reported the incidence of transient ischemic attack, stroke, or stroke death in asymptomatic adults. Two authors independently reviewed and extracted data.

Results.—We included 28 prospective cohort articles that followed a total of 17 913 patients for 67 708 patient-years. Among studies that directly compared patients with and without bruits, the rate ratio for tran- sient ischemic attack was 4.00 (95% CI, 1.8 to 9.0, $P<0.0005$, n=5 studies), stroke was 2.5 (95% CI, 1.8 to 3.5, $P<0.0005$, n=6 studies), and stroke death was 2.7 (95% CI, 1.33 to 5.53, $P=0.002$, n=3 studies). Among the larger pool of studies that provided data on rates, transient ischemic attack rates were 2.6 per 100 patient-years (95% CI, 2.0 to 3.2, $P<0.0005$, n=24 studies) for those with bruits compared with 0.9 per 100 patient-years

(95% CI, 0.2 to 1.6, P=0.02, n=5 studies) for those without carotid bruits. Stroke rates were 1.6 per 100 patient-years (95% CI, 1.3 to 1.9, P<0.0005, n=26 studies) for those with bruits compared with 1.3 per 100 patient-years (95% CI, 0.8 to 1.7, P<0.0005, n=6) without carotid bruits, and death rates were 0.32 (95% CI, 0.20 to 0.44, P<0.005, n=13 studies) for those with bruits compared with 0.35 (95% CI, 0.00 to 0.81, P=0.17, n=3 studies) for those without carotid bruits.

Conclusion.—The presence of a carotid bruit may increase the risk of cerebrovascular disease.

▶ A classic teaching is that the presence of carotid bruits significantly increases risk of myocardial infarction and cardiovascular death. This orientation has been supported by a large recent meta-analysis.[1] The strength of the relationship between cerebrovascular events and carotid bruits is less clear. The Systolic Hypertension in the Elderly study found carotid bruits to be a weak predictor of stroke with relative risk of 1.3.[2] However, the Evans County Study found a stronger relationship with a relative risk of 4.1 for a combined end point of stroke and transient ischemic attack (TIA).[3] Nevertheless, osculation for carotid bruits in asymptomatic patients is not recommended by the US Preventative Services Task Force and the Canadian Task Force.[4,5] The authors sought to investigate if carotid bruit was associated with an increased risk of transient ischemic attack, stroke, or stroke death. Their meta-analysis suggests a higher neurologic risk associated with carotid bruits than is generally appreciated. Patients with carotid bruits have more than 4 times the risk of TIA and over twice the risk for stroke as well as an increased risk of stroke death when compared with patients without carotid bruits. However, the study has several limitations. First, most studies included in the meta-analysis did not report enough information to evaluate the effects of compounding variables. Second, the study tells us nothing about intervening among patients with carotid bruits or that intervention improves outcomes. Also we do not know the degree of stenosis associated with carotid bruits and all strokes and TIAs tracked were not necessarily ipsilateral to the bruits. At the very least, however, carotid bruits appear to identify patients at increased neurologic risk. In conjunction with the known increased risk of cardiac events associated with carotid bruits, it is certainly reasonable to conclude that a carotid bruit identifies patients who require aggressive modification of atherosclerotic risk factors. Listening to the neck may not be such a bad thing!

G. L. Moneta, MD

References

1. Pickett CA, Jackson JL, Hemann BA, Atwood JE. Carotid bruits as a prognostic indicator of cardiovascular death and myocardial infarction: a meta-analysis. *Lancet.* 2008;371:1587-1594.
2. Shorr RI, Johnson KC, Wan JY, et al. The prognostic significance of asymptomatic carotid bruits in the elderly. *J Gen Intern Med.* 1998;13:86-90.
3. Heyman A, Wilkinson WE, Heyden S, et al. Risk of stroke in asymptomatic persons with cervical arterial bruits: a population study in Evans County, Georgia. *N Engl J Med.* 1980;302:838-841.

4. U.S. Preventative Services Task Force. Screening for carotid artery stenosis: U.S. Preventive Services Task Force recommendation statement. *Ann Intern Med.* 2007;147:854-859.

5. Mackey A, Cote R, Battista RN. *Canadian Task Force on the Periodic Health Examination. Canadian Guide to Clinical Preventative Health Care.* Ottawa, Ontario: Health Canada; 1994. 692–704.

Clopidogrel Versus Dipyridamole in Addition to Aspirin in Reducing Embolization Detected With Ambulatory Transcranial Doppler: A Randomized Trial

King A, Bath PMW, Markus HS (St Georges Univ of London, UK; Univ of Nottingham, UK)
Stroke 42:650-655, 2011

Background and Purpose.—After stroke and transient ischemic attack there is a high early risk of recurrent stroke, particularly in large artery disease. It has been suggested more intensive antiplatelet regimens are required, but trial data are lacking. Treatment efficacy can be evaluated using transcranial Doppler detection of embolic signals. Ambulatory transcranial Doppler has recently been developed; prolonged recording may reduce subject numbers required to determine therapeutic efficacy. In a randomized trial (ISRCTN68019845) with blinded end point evaluation, we determined whether treatment with dipyridamole or clopidogrel, in addition to aspirin, was more effective at reducing embolization.

Methods.—Consecutive patients with recent symptomatic carotid stenosis were recruited. Ambulatory transcranial Doppler and platelet aggregometry were performed at baseline and 48 hours. Patients, all on aspirin, were randomized to dipyridamole or clopidogrel. Recordings were analyzed offline masked to subject identity.

Results.—Sixty patients were recruited, 30 in each arm. The primary end point of change in embolic signal frequency did not differ between groups ($P=0.36$). In patients with embolic signals at baseline, there was no difference in reduction in embolic signal frequency: dipyridamole (75.5; SD 17.7%) versus clopidogrel (77.5; SD 20.5%; $P=0.77$). Baseline platelet aggregation was not different between regimens, but at 48 hours, adenosine $5'$-diphosphate aggregation rate (but not collagen) was lower with clopidogrel ($P<0.001$).

Conclusions.—Both dipyridamole and clopidogrel reduced embolization to a similar extent. Embolic signals are strong predictors of future stroke rate in this patient group. Our results suggest these 2 treatment regimens have similar efficacy in early secondary prevention of stroke, although this now needs testing in large Phase III trials.

▶ Patients with transient ischemia attack and stroke secondary to large artery stenosis are felt to be at particularly high risk for early recurrent stroke.[1] Most data analyzing antiplatelet agents in prevention of recurrent stroke are long-term secondary prevention trials. In these settings, the combination of aspirin and dipyridamole is more effective than aspirin but equivalent to clopidogrel alone.[2] The authors postulate that optimal antiplatelet therapy for early secondary prevention may differ from that useful for long-term secondary prevention. In particular, higher risks of bleeding may be acceptable, given the high risk of early recurrent stroke following the initial event. In this study, the authors used detection of embolic signals by ambulatory transcranial Doppler (TCD) as a surrogate end point for clinical neurological events in the prediction of future stroke with symptomatic carotid stenosis.[3] This study was based on a new technique of ambulatory TCD monitoring felt to be more sensitive to embolic signals in patients with carotid stenosis.[4] The data suggest that in patients with acute extracranial cerebral vascular disease, both clopidogrel and dipyridamole will reduce embolization rates detected by TCD to an equal extent when added to aspirin. The data have implications for design of future efficacy trials in that embolic signals detected by TCD have been shown to be a strong independent predictor of stroke rates in patients with extracranial symptomatic cerebral vascular disease.[5] The platelet aggregation studies confirmed the different mechanisms of action of clopidogrel and dipyridamole in reducing platelet aggregation. Nevertheless, the clinical end points with these 2 medications when added to aspirin would be predicated to be the same with respect to secondary prevention of acute symptomatic extracranial carotid artery disease. Clinical efficacy will need to be confirmed in phase III trials.

G. L. Moneta, MD

References

1. Rothwell PM, Buchan A, Johnston SC. Recent advances in management of transient ischaemic attacks and minor ischaemic strokes. *Lancet Neurol.* 2006;5: 323-331.
2. Sacco RL, Diener HC, Yusuf S, et al. Aspirin and extended-release dipyridamole versus clopidogrel for recurrent stroke. *N Engl J Med.* 2008;359:1238-1251.
3. Markus HS, Droste DW, Kaps M, et al. Dual antiplatelet therapy with clopidogrel and aspirin in symptomatic carotid stenosis evaluated using Doppler embolic signal detection: the Clopidogrel and Aspirin for Reduction of Emboli in Symptomatic Carotid Stenosis (CARESS) trial. *Circulation.* 2005;111:2233-2240.
4. Mackinnon AD, Aaslid R, Markus HS. Ambulatory transcranial Doppler cerebral embolic signal detection in symptomatic and asymptomatic carotid stenosis. *Stroke.* 2005;36:1726-1730.
5. King A, Markus HS. Doppler embolic signals in cerebrovascular disease and prediction of stroke risk: a systematic review and meta-analysis. *Stroke.* 2009; 40:3711-3717.

Complex Plaques in the Proximal Descending Aorta: An Underestimated Embolic Source of Stroke

Harloff A, Simon J, Brendecke S, et al (Univ Hosp Freiburg, Germany; et al)
Stroke 41:1145-1150, 2010

Background and Purpose.—To investigate the incidence of retrograde flow from complex plaques (≥4-mm-thick, ulcerated, or superimposed thrombi) of the descending aorta (DAo) and its potential role in embolic stroke.

Methods.—Ninety-four consecutive acute stroke patients with aortic plaques ≥3-mm-thick in transesophageal echocardiography were prospectively included. MRI was performed to localize complex plaques and to measure time-resolved 3-dimensional blood flow within the aorta. Three-dimensional visualization was used to evaluate if diastolic retrograde flow connected plaque location with the outlet of the left subclavian artery, left common carotid artery, or brachiocephalic trunk. Complex DAo plaques were considered an embolic source if retrograde flow reached a supra-aortic vessel that supplied the territory of visible acute and embolic retinal or cerebral infarction.

Results.—Only decreasing heart rate was correlated ($P<0.02$) with increasing flow reversal to the aortic arch. Retrograde flow from complex DAo plaques reached the left subclavian artery in 55 (58.5%), the left common carotid artery in 23 (24.5%), and the brachiocephalic trunk in 13 patients (13.8%). Based on routine diagnostics and MRI of the ascending aorta/aortic arch, stroke etiology was determined in 57 and cryptogenic in 37 patients. Potential embolization from DAo plaques was then identified in 19 of 57 patients (33.3%) with determined and in 9 of 37 patients (24.3%) with cryptogenic stroke.

Conclusions.—Retrograde flow from complex DAo plaques was frequent in both determined and cryptogenic stroke and could explain embolism to all brain territories. These findings suggest that complex DAo plaques should be considered a new source of stroke (Fig 3).

▶ Complex aortic plaques are defined as greater than or equal to 4 mm in thickness or those associated with ulceration or that have mobile thrombi. Such plaques are considered a significant source of stroke. When such plaques are located in the ascending aorta or the aortic arch, embolization can be through antegrade flow from the aorta into a major cerebral vessel. However, the incidence of complex plaques is highest in the proximal descending aorta. Plaques in this location have only previously been considered a source of stroke in the setting of severe aortic valve insufficiency resulting in retrograde flow in the aorta during diastole. However, it now appears that diastolic retrograde flow in the descending thoracic aorta may be common in patients with atherosclerosis and therefore a potentially overlooked mechanism of stroke.[1] The authors hypothesize that retrograde flow in the proximal descending thoracic aorta has the potential to reach all the supra-aortic arteries and, thus, in the setting of a complex descending aorta plaque, may be a previously underappreciated source of stroke. Their data suggest that indeed this is the case and plaques in the descending thoracic aorta beyond the origins of the great vessels should be considered a potential source of stroke (Fig 3). Flow reversal from complex descending thoracic aortic plaques can potentially reach all supra-aortic arteries. Descending thoracic aortic plaques should therefore be assessed in all patients with cryptogenic stroke as a possible source of the stroke. The authors found an 8% incidence of complex descending thoracic aortic plaques

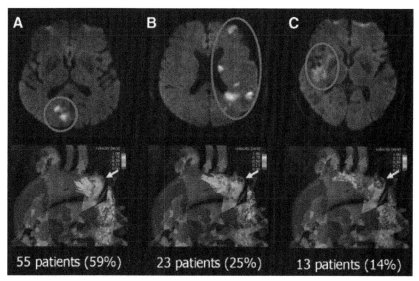

FIGURE 3.—Upper row, Diffusion-weighted cranial MR imaging. Lower row, Time-resolved 3-dimensional particle traces visualize potential embolization pathways from complex plaques in the proximal descending aorta (2-dimensional plane, yellow arrow) to the outlet of the brain-supplying arteries (red arrows). Flow reversal to the LSA potentially causes stroke (red circles) in the posterior circulation (A) or to the CCA, or brachiocephalic trunk potentially causes stroke in the left (B) or right hemisphere (C). The number of patients with potential retrograde embolization into the particular supra-aortic great artery is given in absolute values and in percentages in relation to the 94 patients. For interpretation of the references to color in this figure legend, the reader is referred to web version of this article. (Reprinted from Harloff A, Simon J, Brendecke S, et al. Complex plaques in the proximal descending aorta: An underestimated embolic source of stroke. *Stroke.* 2010;41:1145-1150, with permission from American Heart Association, Inc.)

in patients with determined stroke and 28% in patients with cryptogenic stroke. There was no correlation of retrograde flow with aortic valve insufficiency. These observations clearly contradict previous beliefs that flow reversal in the descending aorta is rare and only present in patients with aortic valve insufficiency. The study demonstrates for the first time that the proximal descending aorta is a potential source for embolic stroke in all brain territories.

G. L. Moneta, MD

Reference

1. Svedlund S, Wetterholm R, Volkmann R, Caidahl K. Retrograde blood flow in the aortic arch determined by transesophageal Doppler ultrasound. *Cerebrovasc Dis.* 2009;27:22-28.

Contemporary Results of Carotid Endarterectomy for Asymptomatic Carotid Stenosis

Woo K, Garg J, Hye RJ, et al (Univ of Southern California, Los Angeles, CA; Scripps Green Hosp, La Jolla, CA; The Southern California Permanente Med Group, San Diego, CA)
Stroke 41:975-979, 2010

Background and Purpose.—The validity of carotid endarterectomy (CEA) for asymptomatic carotid stenosis has been questioned recently due to the increasing effectiveness of medical management. In this study, we evaluated how contemporary outcomes of CEA for asymptomatic carotid stenosis compare with published stroke rates for best medical management.

Methods.—We identified all patients who underwent CEA for asymptomatic carotid stenosis from the 2005, 2006, and 2007 National Surgical Quality Improvement Program (NSQIP) database. Pre-and postoperative variables, including 30-day stroke, death, and myocardial infarction, were analyzed.

Results.—Of 10 423 carotid endarterectomies identified, 5009 were for asymptomatic carotid stenosis. The stroke, death, and myocardial infarction rates of this group were 0.96%, 0.56%, and 0.22%, respectively. If the 0.96% perioperative stroke rate from our contemporary NSQIP analysis is combined with the 5-year stroke risk after CEA of 3.8% from the Asymptomatic Carotid Surgery Trial, the average annual stroke rate is 1%, comparable to the stroke rate of 0.8% for best medical management from the Second Manifestations of Arterial Disease Study trial.

Conclusions.—These contemporary results show that stroke rates with CEA and best medical management for asymptomatic stenosis are similar. Despite limitations, our results emphasize the importance of continuing randomized prospective trials comparing CEA and best medical management for asymptomatic carotid stenosis.

▶ Carotid endarterectomy (CEA) is one of the most common operations performed by vascular surgeons. Overall, 40% to 60% of CEAs are performed for asymptomatic carotid stenosis, and in some areas of the United States, more than 90% of CEAs are performed for asymptomatic stenosis. Statins may reduce risk of stroke by up to 50%.[1,2] Therefore, the current best medical management of asymptomatic patients with significant carotid stenosis includes use of statins and antiplatelet therapy, smoking cessation, and control of hypertension. The authors sought to compare contemporary outcomes of CEA with previously published stroke rates for best medical management of patients with asymptomatic carotid stenosis. A secondary purpose was to establish patient factors that may result in an increased risk of post-CEA morbidity and mortality. The study highlights the increasing scrutiny of the use of CEA for the treatment of asymptomatic patients with carotid artery stenosis. The study was published before the recent 10-year update of the Asymptomatic Carotid Surgery Trial (ACST).[3] Given the results of ACST, the comparison of the National Surgical Quality Improvement Program (NSQIP) data in this article with the Second Manifestations of Arterial Disease Study data loses some of its luster. The results of the ACST should probably be taken more seriously in terms of evaluating the efficacy of CEA for asymptomatic patients with carotid stenosis. The value of this trial lies in the documentation of the stroke, death, and myocardial infarction rates in the NSQIP database. Data indicate that surgeons have become quite good at performing CEA in asymptomatic patients. However, it is also becoming increasingly evident that despite the ability of surgeons to safely perform CEA in the asymptomatic patient, the operation likely has minimal overall benefit from a public health perspective. If surgeons are paying attention to this debate and reading the literature, we should see a decrease in the proportion of patients undergoing CEA for asymptomatic disease.

G. L. Moneta, MD

References

1. Ridker PM, Danielson E, Fonseca FA, et al. Rosuvastatin to prevent vascular events in men and women with elevated C-reactive protein. *N Engl J Med.* 2008;359:2195-2207.
2. Stroke Prevention by Aggressive Reduction in Cholesterol Levels (SPARCL) Investigators. High-dose atorvastatin after stroke or transient ischemic attack. *N Engl J Med.* 2006;355:549-559.
3. Halliday A, Harrison M, Hayter E, et al. 10-year stroke prevention after successful carotid endarterectomy for asymptomatic stenosis (ACST-1): a multicentre randomised trial. *Lancet.* 2010;376:1074-1084.

External Carotid Artery Stenting to Treat Patients With Symptomatic Ipsilateral Internal Carotid Artery Occlusion: A Multicenter Case Series
Xu DS, Abruzzo TA, Albuquerque FC, et al (Northwestern Univ, Chicago, IL; Univ of Cincinnati College of Medicine, OH; Barrow Neurological Inst, Phoenix, AZ; et al)
Neurosurgery 67:314-321, 2010

Background.—The external carotid artery (ECA) anastomoses in many distal territories supplied by the internal carotid artery (ICA) and is an important source of collateral circulation to the brain. Stenosis of the ECA in ipsilateral ICA occlusion can produce ischemic sequelae.

Objective.—To examine the effectiveness of ECA stenting in treating symptomatic ipsilateral ICA occlusion.

Methods.—We retrospectively reviewed patient databases from 5 academic medical centers to identify all individuals who underwent ECA stenting after 1998. For all discovered cases, coinvestigators used a common submission form to harvest relevant demographic information, clinical data, procedural details, and follow-up results for further analysis.

Results.—Twelve patients (median age, 66 years; range, 45-79 years) were identified for our cohort. Vessel disease involvement included severe

ECA stenosis ≥ 70% in 11 patients and ipsilateral ICA occlusion in all patients. Presenting symptoms included signs of transient ischemic attack, stroke, and amaurosis fugax. ECA stenting was associated with preservation of neurological status in 11 patients and resolution of symptoms in 5 patients at a median follow-up time of 26 months (range, 1-87 months; mean, 29 months). Symptomatic in-stent restenosis did not occur within any patient during the follow-up course.

Conclusion.—We found ECA stenting in symptomatic ipsilateral ICA disease to be a potentially effective strategy to preserve neurological function and to relieve ischemic symptoms. Further investigation with larger

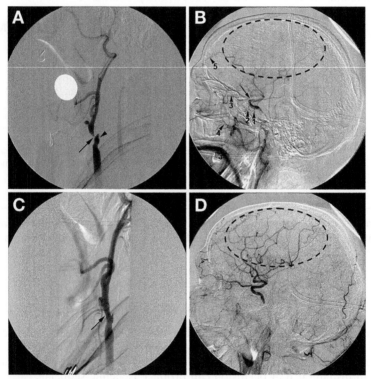

FIGURE 1.—Cerebral angiogram of patient 8. **A,** right common carotid artery angiography demonstrates a 90% stenosis of the right external carotid artery (ECA) origin (arrow) and an ulcerated stump at an occluded right internal carotid artery origin (arrowhead). **B,** angiography of the cranial right ECA territory shows collateral supply to the carotid siphon (arrow) via cavernous branches of the right middle/accessory meningeal artery (arrowhead 1) and the artery of the foramen of rotundum (arrowhead 2) and to the ophthalmic artery (arrowhead 3) via ethmoidal branches of the internal maxillary artery (arrowhead 4) and the palpebral territory of the superficial temporal artery (arrowhead 5). Note the poor opacification of the anterior/middle cerebral artery territories (dashed circle). **C,** repeat angiography of the right ECA origin after angioplasty shows no residual stenosis (arrow). **D,** poststenting angiography of the cranial right ECA territory now shows opacification of the right anterior and middle cerebral artery territories (dashed circle) resulting from improved collateral supply to the internal carotid artery. (Reprinted from Xu DS, Abruzzo TA, Albuquerque FC, et al. External carotid artery stenting to treat patients with symptomatic ipsilateral internal carotid artery occlusion: a multicenter case series. *Neurosurgery.* 2010;67:314-321.)

studies and longer follow-up periods is warranted to elucidate the true indications of this management strategy (Fig 1).

▶ The external carotid artery (ECA) is a significant extracranial-to-intracranial collateral source for the brain when the internal carotid artery (ICA) is occluded. It may contribute, under those circumstances, 10% to 15% of middle cerebral artery blood flow.[1] Chronic neurologic symptoms ipsilateral to the combination of an ICA occlusion and ECA stenosis may be due to emboli originating from the ECA, emboli from a stump of the ICA, or direct reduction of collateral perfusion.[2,3] Although surgical treatment of ECA stenosis is infrequently performed, it is a well-known and well-recognized procedure. However, endovascular management of ECA stenosis with angioplasty and stenting is a rare procedure. (The article actually has more authors [14] than patients [12]!) The results are certainly not a mandate for ECA stenting for apparently symptomatic ECA stenosis (Fig 1). However, there are also no compelling data for open revascularization of the ECA. Revascularization of the ECA, whether by endovascular or open surgical treatment, is supported by nothing more than individual case series. There is certainly no compelling evidence for either approach.

G. L. Moneta, MD

References

1. Fearn SJ, Picton AJ, Mortimer AJ, Parry AD, McCollum CN. The contribution of the external carotid artery to cerebral perfusion in carotid disease. *J Vasc Surg.* 2000;31:989-993.
2. Street DL, Ricotta JJ, Green RM, DeWeese JA. The role of external carotid revascularization in the treatment of ocular ischemia. *J Vasc Surg.* 1987;6:280-282.
3. Nano G, Dalainas I, Casana R, Malacrida G, Tealdi DG. Endovascular treatment of the carotid stump syndrome. *Cardiovasc Intervent Radiol.* 2006;29:140-142.

Limb-shaking transient ischaemic attacks in patients with internal carotid artery occlusion: a case-control study

Persoon S, Kappelle LJ, Klijn CJM (Univ Med Centre Utrecht, The Netherlands)

Brain 133:915-922, 2010

Limb-shaking is a specific clinical feature of transient ischaemic attacks that has been associated with a high-grade stenosis or occlusion of the internal carotid artery. The aim of this study was to describe the clinical characteristics of limb-shaking in patients with internal carotid artery occlusion and to investigate whether patients with limb-shaking have a worse haemodynamic state of the brain than patients with internal carotid artery occlusion without limb-shaking. We included 34 patients (mean age 62 ± 7 years, 82% male) with limb-shaking associated with internal carotid artery occlusion and 68 sex- and age-matched controls with cerebral transient ischaemic attack or minor disabling ischaemic stroke associated with internal carotid artery occlusion, but without limb-shaking. We investigated clinical characteristics, collateral pathways on contrast angiograms and carbon dioxide-reactivity measured by transcranial Doppler. The results showed that limb-shaking usually lasted less than 5 min and was often accompanied by paresis of the involved limb. Compared with controls, patients with limb-shaking more frequently had symptoms precipitated by rising or exercise (odds ratio 14.2, 95% confidence interval 4.2–47.9), more frequently had recurrent ischaemic deficits after documented internal carotid artery occlusion (but before inclusion in the study) (odds ratio 8.2, 95% confidence interval 2.3–29.3), more often had leptomeningeal collaterals (odds ratio 6.8, 95% confidence interval 2.0–22.7), and tended to have a lower carbon dioxide-reactivity (mean 5% ± 16 versus 12% ± 17; odds ratio 0.97 per 1% increase in carbon dioxide-reactivity, 95% confidence interval 0.94–1.00). In conclusion, limb-shaking transient ischaemic attacks in patients with internal carotid artery occlusion can be recognized by their short duration, are often accompanied by paresis and precipitated by rising or exercise and are indicative of an impaired haemodynamic state of the brain.

▶ Case reports have described limb shaking as an unusual clinical feature of transient ischemic attacks (TIA).[1,2] The limb shaking characterizing these TIAs consists of brief, jerky, and coarse involuntary movements involving an arm or a leg and has been associated with high-grade stenosis or occlusion of the internal carotid artery (ICA). An unanswered question is whether patients with high-grade ICA stenosis or occlusion who have limb-shaking TIAs have a worse hemodynamic flow state than patients with ICA stenosis or occlusion who do not have limb-shaking TIAs. Limb shaking as a manifestation of a TIA is relatively unknown to most vascular surgeons. Most of these patients have ICA occlusion; 10% of patients with ICA occlusion will have limb-shaking TIAs. However, some of these patients have high-grade ICA stenosis, rather than occlusion, and therefore are of interest to the peripheral vascular surgeon. It is important to note that this particular form of TIA is likely hemodynamic and not embolic. Patients with limb-shaking TIAs undergoing carotid endarterectomy therefore should perhaps be strongly considered for shunting during the performance of the endarterectomy when technically feasible.

G. L. Moneta, MD

References

1. Klijn CJ, Kappelle LJ, van Huffelen AC, et al. Recurrent ischemia in symptomatic carotid occlusion: prognostic value of hemodynamic factors. *Neurology.* 2000;55: 1806-1812.
2. Firlik AD, Firlik KS, Yonas H. Physiological diagnosis and surgical treatment of recurrent limb shaking: case report. *Neurosurgery.* 1996;39:607-611.

Long-term outcome of symptomatic severe ostial vertebral artery stenosis (OVAS)
Karameshev A, Schroth G, Mordasini P, et al (Univ of Bern, Switzerland)
Neuroradiology 52:371-379, 2010

Introduction.—The optimal management of patients with symptomatic severe ostial vertebral artery stenosis (OVAS) is currently unclear. We analyzed the long-term outcome of consecutive patients with OVAS who received either medical treatment (MT) or vertebral artery stenting (VAS).

Methods.—Thirty-nine (>70%) patients with severe OVAS were followed for a mean period of 2.8 years. The decision for VAS ($n=10$) or MT ($n=29$) was left to the clinician. The Kaplan—Meier method was used to assess the risk of recurrent stroke, transient ischemic attack (TIA), or death over the study period.

Results.—Patients in the VAS group were significantly younger and more likely to have bilateral VA disease ($P=0.04$ and $P=0.02$). VAS was successfully performed in all ten patients. The periprocedural risk within 30 days was 10% (one TIA). The overall restenosis rate was 10%. One restenosis occurred after 9 months in a patient treated with bare-metal stent. At 4 years of follow-up, VAS showed a nonsignificant trend toward a lower risk for the combined endpoint of TIA and stroke in posterior circulation compared to medical treatment (10% vs. 45%, $P=0.095$; relative risk (RR)=0.24, 95% confidence interval (CI) 0.031—1.85). Patients with bilateral VA disease had a significantly lower recurrence risk after VAS compared with medical treatment (0% vs. 91% at 4 years, $P=0.004$; RR 0.10, 95% CI 0.022—0.49)

Conclusion.—VAS was performed without permanent complications in this small series of patients with symptomatic severe OVAS. The long-term benefit seems to be confined to patients with bilateral but not to those with unilateral VA disease.

▶ About 25% of all strokes are posterior circulation strokes.[1] Of posterior circulation strokes, 20% to 25% are associated with a severe ostial stenosis or occlusion of the vertebral artery (VA).[2] Treatment of VA stenosis can be medical management alone, surgical bypass, transposition of the VA, or endovascular management. Endovascular management of VA stenosis is infrequently reported with only 1 randomized trial.[3] Carotid and Vertebral Artery Transluminal Angioplasty Study, however, enrolled only 16 patients with VA stenosis. An additional trial, the Vertebral Artery Stenting trial, may be under way.[4] Results, however, are unlikely to be available for many years. This study does not really help much in deciding how to manage patients with VA stenosis. It is too small to draw any meaningful conclusion about the efficacy of VA stenting for treatment of ostial VA stenosis. The study was not randomized and the patients were highly selected for treatment. Clearly the study does not provide sufficient data to justify a widespread approach to endovascular management of VA stenosis. Medical management remains the mainstay for patients with symptomatic VA stenosis with intervention by either open or endovascular techniques reserved for highly selected patients, using what amounts to really no more than best-guess criteria.

G. L. Moneta, MD

References

1. Bogousslavsky J, Van Melle G, Regli F. The Lausanne Stroke Registry: analysis of 1,000 consecutive patients with first stroke. *Stroke*. 1988;19:1083-1092.
2. Wityk RJ, Chang HM, Rosengart A, et al. Proximal extracranial vertebral artery disease in the New England Medical Center Posterior Circulation Registry. *Arch Neurol*. 1998;55:470-478.
3. Coward LJ, McCabe DJ, Ederle J, Featherstone RL, Clifton A, Brown MM. Long-term outcome after angioplasty and stenting for symptomatic vertebral artery stenosis compared with medical treatment in the Carotid And Vertebral Artery Transluminal Angioplasty Study (CAVATAS): a randomized trial. *Stroke*. 2007; 38:1526-1530.
4. Compter A, van der Worp HB, Schonewille WJ, et al. VAST: Vertebral Artery Stenting Trial. Protocol for a randomised safety and feasibility trial. *Trials*. 2008;9:65.

New ischemic brain lesions on MRI after stenting or endarterectomy for symptomatic carotid stenosis: a substudy of the International Carotid Stenting Study (ICSS)

Bonati LH, for the ICSS-MRI study group (Univ Hosp Basel, Switzerland; et al)
Lancet Neurol 9:353-362, 2010

Background.—The International Carotid Stenting Study (ICSS) of stenting and endarterectomy for symptomatic carotid stenosis found a higher incidence of stroke within 30 days of stenting compared with endarterectomy. We aimed to compare the rate of ischaemic brain injury detectable on MRI between the two groups.

Methods.—Patients with recently symptomatic carotid artery stenosis enrolled in ICSS were randomly assigned in a 1:1 ratio to receive carotid artery stenting or endarterectomy. Of 50 centres in ICSS, seven took part in the MRI substudy. The protocol specified that MRI was done 1−7 days before treatment, 1−3 days after treatment (post-treatment scan), and 27−33 days after treatment. Scans were analysed by two or three investigators who were masked to treatment. The primary endpoint was the presence of at least one new ischaemic brain lesion on diffusion-weighted imaging (DWI) on the post-treatment scan. Analysis was per protocol. This is a substudy of a registered trial, ISRCTN 25337470.

Findings.—231 patients (124 in the stenting group and 107 in the endarterectomy group) had MRI before and after treatment. 62 (50%) of 124 patients in the stenting group and 18 (17%) of 107 patients in the endarterectomy group had at least one new DWI lesion detected on post-treatment scans done a median of 1 day after treatment (adjusted odds ratio [OR] 5·21, 95% CI 2·78−9·79; p<0·0001). At 1 month, there were changes on fluid-attenuated inversion recovery sequences in 28 (33%) of 86 patients in the stenting group and six (8%) of 75 in the endarterectomy group (adjusted OR 5·93, 95% CI 2·25—15·62; p=0·0003). In patients treated at a centre with a policy of using cerebral protection devices, 37 (73%) of 51 in the stenting group and eight (17%) of 46 in the endarterectomy group had at least one new DWI lesion on post-treatment scans (adjusted OR 12·20, 95% CI 4·53—32·84), whereas in those treated at a centre with a policy of unprotected stenting, 25 (34%) of 73 patients in the stenting group and ten (16%) of 61 in the endarterectomy group had new lesions on DWI (adjusted OR 2·70, 1·16—6·24; interaction p=0·019).

Interpretation.—About three times more patients in the stenting group than in the endarterectomy group had new ischaemic lesions on DWI on post-treatment scans. The difference in clinical stroke risk in ICSS is therefore unlikely to have been caused by ascertainment bias. Protection devices did not seem to be effective in preventing cerebral ischaemia during stenting. DWI might serve as a surrogate outcome measure in future trials of carotid interventions (Figs 2 and 4).

▶ The International Carotid Stenting Study (ICSS) randomized patients with symptomatic carotid artery stenosis to either carotid stenting or carotid

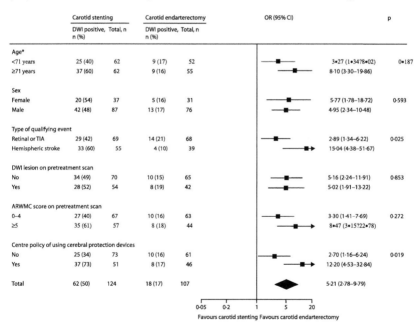

FIGURE 2.—New DWI lesions on post-treatment scans in patient subgroups. Data are numbers of patients (%) with new DWI lesions on post-treatment scans (DWI positive) and total numbers of patients per treatment group. Squares and horizontal lines are adjusted odds ratios (OR) and 95% CIs. The diamond represents the overall adjusted OR and 95% CI. All OR and interaction p values are adjusted for interval between treatment and post-treatment scan. *Dichotomised at the rounded median age of the study population. DWI=diffusion-weighted imaging. ARWMC=age-related white matter changes. (Reprinted from Bonati LH, for the ICSS-MRI study group. New ischemic brain lesions on MRI after stenting or endarterectomy for symptomatic carotid stenosis: a substudy of the International Carotid Stenting Study (ICSS). *Lancet Neurol.* 2010;9:353-362, with permission from Elsevier.)

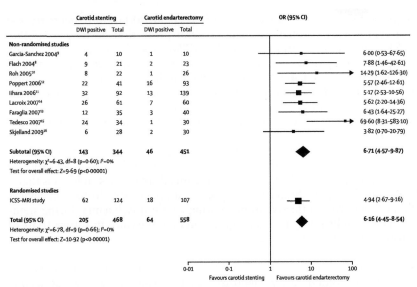

FIGURE 4.—Meta-analysis of studies comparing ischaemic lesions on DWI after carotid stenting versus carotid endarterectomy. Mantel-Haenszel fixed effect model comparing the proportions of patients with hyperintense DWI lesions after stenting versus endarterectomy in nine non-randomised studies, and in the ICSS-MRI study. Data are numbers of patients with new DWI lesions on post-treatment scans (DWI positive) and total numbers of patients in studies. Squares and horizontal lines are odds ratios (OR) and 95% CIs, with size of squares representing study weight. Diamonds represent aggregate OR and 95% CI. DWI=diffusion-weighted imaging. (Reprinted from Bonati LH, for the ICSS-MRI study group. New ischemic brain lesions on MRI after stenting or endarterectomy for symptomatic carotid stenosis: a substudy of the International Carotid Stenting Study (ICSS). *Lancet Neurol.* 2010;9:353-362, with permission from Elsevier.)

endarterectomy.[1] Using intention-to-treat analysis, the results of the study demonstrate that the risk of procedural stroke, death, or myocardial infarction within the first 120 days following randomization was significantly higher with stenting than with surgery (8.5% vs 5.2%, $P = .006$). At 30 days, per protocol analysis, the risk of stroke, myocardial infarction, or death was also higher (7.4% vs 4.0%, $P = .003$). This was primarily attributed to a higher number of nondisabling strokes in the stenting group (36 vs 11 within 30 days). Of the 50 centers that participated in the ICSS study, 7 took part in an MRI substudy, the results of which were reported in this article and indicate far more diffusion-weighted imaging (DWI) lesions with stenting than with endarterectomy (Fig 2). Previous nonrandomized studies have also suggested higher rates of postprocedural ischemic lesions detected on DWI after stenting than after endarterectomy. As shown in Fig 4, a meta-analysis of these studies indicated that the odds ratio of new ischemic lesion after treatment was 6.71 (95% CI 4.57-9.87), favoring endarterectomy. The authors' odds ratio of 5.21 is very similar to that obtained from the meta-analysis. The clinical significance of DWI lesions in the long run is unknown but is postulated to eventually lead to cognitive decline and dementia.[2] Of particular interest is the apparent lack of protection against DWI lesions afforded by cerebral protection devices. One might postulate, given the relative odds ratios for DWI lesions with and without protection devices, that protection devices actually increase the risk of DWI lesions. There are a number of reasons why cerebral protection devices may have been ineffective in this study. For instance, all protection devices in this study were of the filter type, and conclusions about other types of devices cannot be made. Another possible conclusion is that cerebral protection during carotid artery stenting is another idea that seems good but does not hold up to proper scrutiny when one actually examines data collected by unbiased observers.

G. L. Moneta, MD

References

1. International Carotid Stenting Study investigators, Ederle J, Dobson J, Featherstone RL, et al. Carotid artery stenting compared with endarterectomy in patients with symptomatic carotid stenosis (International Carotid Stenting Study): an interim analysis of a randomised controlled trial. *Lancet.* 2010;375: 985-997.
2. Pendlbury ST, Rothwell PM. Prevalence, incidence, and factors associated with pre-stroke and post-stroke dementia: a systematic review and meta-analysis. *Lancet Neurol.* 2009;8:1006-1018.

Perioperative Ischemic Complications of the Brain After Carotid Endarterectomy
Hebb MO, Heiserman JE, Forbes KPN, et al (St Joseph's Hosp and Med Ctr, Phoenix, AZ)
Neurosurgery 67:286-294, 2010

Background.—The potential morbidity of cerebral ischemia after carotid endarterectomy (CEA) has been recognized, but its reported incidence varies widely.

Objective.—To prospectively evaluate the development of cerebral ischemic complications in patients treated by CEA at a high-volume cerebrovascular center.

Methods.—Fifty patients with moderate or severe carotid stenosis awaiting CEA were studied with perioperative diffusion-weighted imaging of the brain and standardized neurological evaluations. Microsurgical CEA was performed by 1 of 2 vascular neurosurgeons. Radiological studies were evaluated by faculty neuroradiologists who were blinded to the details of the clinical situation.

Results.—Preoperative diffusion-weighted imaging studies were performed within 24 hours of surgery. A second study was obtained within 24 (92% of patients), 48 (4% of patients), or 72 (4% of patients) hours after surgery. Intraluminal shunting was used in 1 patient (2%), and patch angioplasty was used in 2 patients (4%). No patient had diffusion-weighted imaging evidence of procedure-related cerebral ischemia. Non-ischemic complications consisted of postoperative confusion in an 87-year-old man with a urinary tract infection and a marginal mandibular nerve paresis in another patient. Radiological studies were normal in both patients.

Conclusion.—CEA is a relatively safe procedure that may be performed with an acceptable risk of cerebral ischemia in select patients. The low rate of ischemic complications associated with CEA sets a standard to which other carotid revascularization techniques should be held. The current results are presented with a discussion of the senior author's preferred surgical technique and a brief review of the literature.

▶ Carotid endarterectomy is perhaps the most well-studied operative procedure— certainly the most well-studied operative procedure in vascular surgery. It is known that with carotid artery stenting, the incidence of cerebral infarction that is asymptomatic but detected by magnetic resonance diffusion-weighted imaging (MR DWI) can be quite high and can exceed 50% even when cerebral protection devices are used. The authors present a small series of carotid endarterectomies in which the patients were evaluated postoperatively both clinically and with routine MR DWI. There are of course a number of limitations to interpretation of the data here. First of all, it is highly unlikely many vascular surgeons use the technique for carotid endarterectomy described in the article. Two-thirds of the patients were asymptomatic and therefore likely are at low risk for any postoperative ischemic complication. Nevertheless, the series does demonstrate that it is possible to perform carotid endarterectomy with a rate of new DWI-detected lesions following the procedure that is unlikely to be matched anytime in the near future by carotid artery stenting.

G. L. Moneta, MD

Prevalence of Asymptomatic Carotid Artery Stenosis in the General Population: An Individual Participant Data Meta-Analysis
de Weerd M, Greving JP, Hedblad B, et al (Univ Med Ctr Utrecht, The Netherlands; Lund Univ, Malmö, Sweden; et al)
Stroke 41:1294-1297, 2010

Background and Purpose.—In the discussion on the cost-effectiveness of screening, precise estimates of severe asymptomatic carotid stenosis are vital. Accordingly, we assessed the prevalence of moderate and severe asymptomatic carotid stenosis by age and sex using pooled cohort data.

Methods.—We performed an individual participant data meta-analysis (23 706 participants) of 4 population-based studies (Malmö Diet and Cancer Study, Tromsø Carotid Atherosclerosis Progression Study, and Cardiovascular Health Study). Outcomes of interest were asymptomatic moderate ($\geq50\%$) and severe carotid stenosis ($\geq70\%$).

Results.—Prevalence of moderate asymptomatic carotid stenosis ranged from 0.2% (95% CI, 0.0% to 0.4%) in men aged <50 years to 7.5% (5.2% to 10.5%) in men aged ≥80 years. For women, this prevalence increased from 0% (0% to 0.2%) to 5.0% (3.1% to 7.5%). Prevalence

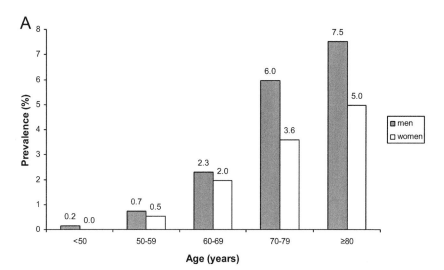

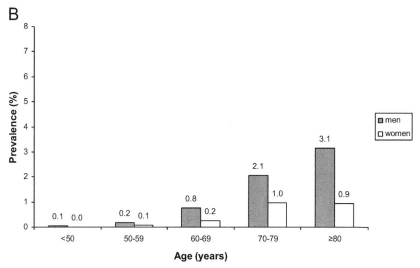

FIGURE 1.—Age- and sex-specific prevalence estimates of moderate (A) and severe ACAS (B) in men and women. (Reprinted from de Weerd M, Greving JP, Hedblad B, et al. Prevalence of asymptomatic carotid artery stenosis in the general population: an individual participant data meta-analysis. *Stroke.* 2010;41:1294-1297, with permission from American Heart Association, Inc.)

of severe asymptomatic carotid stenosis ranged from 0.1% (0.0% to 0.3%) in men aged <50 years to 3.1% (1.7% to 5.3%) in men aged ≥80. For women, this prevalence increased from 0% (0.0% to 0.2%) to 0.9% (0.3% to 2.4%).

Conclusions.—The prevalence of severe asymptomatic carotid stenosis in the general population ranges from 0% to 3.1%, which is useful

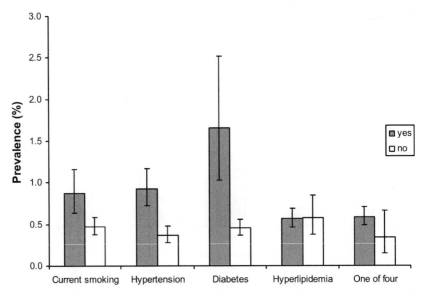

FIGURE 2.—Prevalence of severe stenosis in subgroups. (Reprinted from de Weerd M, Greving JP, Hedblad B, et al. Prevalence of asymptomatic carotid artery stenosis in the general population: an individual participant data meta-analysis. *Stroke*. 2010;41:1294-1297, with permission from American Heart Association, Inc.)

information in the discussion on the cost-effectiveness of screening (Figs 1 and 2).

▶ The effectiveness of screening programs for a disease reflects the prevalence of the disease in the screened population, the cost of screening, the impact of potential interventions as a result of screening, and cost-effectiveness of any potential intervention. With these considerations, there is ongoing debate as to the effectiveness of screening for internal carotid artery (ICA) stenosis. Screening for asymptomatic carotid stenosis has not been endorsed by the US Preventative Health Services Task Force. There are no data here that should lead that group to change its opinion. Until one is older than 70 years (Fig 1), the prevalence of high-grade asymptomatic carotid stenosis is less than 2% (Fig 1) and no comorbidity increases that prevalence beyond 2% (Fig 2). Whereas it is clear that the prevalence of severe asymptomatic ICA stenosis does increase with age and risk factors, the prevalence is still low. Given the relatively benign natural history of asymptomatic ICA stenosis, it is highly unlikely that, based on these data, screening for asymptomatic high-grade ICA stenosis would ever be clinically effective or cost effective in any patient subgroup.

G. L. Moneta, MD

Risk of Early Carotid Endarterectomy for Symptomatic Carotid Stenosis

Brinjikji W, Rabinstein AA, Meyer FB, et al (Mayo Clinic, Rochester, MN)
Stroke 41:2186-2190, 2010

Background and Purpose.—The purpose of this study was to determine and compare the rate of stroke, myocardial infarction, and death in patients undergoing early and late carotid endarterectomy (CEA) after a symptomatic event and in asymptomatic patients.

Methods.—We conducted a retrospective analysis of all CEAs performed in the Department of Neurosurgery between January 2004 and May 2009. Patients were divided into 3 groups: Group 1, asymptomatic patients; Group 2, symptomatic patients operated on >2 weeks after their transient ischemic attack or stroke; and Group 3, symptomatic patients operated on ≤2 weeks of their transient ischemic attack or stroke. Primary outcomes were any myocardial infarction, stroke, or death occurring within 30 days postoperatively. The secondary end point was transient ischemic attack within 30 days postoperatively.

Results.—Five hundred thirty-two CEAs were performed on 507 patients during the study period. Thirty-day follow-up was available for 500 patients with 525 CEAs. Groups 1, 2, and 3 consisted of 278, 105, and 142 CEAs, respectively. In total, 12 patients had primary outcomes. In Group 1, 5 patients had primary outcomes of stroke, myocardial infarction, or death (1.8%); in Group 2, 1 patient had primary outcomes (1.0%); and in Group 3, 6 patients had primary outcomes (4.2%). There was no significant difference in the rate of primary outcomes among the 3 groups (*P*=0.17) or when Groups 2 and 3 were compared (*P*=0.24).

Conclusions.—Although the perioperative risk of transient ischemic attacks, stroke, death, and myocardial infarction is slightly higher in symptomatic patients operated on early, CEA can be done with an acceptable risk in properly selected symptomatic patients within 2 weeks of their transient ischemic attack or stroke.

▶ Current guidelines from the American Academy of Neurology and American Heart Association indicate patients with symptomatic carotid stenosis should preferentially undergo carotid endarterectomy (CEA) within 2 weeks of the symptomatic event.[1,2] However, for referral and logistical reasons, many patients are not operated within the recommended 2-week period. In addition, traditional surgical wisdom has shied away from acute operation, especially in stroke patients, for fear of a higher incidence of complications.[3]

The authors examined their institutional experience with CEA over a 5-year period with particular analysis of symptomatic patients operated on within 2 weeks of their symptom. Symptomatic patients were not considered for early CEA if they had an infarct involving more than one-third of the middle cerebral artery territory or a patient had a fixed disabling deficit or unstable medical condition. When those conditions were not present, patients were operated on soon after evaluation irrespective of the interval from the symptomatic event. The authors felt delays were usually related to delayed referral after symptom onset. This study has all the limitations of a single-institution retrospective review. Nevertheless, the results are consistent with what one would hope, given current guidelines. The biggest problem, of course, is ensuring that patients in groups 2 and 3 did in fact differ primarily by referral pattern and not by other more pertinent medical conditions. The percentage of patients presenting with stroke in group 2 was similar to that in group 3 (36.2% vs 35.2%), but we really don't know whether the severity of the strokes was the same and whether their pre- and postoperative management was the same. Nevertheless, given studies that have indicated a relative high rate of repeat events shortly after the initial event and the reasonably good results in group 3 patients, this study lends further support to a policy of performance of CEA in selected patients shortly after the onset of a neurologic symptom.

G. L. Moneta, MD

References

1. Chaturvedi S, Bruno A, Feasby T, et al. Carotid endarterectomy–an evidence-based review: report of the Therapeutics and Technology Assessment Subcommittee of the American Academy of Neurology. *Neurology.* 2005;65:794-801.
2. Sacco RL, Adams R, Albers G, et al. Guidelines for prevention of stroke in patients with ischemic stroke or transient ischemic attack: a statement for healthcare professionals from the American Heart Association/American Stroke Association Council on Stroke: co-sponsored by the Council on Cardiovascular Radiology and Intervention: the American Academy of Neurology affirms the value of this guideline. *Stroke.* 2006;37:577-617.
3. Naylor AR. Time is brain! *Surgeon.* 2007;5:23-30.

Safety of Stenting and Endarterectomy by Symptomatic Status in the Carotid Revascularization Endarterectomy Versus Stenting Trial (CREST)

Silver FL, for the CREST Investigators (Univ of Toronto, Ontario, Canada; et al)
Stroke 42:675-680, 2011

Background and Purpose.—The safety of carotid artery stenting (CAS) and carotid endarterectomy (CEA) has varied by symptomatic status in previous trials. The Carotid Revascularization Endarterectomy Versus Stenting Trial (CREST) data were analyzed to determine safety in symptomatic and asymptomatic patients.

Methods.—CREST is a randomized trial comparing safety and efficacy of CAS versus CEA in patients with high-grade carotid stenoses. Patients were defined as symptomatic if they had relevant symptoms within 180 days of randomization. The primary end point was stroke, myocardial infarction, or death within the periprocedural period or ipsilateral stroke up to 4 years.

Results.—For 1321 symptomatic and 1181 asymptomatic patients, the periprocedural aggregate of stroke, myocardial infarction, and death did not differ between CAS and CEA (5.2% versus 4.5%; hazard ratio, 1.18; 95% CI, 0.82 to 1.68; P=0.38). The stroke and death rate was higher for CAS versus CEA (4.4% versus 2.3%; hazard ratio, 1.90; 95% CI, 1.21

to 2.98; $P=0.005$). For symptomatic patients, the periprocedural stroke and death rates were 6.0% ± 0.9% for CAS and 3.2% ± 0.7% for CEA (hazard ratio, 1.89; 95% CI, 1.11 to 3.21; $P=0.02$). For asymptomatic patients, the stroke and death rates were 2.5% ± 0.6% for CAS and 1.4% ± 0.5% for CEA (hazard ratio, 1.88; 95% CI, 0.79 to 4.42; $P=0.15$). Rates were lower for those aged <80 years.

Conclusions.—There were no significant differences between CAS versus CEA by symptomatic status for the primary CREST end point. Periprocedural stroke and death rates were significantly lower for CEA in symptomatic patients. However, for both CAS and CEA, stroke and death rates were below or comparable to those of previous randomized trials and were within the complication thresholds suggested in current guidelines for both symptomatic and asymptomatic patients.

▶ This is a secondary analysis of the Carotid Revascularization Endarterectomy Versus Stenting Trial (CREST). CREST investigated the safety and efficacy of carotid artery stenting (CAS) versus carotid endarterectomy (CEA) in patients with high-grade carotid stenosis. Every reasonable analysis of government-sponsored randomized trials, including this one, continues to indicate that CEA is superior to CAS for treatment of patients with symptomatic carotid stenosis if the goal of the procedure is to prevent stroke. Very significant questions remain about the treatment of asymptomatic patients. The majority of patients undergoing carotid intervention in the United States do so for asymptomatic carotid stenosis. And yet, we really do not know the natural history of this disease in the modern era, with more advanced antiplatelet medications, statin medications, and better blood pressure control available now than 20 years ago. However, these medications will only be effective if the patients take them. What is needed is a 3-arm trial in asymptomatic patients with carotid artery stenosis: medical management alone versus medical management combined with CEA versus medical management combined with CAS. Given the anticipated number of events, the number of patients required and the number of centers required will likely be large. However, given the demographics of carotid interventions in the United States, the potential public health and economic impact of the results of such a trial would likely be felt immediately.

G. L. Moneta, MD

Short-term outcome after stenting versus endarterectomy for symptomatic carotid stenosis: a preplanned meta-analysis of individual patient data
Carotid Stenting Trialists' Collaboration (Univ Hosp Basel, Switzerland; London School of Hygiene and Tropical Medicine, UK; Univ Med Centre Utrecht, Netherlands; et al)
Lancet 376:1062-1073, 2010

Background.—Results from randomised controlled trials have shown a higher short-term risk of stroke associated with carotid stenting than with carotid endarterectomy for the treatment of symptomatic carotid stenosis. However, these trials were underpowered for investigation of whether carotid artery stenting might be a safe alternative to endarterectomy in specific patient subgroups. We therefore did a preplanned meta-analysis of individual patient data from three randomised controlled trials.

Methods.—Data from all 3433 patients with symptomatic carotid stenosis who were randomly assigned and analysed in the Endarterectomy versus Angioplasty in Patients with Symptomatic Severe Carotid Stenosis (EVA-3S) trial, the Stent-Protected Angioplasty versus Carotid Endarterectomy (SPACE) trial, and the International Carotid Stenting Study (ICSS) were pooled and analysed with fixed-effect binomial regression models adjusted for source trial. The primary outcome event was any stroke or death. The intention-to-treat (ITT) analysis included all patients and outcome events occurring between randomisation and 120 days thereafter. The per-protocol (PP) analysis was restricted to patients receiving the allocated treatment and events occurring within 30 days after treatment.

Findings.—In the first 120 days after randomisation (ITT analysis), any stroke or death occurred significantly more often in the carotid stenting group (153 [8·9%] of 1725) than in the carotid endarterectomy group (99 [5·8%] of 1708, risk ratio [RR] 1·53, [95% CI 1·20-1·95], p=0·0006; absolute risk difference 3·2 [1·4-4·9]). Of all subgroup variables assessed, only age significantly modified the treatment effect: in patients younger than 70 years (median age), the estimated 120-day risk of stroke or death was 50 (5·8%) of 869 patients in the carotid stenting group and 48 (5·7%) of 843 in the carotid endarterectomy group (RR 1·00 [0·68-1·47]); in patients 70 years or older, the estimated risk with carotid stenting was twice that with carotid endarterectomy (103 [12·0%] of 856 vs 51 [5·9%] of 865, 2·04 [1·48-2·82], interaction p=0·0053, p=0·0014 for trend). In the PP analysis, risk estimates of stroke or death within 30 days of treatment among patients younger than 70 years were 43 (5·1%) of 851 patients in the stenting group and 37 (4·5%) of 821 in the endarterectomy group (1·11 [0·73-1·71]); in patients 70 years or older, the estimates were 87 (10·5%) of 828 patients and 36 (4·4%) of 824, respectively (2·41 [1·65-3·51]; categorical interaction p=0·0078, trend interaction p=0·0013].

Interpretation.—Stenting for symptomatic carotid stenosis should be avoided in older patients (age ≥70 years), but might be as safe as endarterectomy in younger patients (Figs 2 and 4).

▶ The Stenting and Angioplasty with Protection in Patients at High Risk for Endarterectomy trial[1] suggested carotid endarterectomy (CEA) and carotid artery stenting (CAS) provided equivalent results in patients with high-grade internal carotid artery (ICA) stenosis at high risk for surgery. However, the trial was hampered by recruitment difficulties, and most of the patients had asymptomatic ICA stenosis. However, 3 large government-sponsored European trials, the Endarterectomy versus Angioplasty in Patients with Symptomatic Severe Carotid Stenosis (EVA-3S) trial, the Stent-protected Angioplasty versus Carotid

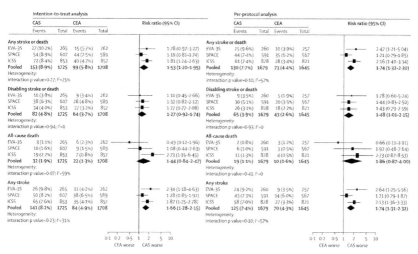

FIGURE 2.—Forest plot of risk ratios of major outcome events in trials and in pooled analysis. Data are number or number (%), unless otherwise indicated. Percentages are number of events divided by number of patients. Squares and horizontal bars represent within-trial treatment risk ratios and 95% CIs, respectively, with carotid endarterectomy (CEA) as the reference group, on a log scale. The size of squares represents study weight. Diamonds represent pooled risk ratios and 95% CIs, adjusted for source trial. In the investigation of heterogeneity, the interaction p value represents the significance of the interaction between source trial and treatment effect in the regression model (likelihood ratio test); a significant p value suggests heterogeneity. The estimate of I^2 was based on summary statistics from each trial and represents the percentage of the total variation in estimated treatment effects across trials better accounted for by heterogeneity rather than by chance. CAS=carotid stenting. EVA-3S=Endarterectomy versus Angioplasty in Patients with Symptomatic Severe Carotid Stenosis. SPACE=Stent-Protected Angioplasty versus Carotid Endarterectomy. ICSS=International Carotid Stenting Study. (Reprinted from The Lancet, Carotid Stenting Trialists' Collaboration. Short-term outcome after stenting versus endarterectomy for symptomatic carotid stenosis: a preplanned meta-analysis of individual patient data. *Lancet.* 2010;376:1062-1073. Copyright 2010, with permission from Elsevier.)

Endarterectomy (SPACE) trial, and the International Carotid Stenting Study (ICSS), evaluated symptomatic patients considered to be at standard surgical risk. These trials indicated a higher periprocedural risk of stroke with stenting than with endarterectomy. However, the number of patients in each trial was insufficient to establish the relative merits of stenting versus endarterectomy in particular patient subgroups. The investigators of EVA-3S, SPACE, and ICSS therefore established the Carotid Stenting Trialists' Collaboration anticipating a preplanned meta-analysis of individual patient data from these 3 trials. They sought to compare the safety and efficacy of CEA and CAS in predefined subgroups of patients through this meta-analysis. The European investigators showed significant insight in the planning of this preplanned meta-analysis. These data, in combination with the recently reported Carotid Revascularization Endarterectomy versus Stenting Trial data, strongly suggest that CEA is the preferred treatment for patients with symptomatic carotid stenosis who are aged 70 years or older (Figs 2 and 4). It is important to remember, however, that the data apply only to symptomatic standard surgical risk patients. They are only short-term data, and the relative efficacy of the 2 procedures for

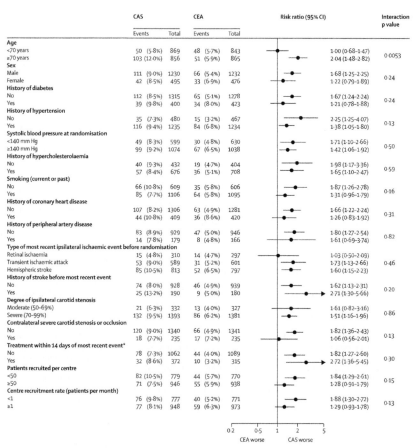

FIGURE 4.—Treatment risk ratios of any stroke or death within 120 days of randomisation in patient subgroups. Data are number or number (%), unless otherwise indicated. Percentages are number of events divided by number of patients. Analysis was by intention to treat. Dots and horizontal bars represent treatment risk ratios and 95% CIs within subgroups, respectively, with carotid endarterectomy (CEA) as the reference group, on a log scale. Risk ratios and interaction p values (categorical interaction) were adjusted for source trial. Patients with missing subgroup data were excluded from subgroup analysis (for details of missing data see webappendix pp 2–4). *Risk ratio of any stroke or death within 30 days of treatment in patients receiving the randomly allocated treatment (per-protocol analysis). CAS=carotid stenting. (Reprinted from The Lancet, Carotid Stenting Trialists' Collaboration. Short-term outcome after stenting versus endarterectomy for symptomatic carotid stenosis: a preplanned meta-analysis of individual patient data. *Lancet*. 2010;376:1062-1073. Copyright 2010, with permission from Elsevier.)

long-term stroke prevention, both in symptomatic and asymptomatic patients, is less clear.

G. L. Moneta, MD

Reference

1. Yadav JS, Wholey MH, Kuntz RE, et al. Protected carotid-artery stenting versus endarterectomy in high-risk patients. *N Engl J Med*. 2004;351:1493-1501.

Oxidized LDL in human carotid plaques is related to symptomatic carotid disease and lesion instability

Sigala F, Kotsinas A, Savari P, et al (Univ of Athens, Greece)
J Vasc Surg 52:704-713, 2010

Background.—Oxidative stress is an important determinant in atherosclerosis development. Various markers of oxidative stress, such as oxidation of low-density lipoprotein (LDL), nitrosative stress, lipid peroxidation, and protein oxidation, have been implicated in the initiation and/or progression of atherosclerosis, but their association with plaque erosion and symptomatic carotid disease has not been fully defined. In addition, certain oxidative markers have been shown in various models to promote plaque remodeling through matrix metalloproteinase (MMP) activation.

Objective.—To perform a global investigation of various oxidative stress markers and assess for potential relationships with destabilization and symptomatic development in human carotid plaques.

Methods.—Thirty-six patients undergoing endarterectomy were evaluated and compared with 20 control specimens obtained at the time of autopsy. Differences between stable and unstable plaques, symptomatic and asymptomatic patients, and ≥90% and <90% stenosis were evaluated. Oxidized LDL (ox-LDL), nitrotyrosine (NT), malondialdehyde (MDA), and protein carbonyls (PCs) levels were determined in atheromatic plaques homogenates by corresponding biochemical assays. Immunohistochemical (IHC) analysis was also employed to determine the percentage and topological distribution of cells expressing NT and metalloproteinase-9 (MMP-9) in serial sections from corresponding atheromatic plaques. MMP-9 expression was further verified using Western blot analysis.

Results.—Ox-LDL was increased in symptomatic patients ($P < .05$). Also, ox-LDL and NT levels were significantly higher in unstable versus stable carotid plaques ($P < .05$, respectively). Furthermore, IHC serial section analysis, corroborated by statistical analysis, showed a topological and expressional correlation between NT and MMP-9 ($P < .05$). MDA and PCs levels, although increased in carotid plaques, did not distinguish stable from unstable carotid plaques as well as symptomatic from asymptomatic patients with various degrees of stenosis.

Conclusion.—All types of investigated oxidative stress markers were significantly increased in human carotid plaques, but only ox-LDL levels were associated with clinical symptoms, while peroxynitrite products and MMP-9 were specifically related to plaque instability.

▶ The identification of carotid plaques at risk for plaque rupture potentially leading to stroke has been evaluated using various noninvasive techniques with variable results. However, the actual plaque biochemistry involving the inflammatory cascade and oxidative pathways leading to plaque instability is poorly defined. It is well known that oxidative stress is an important event that leads to oxidation of various molecules including lipoproteins, lipids, and proteins that are necessary for atherosclerotic plaque to form. Specifically, peroxynitrite (the reaction product between nitric oxide and superoxide anion radicals) and malondialdehyde (the product from lipid peroxidation) are powerful low-density lipoprotein (LDL) oxidants, which generate modified LDL with increased atherogenic potential, and oxidized LDL (oxLDL) can lead to further oxidation of other molecules. This particular study evaluates oxidative metabolites in carotid plaques from patients with and without symptoms. The study also classifies plaques as stable or unstable by histopathology. In addition, the study uses 20 control carotid arteries from cadavers that are age and sex matched. The biomolecules that were measured to assess oxidative stressed metabolites included the level of oxLDL, nitrosative stress (measuring nitrotyrosine levels, a byproduct of reaction from peroxynitrite), lipid peroxidation (measuring malondialdehyde levels), and protein oxidation (by measuring protein carbonyls). Also, matrix metalloproteinases have been implicated in plaque instability and may be activated by oxidative molecules. The major finding of the study found an increased oxLDL in symptomatic patients ($P < .05$) versus asymptomatic patients and significantly increased oxLDL in unstable plaques versus stable plaques of control carotid artery. Also, oxLDL and nitrotyrosine levels were significantly higher in unstable versus stable carotid plaques ($P < .05$, respectively), but the nitrotyrosine levels were similar between patients with or without symptoms but significantly elevated compared with control. Matrix metalloproteinase (MMP)-9 expression levels were found significantly increased in unstable plaques in comparison to the stable ones and on immunohistochemistry colocalized with areas of intense staining for nitrotyrosine. In addition, both stable and unstable plaques had higher MMP-9 protein levels than control carotid. Although both malondialdehyde and protein carbonyls were elevated in diseased carotid plaques compared with controls, there were no differences between stable and unstable plaques or symptomatic and asymptomatic patients. The interesting aspect of this study is that markers of oxidative stress are present in carotid plaques and oxLDL and nitrotyrosine levels distinguish symptomatic and asymptomatic, as well as unstable and stable plaques. These findings suggest that potential markers can be used to identify carotid plaques at risk for rupture and provide an avenue to assess if certain drugs such as statins can have an effect on the stability of the plaques as measured by oxidative stress markers. The limitations of this study are that the number of plaques studied was small with a total of 36 (19 symptomatic, 17 asymptomatic). However, the information presented will set a precedent for future studies in carotid plaque inflammation and plaque stability.

J. D. Raffetto, MD

Transatlantic Debate. Asymptomatic Carotid Artery Stenosis—Medical Therapy Alone Versus Medical Therapy Plus Carotid Endarterectomy or Stenting
Schneider PA, Naylor AR (Kaiser Foundation Hosp, Honolulu, HI; Leicester Royal Infirmary LE2 7LX, UK)
Eur J Vasc Endovasc Surg 40:274-281, 2010

Background.—In the 1970s the Asymptomatic Carotid Atherosclerosis Study (ACAS) and the Asymptomatic Carotid Surgery Trial (ACST) found that carotid endarterectomy (CEA) prevented stroke in asymptomatic patients with 60% to 99% stenosis. These findings led the American Heart Association (AHA) to recommend that CEA be done for highly selected patients with high-grade asymptomatic stenosis. A debate rages as to whether CEA or stents are best or medical treatment is sufficient.

CEA Plus Medical Therapy.—Most asymptomatic patients with carotid stenosis of 60% to 99% are best treated by repairing the stenosis; leaving it can cause preventable strokes. Used judiciously with the best medical therapy (BMT) and done well, carotid repair offers lifelong protection against stroke-related death and disability. Practitioners performing carotid repair for their own benefit and not to benefit the patient should refrain from CEA or stenting. BMT reduces strokes in some populations, but has not been well tested in low-risk patients with significant asymptomatic carotid stenosis. Patching and medical management both contribute positively to the outcomes with repair. The use of antiplatelet agents and statin has improved the safety of repair by up to 50%. Research is needed to identify which patients are most likely to benefit from repair plus BMT and which patients are less likely to benefit. Patients who have significant carotid stenosis remain at risk for stroke until the stenosis is removed. They also suffer the psychological effects of living with a threatening lesion. Any negative effects of repair are apparent within 30 days, whereas the risks of using BMT alone develop only with time. No level 1 evidence supports using BMT alone.

Medical Therapy Alone.—Determining which asymptomatic patients need more than medical therapy has been left up to the physicians. This makes it difficult to introduce changes in the current practice of using CEA for all asymptomatic patients with stenosis because it significantly reduces stroke risk. Data from the ACAS and ACST studies show that nearly 90% of medically treated patients were not destined to have a stroke within 5 years. Treating everyone who fulfills the ACAS criteria with a 2.3% procedural risk will not prevent 95% of the strokes, those 70% unrelated to carotid disease and the strokes of carotid origin that do not involve significant stenosis. In addition, 15% to 20% first exhibit a transient ischemic attack (TIA). If CEA reduces stroke by 50%, only about five strokes will be prevented but many patients will undergo an unnecessary procedure. Such procedures cost US health care providers about $2.1 billion annually. In addition, for medically treated patients the annual risk of stroke has fallen significantly over the past 15 years. The 1995

5-year risk of any stroke was 17.5%, which fell to 11.8% after 5 years, then to 7.2% after 5 more years. The average annual risk of any stroke has fallen from 60% to 1.4% since the ACAS was published, with ipsilateral stroke risk falling from 67% to 0.7%.

Conclusions.—Research is needed to pit BMT plus repair against BMT alone. However, this will require about a decade to plan and conduct, so decisions must be made now about how to manage patients who are asymptomatic but have significant carotid stenosis. With medical therapy alone the risk of stroke has fallen significantly, making about 94% of interventions in asymptomatic patients unneeded.

▶ In this debate between 2 individuals with very different opinions regarding carotid endarterectomy in asymptomatic carotid stenosis, an outstanding review of the literature and an enlightening example of different interpretations of the same trials are evident. Dr Schneider makes the case for carotid endarterectomy along with best medical therapy (BMT) for asymptomatic high-grade carotid stenosis and identifies several key trials that support his viewpoint. He cites the Asymptomatic Carotid Atherosclerosis Study (ACAS) and the Asymptomatic Carotid Surgery Trial (ACST) studies, which demonstrated the decreased rate of stroke by 50% at 5 years. In addition, he argues that repair is front loaded with most complications occurring in the first 30 days, while BMT is pay-as-you-go, with risks becoming evident over the remainder of the patient's life. He also cites the lack of level 1 evidence supporting the BMT alone for treating this issue and the actual difficulty in compliance with a medical regimen.

Dr Naylor argues the point that patients with asymptomatic carotid stenosis were validated by groups such as the American Heart Association and their recommendations have been generalized by others and taken to mean "CEA is appropriate in asymptomatic patients with 60–99% stenosis" and the original phrase that was included in their recommendation "highly selected patients" was never clarified. In addition, he goes on to note that ACAS with a 2.3% procedural risk only prevents 59 strokes per 1000 carotid endarterectomies and that 90% of patients who were medically treated in ACAS/ACST were never destined to suffer a stroke over 5 years. In studies supporting BMT, he cites the meta-analysis of Abbott, who found that the annual risk of stroke has declined over the last 20 years and believes this finding can be attributed to improvements of BMT (high-dose statins).

These arguments represent different background and cultural viewpoints on this disease process and each has valid points. Both authors make a strong argument for their stance, and it is likely the truth lies somewhere between both of these disparate opinions.

N. Singh, MD

15 Vascular Trauma

Blunt Thoracic Aortic Injuries: An Autopsy Study
Teixeira PGR, Inaba K, Barmparas G, et al (Univ of Southern California, Los Angeles, CA)
J Trauma 70:197-202, 2011

Objective.—The objective of this study was to identify the incidence and patterns of thoracic aortic injuries in a series of blunt traumatic deaths and describe their associated injuries.

Methods.—All autopsies performed by the Los Angeles County Department of Coroner for blunt traumatic deaths in 2005 were retrospectively reviewed. Patients who had a traumatic thoracic aortic (TTA) injury were compared with the victims who did not have this injury for differences in baseline characteristics and patterns of associated injuries.

Results.—During the study period, 304 (35%) of 881 fatal victims of blunt trauma received by the Los Angeles County Department of Coroner underwent a full autopsy and were included in the analysis. The patients were on average aged 43 years ±21 years, 71% were men, and 39% had a positive blood alcohol screen. Motor vehicle collision was the most common mechanism of injury (50%), followed by pedestrian struck by auto (37%). A TTA injury was identified in 102 (34%) of the victims. The most common site of TTA injury was the isthmus and descending thoracic aorta, occurring in 67 fatalities (66% of the patients with TTA injuries). Patients with TTA injuries were significantly more likely to have other associated injuries: cardiac injury (44% vs. 25%, $p = 0.001$), hemothorax (86% vs. 56%, $p < 0.001$), rib fractures (86% vs. 72%, $p = 0.006$), and intra-abdominal injury (74% vs. 49%, $p < 0.001$) compared with patients without TTA injury. Patients with a TTA injury were significantly more likely to die at the scene (80% vs. 63%, $p = 0.002$).

Conclusion.—Thoracic aortic injuries occurred in fully one third of blunt traumatic fatalities, with the majority of deaths occurring at the scene. The risk for associated thoracic and intra-abdominal injuries is significantly increased in patients with thoracic aortic injuries.

▶ Over the last several years, there have been paradigm shifts in the management of blunt thoracic aortic trauma. These changes included more widespread imaging using CT scanning, aggressive blood pressure control of patients who reach the hospital alive, delayed treatment of thoracic aortic injuries, and more frequent use of endovascular techniques for repair of blunt thoracic trauma. These changes appear to have resulted over the last decade in a decline in mortality rate from about 22% to 13% for patients with thoracic aortic injuries who reach the hospital alive.[1] The authors point out, however, that many patients with blunt thoracic injury cannot benefit from these advantages because they die at the scene of the trauma. To develop some sense of the magnitude of this problem, the authors analyzed autopsy findings in a series of blunt traumatic fatalities. It is not surprising that the authors found that most patients with thoracic aortic injury die at the scene of the trauma. These patients often have multiple injuries, and it is impossible from these data to discern whether the thoracic aortic injury was the actual cause of death or was in fact merely a marker of the magnitude of the trauma and severity of associated injuries. It is likely that there is some truth to both options. It is important to note that motor vehicle accidents serve as the greatest source of thoracic aortic injury. The authors point out that despite advances in automotive and safety engineering, the prevalence of blunt thoracic aortic injury in motor vehicle accidents does not seem to have been impacted by these engineering advances. The association of thoracic aortic injury with motor vehicle accidents appears very similar to that identified by Parmley et al 50 years ago.[2] However, the data cannot answer the question of whether engineering advances may have reduced the fatality rate of blunt aortic thoracic trauma without affecting the prevalence of thoracic aortic injury as a consequence of motor vehicle trauma.

G. L. Moneta, MD

References

1. Demetriades D, Velmahos GC, Scalea TM, et al. Diagnosis and treatment of blunt thoracic aortic injuries: changing perspectives. *J Trauma*. 2008;64:1415-1418.
2. Parmley LF, Mattingly TW, Manion WC, Jahnke EJ Jr. Nonpenetrating traumatic injury of the aorta. *Circulation*. 1958;17:1086-1101.

Blunt Traumatic Thoracic Aortic Injuries: Early or Delayed Repair—Results of an American Association for the Surgery of Trauma Prospective Study
Demetriades D, Velmahos GC, Scalea TM, et al (American Association for the Surgery of Trauma, Los Angeles, CA)
J Trauma 66:967-973, 2009

Background.—The traditional approach to stable blunt thoracic aortic injuries (TAI) is immediate repair, with delayed repair reserved for patients with major associated injuries. In recent years, there has been a trend toward delayed repair, even in low-risk patients. This study evaluates the current practices in the surgical community regarding the timing of aortic repair and its effects on outcomes.

Methods.—This was a prospective, observational multicenter study sponsored by the American Association for the Surgery of Trauma. The study included patients with blunt TAI scheduled for aortic repair by open or endovascular procedure. Patients in extremis and those managed without aortic repair were excluded. The data collection included demographics, initial clinical presentation, Injury Severity Scores, type and site of aortic injury, type of aortic repair (open or endovascular repair), and time from injury to aortic repair. The study patients were divided into an early repair (≤24hours) and delayed repair groups (>24 hours). The outcome variables included survival, ventilator days, intensive care unit (ICU) and hospital lengths of stay, blood transfusions, and complications. The outcomes in the two groups were compared with multivariate analysis after adjusting for age, Glasgow Coma Scale, hypotension, major associated injuries, and type of aortic repair. A second multivariate analysis compared outcomes between early and delayed repair, in patients with and patients without major associated injuries.

Results.—There were 178 patients with TAI eligible for inclusion and analysis, 109 (61.2%) of which underwent early repair and 69 (38.8%) delayed repair. The two groups had similar epidemiologic, injury severity, and type of repair characteristics. The adjusted mortality was significantly higher in the early repair group (adjusted OR [95% CI] 7.78 [1.69−35.70], adjusted p value = 0.008). The adjusted complication rate was similar in the two groups. However, delayed repair was associated with significantly longer ICU and hospital lengths of stay. Analysis of the 108 patients without major associated injuries, adjusting for age, Glasgow Coma Scale, hypotension, and type of aortic repair, showed that in early repair there was a trend toward higher mortality rate (adjusted OR 9.08 [0.88−93.78], adjusted p value = 0.064) but a significantly lower complication rate (adjusted OR 0.4 [0.18−0.96], adjusted p value 0.040) and shorter ICU stay (adjusted p value = 0.021) than the delayed repair group. A similar analysis of the 68 patients with major associated injuries, showed a strong trend toward higher mortality in the early repair group (adjusted OR 9.39 [0.93−95.18], adjusted p value = 0.058). The complication rate was similar in both groups (adjusted p value = 0.239).

Conclusions.—Delayed repair of stable blunt TAI is associated with improved survival, irrespective of the presence or not of major associated injuries. However, delayed repair is associated with a longer length of ICU stay and in the group of patients with no major associated injuries a significantly higher complication rate.

▶ A number of individual case series over the past several years have suggested that blunt traumatic thoracic aortic injury can be effectively managed with delayed repair. The stimulus for delayed repair undoubtedly resulted from dissatisfaction with the results of emergent operation, the greater availability of endografts, and more widespread use of beta-blockers in the management of thoracic aortic trauma. This study reports data from the American Association for the Surgery of Trauma multicenter registry of 18 participating trauma centers. The literature on delayed versus urgent repair to blunt thoracic aortic injuries is mixed. Previous studies have reported improved results with delayed repair, but others have been unable to demonstrate benefit. Delayed repair appeared to be safe but perhaps is associated with longer hospital lengths of stay and higher direct costs than earlier repair. Overall, previous studies, and this study, suggest that there is a survival advantage of delayed repair. Patients with major associated injuries seem to benefit most with delayed repair with demonstrated improved survival and no increased systemic complications at the expense of a longer length of stay than early repair. The data support delayed repair in all patients with blunt thoracic aortic injuries irrespective of risk factors. Patients with major associated injuries are most likely to benefit from delayed repair.

G. L. Moneta, MD

Blunt Vertebral Artery Injuries in the Era of Computed Tomographic Angiographic Screening: Incidence and Outcomes From 8292 Patients

Berne JD, Norwood SH (East Texas Med Ctr, Tyler)
J Trauma 67:1333-1338, 2009

Introduction.—Blunt injuries to the vertebral artery (BVI) are rare. Recent improvements in the multidetector computer tomography (MDCT) technology and increased use of screening protocols have led to a greater number of these injuries identified. Well-defined treatment recommendations are still lacking, and it is unclear whether screening and treatment lead to improved outcome.

Methods.—All patients who met predefined screening criteria were screened for BVI with a MDCT angiogram (MDCT-A). All patients identified with BVI were treated based on injury grade and associated injuries. Hospital course, morbidity, mortality, and follow-up were recorded and analyzed.

Results.—A total of 8292 patients were admitted for blunt injuries during this time period. Forty-four patients were found to have 47 BVI (three bilateral). Pharmacologic treatment with anticoagulants (AC)—heparin and warfarin—or an antiplatelet agent—clopidogrel and aspirin—was initiated in 37 patients (84%). Angiographic coiling was performed in eight patients (18%), and two (5%) had endovascular stents placed. Four patients developed signs of cerebral ischemia (9%), of whom three died and one recovered completely. Overall mortality rate was 16% (7/44). BVI-related mortality occurred in three patients (7%). Of these, two patients had bilateral vertebral artery occlusion or transaction, and death was considered nonpreventable. One death occurred in a patient with a unilateral vertebral dissection developed a posterior circulation infarct. Anticoagulation was felt to be contraindicated in this patient initially due to intracranial hemorrhage. This was deemed the only potentially preventable BVI-related mortality. Annual BVI-related mortality rate in the 4 years before initiating the screening protocol was 0.75 cases per year. During this study period, it was 0.57 cases per year.

Conclusion.—Under an aggressive screening and individualized treatment protocol for BVI, we had very few potentially preventable BVI-related strokes and deaths. We are unable to conclude; however, based on historical controls that either screening or treatment improved overall outcome.

▶ When patients are screened aggressively for blunt vertebral artery injury (BVI), the incidence following appears to be 0.49% to 0.71%.[1,2] This rate of identification of BVI appears to be higher than the prescreening era where approximately 0.1% of patients with blunt injuries were identified with BVI.[3] Stroke rates associated with BVI have been reported at 24% with BVI mortality rates of 8%.[4] Clearly, if one looks for BVIs, they can be found. In this study, criteria for screening included basilar skull fractures, cervical spine injuries, severe facial fractures, cervical hematomas, or cervical abrasions, as well as GCS ≤ 8 and lateralizing neurologic signs and mechanism of hanging for the injury. All patients had a high-speed deceleration incident or blunt cervical trauma. In this study, 86.4% of the patients were identified based on screening criteria alone. Patients overall did well with only one possibly preventable death from BVI. Strictly speaking, however, one cannot conclude that screening for BVI in itself results in decreased neurologic morbidity and mortality as there is no control group. What this study tells us is that patients with BVI identified through screening and treated with a variety of modalities will have low neurologic morbidity and mortality. Whether that treatment was necessary to provide that low neurologic morbidity and mortality is unknown.

G. L. Moneta, MD

References

1. Miller PR, Fabian TC, Croce MA, et al. Prospective screening for blunt cerebrovascular injuries: analysis of diagnostic modalities and outcomes. *Ann Surg.* 2002;236:386-393.
2. Berne JD, Reuland KS, Villarreal DH, McGovern TM, Rowe SA, Norwood SH. Sixteen-slice multi-detector computed tomographic angiography improves the accuracy of screening for blunt cerebrovascular injury. *Trauma.* 2006;60: 1204-1219.
3. Thibodeaux LC, Hearn AT, Peschiera JL, et al. Extracranial vertebral artery dissection after trauma: a 5-year review. *Br J Surg.* 1997;84:94.
4. Biffl WL, Moore EE, Elliott JP, et al. The devastating potential of blunt vertebral arterial injuries. *Ann Surg.* 2000;231:672-681.

Damage Control Techniques for Common and External Iliac Artery Injuries: Have Temporary Intravascular Shunts Replaced the Need for Ligation?
Ball CG, Feliciano DV (Emory Univ School of Medicine, Atlanta, GA)
J Trauma 68:1117-1120, 2010

Background.—Trauma to the common or external iliac arteries has a mortality rate of 24% to 60%. "Damage control" options for these severely injured vessels are either ligation or temporary intravascular shunts (TIVSs). Complications of ligation include a 50% amputation rate and up to 90% mortality. The primary goal of this study was to identify the consequences of using ligation versus TIVS for common or external iliac artery injuries in damage control scenarios.

Methods.—All patients with injuries to an iliac artery (1995–2008) at a Level I trauma center were reviewed. Demographics and outcomes were analyzed using standard statistical methodology.

Results.—Iliac artery injuries were present in 88 patients (71 external and 17 common; 72% penetrating; median Injury Severity Score, 25; mean hospital stay, 28 days). Most nonsurvivors (73%) died of refractory shock within the first 24 hours after presenting with hemodynamic instability (66%). Ligation was required in one (6%) common and 14 (20%) external iliac arteries. TIVS was used in two (12%) common and five (7%) external iliac arteries. Patients requiring ligation (1995–2005) or TIVS (2005–2008) for their common or external iliac arteries had similar demographics and injuries ($p > 0.05$). Compared with patients who underwent ligation, patients receiving TIVS required fewer amputations (47% vs. 0%) and fasciotomies (93% vs. 43%; $p < 0.05$). Mortality in the ligation group was 73%, versus 43% in the TIVS cohort.

Conclusions.—TIVSs have replaced ligation as the primary damage control procedure for injuries to common and external iliac arteries. As a result, the high incidence of subsequent amputation has been virtually eliminated. With increased TIVS experience, an improvement in survival is likely.

▶ Iliac artery trauma is highly lethal, with mortality rates ranging from 24% to 60%.[1] Traditional damage control for iliac artery injuries has been ligation and was associated with a 50% amputation and up to 90% mortality rate. The goal of this study was to identify the consequences of using ligation versus temporary intravascular shunt (TIVS) for common or external iliac artery injuries in damage control scenarios. TIVSs have long been used as a method of temporarily restoring arterial circulation in patients with peripheral arterial injuries distal to the axillary crease and inguinal ligament. Their use, and particularly prolonged use, for maintaining arterial circulation after injuries at other sites is less frequent. The article indicates that a major vascular injury within the abdomen does not necessarily need to be acutely repaired in damage control situations. A shunt can be placed and the patient resuscitated appropriately, coagulopathy corrected, and the patient brought back to the operating room for interval repair of vascular and other associated injuries. Of course, the overall number of patients is small, but the use of temporary shunts for selected cases of iliac artery injury appears reasonable and may result in a reduced rate of amputation and perhaps improved survival as well.

G. L. Moneta, MD

Reference

1. Dente CJ, Feliciano DV. *Trauma.* 6th ed. New York: McGraw-Hill Medical; 2008. 737–757.

Early outcomes of deliberate nonoperative management for blunt thoracic aortic injury in trauma
Caffarelli AD, Mallidi HR, Maggio PM, et al (Stanford Univ School of Medicine, CA)
J Thorac Cardiovasc Surg 140:598-605, 2010

Objective.—Traumatic blunt aortic injury has traditionally been viewed as a surgical emergency, whereas nonoperative therapy has been reserved for nonsurgical candidates. This study reviews our experience with deliberate, nonoperative management for blunt thoracic aortic injury.

Methods.—A retrospective chart review with selective longitudinal follow-up was conducted for patients with blunt aortic injury. Surveillance imaging with computed tomography angiography was performed. Nonoperative patients were then reviewed and analyzed for survival, evolution of aortic injury, and treatment failures.

Results.—During the study period, 53 patients with an average age of 45 years (range, 18–80 years) were identified, with 28% presenting to

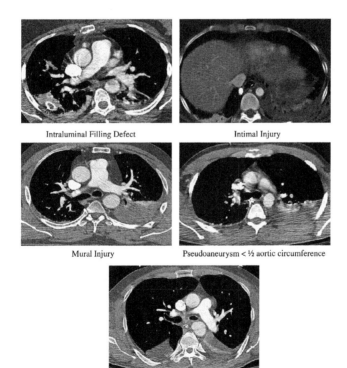

Intraluminal Filling Defect   Intimal Injury

Mural Injury   Pseudoaneurysm < ½ aortic circumference

Pseudoaneurysm > ½ aortic circumference

FIGURE 1.—Computed tomography grading. (Reprinted from the Journal of Thoracic and Cardiovascular Surgery, Caffarelli AD, Mallidi HR, Maggio PM, et al. Early outcomes of deliberate nonoperative management for blunt thoracic aortic injury in trauma. *J Thorac Cardiovasc Surg.* 2010;140:598-605. Copyright 2010 with permission from The American Association for Thoracic Surgery.)

Year	2001	2002	2003	2004	2005	2006	2007	2008
Non-OP	1	2	1	0	5	5	14	1
Operative	4	2	6	9	1	2	0	0
stent	1	1	6	6	0	1	-	-
open	3	1	0	3	1	1	-	-

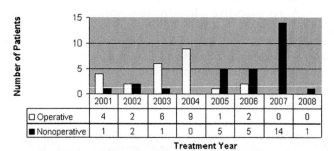

Operative vs Non-Operative Management by Years

Treatment Year	2001	2002	2003	2004	2005	2006	2007	2008
☐ Operative	4	2	6	9	1	2	0	0
■ Nonoperative	1	2	1	0	5	5	14	1

FIGURE 2.—Operative versus nonoperative management by year. (Reprinted from the Journal of Thoracic and Cardiovascular Surgery, Caffarelli AD, Mallidi HR, Maggio PM, et al. Early outcomes of deliberate nonoperative management for blunt thoracic aortic injury in trauma. *J Thorac Cardiovasc Surg.* 2010;140:598-605. Copyright 2010 with permission from The American Association for Thoracic Surgery.)

the Stanford University School of Medicine emergency department and 72% transferred from outside hospitals. Of the 53 patients, 29 underwent planned, nonoperative management. Of the 29 nonoperative patients, in-hospital survival was 93% with no aortic deaths in the remaining patients. Survival was 97% at a median of 1.8 years (range, 0.9—7.2 years). One patient failed nonoperative management and underwent open repair. Serial imaging was performed in all patients (average = 107 days; median, 31 days), with 21 patients having stable aortic injuries without progression and 5 patients having resolved aortic injuries.

Conclusions.—This experience suggests that deliberate, nonoperative management of carefully selected patients with traumatic blunt aortic injury may be a reasonable alternative in the polytrauma patient; however, serial imaging and long-term follow-up are necessary (Figs 1 and 2).

▶ Early operative repair has been the standard for management of blunt thoracic aortic injuries. However, in recent years delayed repair in selected patients has also become accepted. In this article, the authors go an additional step further and report deliberate nonoperative management of blunt thoracic aortic injury. They note that over the last decade with improved prehospital care and improved imaging studies, patients arrive at the hospital with a spectrum of thoracic aortic injury. Whereas it has now become common to treat blunt thoracic aortic injury with thoracic endovascular aortic repair (TEVAR), the authors have expressed reluctance to implant endografts in young patients with perhaps 50 to 60 more years of life expectancy. They have now increasingly adopted a deliberate strategy of nonoperative management of selected patients with blunt thoracic aortic injury (Fig 2). Their strategy includes aggressive negative inotropic therapy, serial imaging (Fig 1), and close clinical observation. In this report, they present very favorable short-term results of deliberate nonoperative management of blunt thoracic aortic injury. Also with this report, another so-called principle of trauma management has now come under question. Fifteen years ago, anyone advocating delayed and now even nonoperative management of thoracic aortic injury would have been booted from the room. The Stanford surgeons are to be congratulated for their continued contributions to the management of thoracic aortic disease and their willingness to look at the patients in their practice and, based on these observations, to then buck the current trend to reflexively treat thoracic aortic injuries with TEVAR. Of course, this is one practice where almost 75% of the patients with thoracic injury were received as transfers. However, this is also likely the case in most centers that treat thoracic aortic injuries, and one can strongly suspect that the authors' observations will be transferable to other centers as well.

G. L. Moneta, MD

16 Nonatherosclerotic Conditions

Effect of celiprolol on prevention of cardiovascular events in vascular Ehlers-Danlos syndrome: a prospective randomised, open, blinded-endpoints trial

Ong K-T, Perdu J, De Backer J, et al (Hôpital Européen Georges Pompidou, Paris, France; Ghent Univ Hosp, Belgium; et al)

Lancet 376:1476-1484, 2010

Background.—Vascular Ehlers-Danlos syndrome is a rare severe disease that causes arterial dissections and ruptures that can lead to early death. No preventive treatment has yet been validated. Our aim was to assess the ability of celiprolol, a β_1-adrenoceptor antagonist with a β_2-adrenoceptor agonist action, to prevent arterial dissections and ruptures in vascular Ehlers-Danlos syndrome.

Methods.—Our study was a multicentre, randomised, open trial with blinded assessment of clinical events in eight centres in France and one in Belgium. Patients with clinical vascular Ehlers-Danlos syndrome were randomly assigned to 5 years of treatment with celiprolol or to no treatment. Randomisation was done from a centralised, previously established list of sealed envelopes with stratification by patients' age (≤ 32 years or >32 years). 33 patients were positive for mutation of collagen 3A1 (*COL3A1*). Celiprolol was uptitrated every 6 months by steps of 100 mg to a maximum of 400 mg twice daily. The primary endpoints were arterial events (rupture or dissection, fatal or not). This study is registered with ClinicalTrials.gov, number NCT00190411.

Findings.—53 patients were randomly assigned to celiprolol (25 patients) or control groups (28). Mean duration of follow-up was 47 (SD 5) months, with the trial stopped early for treatment benefit. The primary endpoints were reached by five (20%) in the celiprolol group and by 14 (50%) controls (hazard ratio [HR] $0 \cdot 36$; 95% CI $0 \cdot 15 - 0 \cdot 88$; $p = 0 \cdot 040$). Adverse events were severe fatigue in one patient after starting 100 mg celiprolol and mild fatigue in two patients related to dose uptitration.

Interpretation.—We suggest that celiprolol might be the treatment of choice for physicians aiming to prevent major complications in patients with vascular Ehlers-Danlos syndrome. Whether patients with similar clinical presentations and no mutation are also protected remains to be established.

▶ Ehlers-Danlos syndrome is a heterogeneous group of connective tissue disorders. It results from heterogeneous mutations in the COL3A1 gene, which causes structural defects in the pro1(III) chain of collagen type III. The vascular form of Ehlers-Danlos is the most severe form of the syndrome. This form is autosomal dominant. The median survival is 40 to 50 years, and major complications include vascular dissection or rupture of hollow organs (uterus, intestine). Initial complications are usually seen by 20 years of age, and by 40 years of age, 90% of patients have had a major event.

Patients with vascular Ehlers-Danlos syndrome have decreased intima-media thickness (IMT).[1] Decreases in IMT may lead to decreased resistance to mechanical stress and have led the authors to propose that treatment with celiprolol may prevent the vascular events associated with Ehlers-Danlos syndrome. Celiprolol reduces heart rate and mean and pulsatile pressures in patients with essential hypertension and therefore theoretically could decrease continuous and pulsatile mechanical stresses on weakened collagen fibers in the arterial wall of patients with Ehlers-Danlos syndrome. The trial suggests benefit of prevention of major complications of Ehlers-Danlos syndrome in patients with a clinical diagnosis of the syndrome. Subgroup analysis indicates equal benefit in patients with and without proven COL3A1 mutation. Most of the patients in this study were normotensive at inclusion. The authors found that celiprolol did not decrease brachial systolic or diastolic pressures or heart rate, making it unlikely that the protective effect of celiprolol was mediated through blood pressure lowering. The authors postulated that the mechanism of action of celiprolol in Ehlers-Danlos syndrome may be through an effect on transforming growth factor β and collagen synthesis. Results of the study must be interpreted with caution, as not all patients in the study were positive for proven genetic mutations associated with Ehlers-Danlos syndrome. Nevertheless, all included patients met the clinical criteria for Ehlers-Danlos syndrome and the results in the mutation-positive and mutation-negative patients were similar, although that analysis was not prespecified in the study design.

G. L. Moneta, MD

Reference

1. Boutouyrie P, Germain DP, Fiessinger JN, Laloux B, Perdu J, Laurent S. Increased carotid wall stress in vascular Ehlers-Danlos syndrome. *Circulation*. 2004;109: 1530-1535.

Evaluation for Clinical Predictors of Positive Temporal Artery Biopsy in Giant Cell Arteritis

Rieck KL, Kermani TA, Thomsen KM, et al (Mayo Clinic, Rochester, MN)
J Oral Maxillofac Surg 69:36-40, 2011

Purpose.—To examine the clinical predictors of a positive temporal artery biopsy (TAB) among patients suspected of having giant cell arteritis. *Patients and Methods.*—We conducted a retrospective study of all consecutive patients who underwent TAB by a single surgeon (K.L.R.) at the Department of Oral Maxillofacial Surgery from April 30, 2002, to June 29, 2006. The medical records were reviewed for the clinical symptoms, laboratory findings, biopsy results, and final diagnosis. The variables of interest as predictors of positive biopsy findings were analyzed using logistic regression analysis.

Results.—During the study period, 82 patients underwent TAB. Histologic evidence of arteritis was present in 22 patients (26.8%). Two (2.4%) were diagnosed with giant cell arteritis clinically but had negative TAB findings. The patients presenting with weight loss or jaw claudication were more likely to have a positive TAB finding (odds ratio 4.50, 95% confidence interval 1.45 to 13.93; and odds ratio 3.71, 95% confidence interval 1.28 to 10.76, respectively). No laboratory findings were predictive of a positive TAB finding. Prednisone use before TAB also was not associated with a decreased likelihood of a positive finding.

Conclusions.—Patients suspected of having giant cell arteritis were more likely to have a positive TAB finding if they presented with weight loss or jaw claudication. In the present series, corticosteroid therapy before biopsy did not affect the rate of positive TAB findings.

▶ Temporal arteritis (TA) is the most common systemic vasculitis in adults older than 50 years. Patients are most likely to present with tenderness of the scalp or new onset of headache. Others present with predominately constitutional symptoms, such as weight loss, fatigue, or fever. Pain with mastication is present in 50% of cases.[1] Ocular manifestations of TA are common and include decreased vision, diplopia, and amaurosis fugax. Up to 20% of patients may develop irreversible visual loss from optic nerve ischemia. The diagnosis of TA can be difficult, and although elevated inflammatory markers, such as erythrocyte sedimentation rate and C-reactive protein, are frequently seen in patients with temporal arteritis, they are not specific. An abnormal finding on temporal artery biopsy is, however, a part of the American College of Rheumatology criteria for diagnosis of TA.[2] However, up to two-thirds of temporal artery biopsies are negative. It would, therefore, be useful to determine which clinical parameters most likely correlate with TA to identify patients who will most likely benefit from treatment while waiting to undergo temporal artery biopsy.[3] High doses of corticosteroids are used in the initial treatment of TA. Such drugs are not benign in elderly patients, and for logistical and referral reasons, temporal artery biopsy and the results of that biopsy may not be available as rapidly as desirable. If one does not wish to treat all patients suspected of TA prior to the biopsy results, the study provides some guidance for patients who are at highest risk for actually having a positive biopsy. Pain with mastication and weight loss appear to be more important parameters in predicting temporal artery biopsy positivity than laboratory markers of information. It is also useful to know that beginning prednisone therapy based on clinical parameters will not decrease the likelihood of a positive temporal artery biopsy.

G. L. Moneta, MD

References

1. Salvarani C, Cantini F, Hunder GG. Polymyalgia rheumatica and giant-cell arteritis. *Lancet.* 2008;372:234-245.
2. Hunder GG, Bloch DA, Michel BA, et al. The American College of Rheumatology 1990 criteria for the classification of giant cell arteritis. *Arthritis Rheum.* 1990;33: 1122-1128.
3. Younge BR, Cook BE Jr, Bartley GB, Hodge DO, Hunder GG. Initiation of glucocorticoid therapy: before or after temporal artery biopsy? *Mayo Clin Proc.* 2004; 79:483-491.

How Do the Type and Location of a Vascular Malformation Influence Growth in Klippel-Trénaunay Syndrome?

Funayama E, Sasaki S, Oyama A, et al (Hokkaido Univ Graduate School of Medicine, Sapporo, Japan; Tonan Hosp, Sapporo, Japan)
Plast Reconstr Surg 127:340-346, 2011

Background.—Although Klippel-Trénaunay syndrome is a mixed vascular malformation characterized by abnormal growth in the extremities, no uniform diagnostic criteria have been established because of the variety in its manifestation. Consequently, no anatomical analysis based on a comparison study has been reported. In this study, the authors determine the frequency of various vascular malformations and abnormal growth and assess any statistical relationship between vascular malformation type/location and abnormal growth in terms of length and girth.

Methods.—Thirty-five patients with Klippel-Trénaunay syndrome satisfying the criteria proposed by Oduber et al. in 2008 were enrolled. The type and location of the vascular malformation and abnormal circumferential growth were assessed by magnetic resonance imaging and ultrasonography. Bone girth was assessed by axial magnetic resonance imaging/computed tomography. Plain radiographs of the long bones were used to measure growth in length.

Results.—The spectrum of vascular types was similar to that in previous reports. There was no significant association between leg length and vascular malformation type or location. Leg bone circumferential hypoplasia was observed in 50 percent of cases and was significantly related to the presence of intramuscular lesions. A single venous malformation in the subcutaneous tissue was significantly associated with the presence of subcutaneous hypertrophy. Patients with intramuscular lymphatic malformations had a significantly higher frequency of muscle hypoplasia.

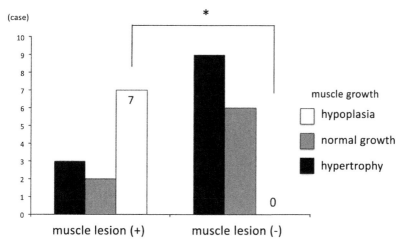

FIGURE 2.—Of 29 lower leg Klippel-Trénaunay syndrome patients, 27 had abnormal circumferential growth. The presence of vascular malformations in muscle was significantly associated with muscle hypoplasia (*p = 0.00089). (Reprinted from Funayama E, Sasaki S, Oyama A, et al. How do the type and location of a vascular malformation influence growth in Klippel-Trénaunay syndrome? *Plast Reconstr Surg.* 2011;127:340-346, http://lww.com.)

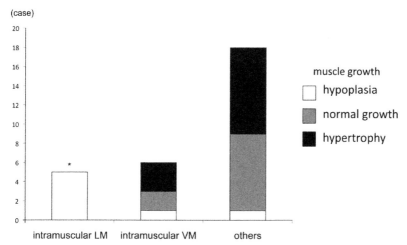

FIGURE 3.—Abnormal circumferential growth in 29 Klippel-Trénaunay syndrome patients with lower leg lesions was analyzed according to the type of intramuscular vascular malformation. Intramuscular lymphatic malformation was significantly correlated with muscle hypoplasia (*p = 0.015). The patient with no deep vascular lesions had only capillary malformations. One case presented with treated tufted angioma and subcutaneous venous malformations. *LM*, lymphatic malformation; *VM*, venous malformation. (Reprinted from Funayama E, Sasaki S, Oyama A, et al. How do the type and location of a vascular malformation influence growth in Klippel-Trénaunay syndrome? *Plast Reconstr Surg.* 2011;127:340-346, http://lww.com.)

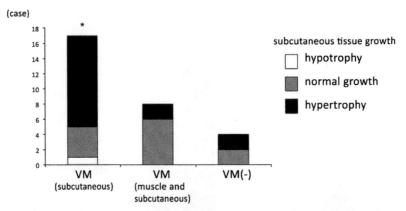

FIGURE 4.—Abnormal circumferential soft-tissue growth in 29 Klippel-Trénaunay syndrome patients with lower leg lesions was analyzed according to the location of the venous malformation (subcutaneous tissue/both subcutaneous tissue and muscle/none). No patient had venous malformations in muscle alone. Venous malformations in subcutaneous tissue alone, but not in both subcutaneous tissue and muscle, were significantly associated with hypertrophy of the subcutaneous tissue (*$p = 0.032$). VM, venous malformation. (Reprinted from Funayama E, Sasaki S, Oyama A, et al. How do the type and location of a vascular malformation influence growth in Klippel-Trénaunay syndrome? *Plast Reconstr Surg.* 2011;127:340-346, http://lww.com.)

Conclusion.—The type and location of certain vascular malformations were significantly associated with abnormal subcutaneous tissue, muscle, and bone growth.

▶ Klippel-Trénaunay (KT) syndrome is a mixed vascular malformation with a combination of capillary nevus, early-onset varicosities, and hypertrophy of tissues and bones of the affected limb. The syndrome has a wide variety of manifestations, and different authors describing KT syndrome use different diagnostic criteria. Oduber et al,[1] in 2008, proposed restrictive diagnostic criteria for KT syndrome. They categorized manifestations of KT syndrome into 2 groups. Group A consists of venous and capillary malformations, and group B is defined by abnormal growth of the affected limb in terms of length or girth. The authors' use of the categorization criteria of Oduber et al is useful, as it provides a precise description of the patients in the study. Their observations that certain patterns of malformation influence patterns of subcutaneous or muscle hypertrophy (Figs 2, 3, and 4) may provide a starting point for determining what elements of a vascular malformation should be treated to maximize patient function in the long term by normalizing muscle mass or decreasing subcutaneous hypertrophy.

G. L. Moneta, MD

Reference

1. Oduber CE, van der Horst CM, Hennekam RC. Klippel-Trenaunay syndrome: diagnostic criteria and hypothesis on etiology. *Ann Plast Surg.* 2008;60:217-223.

Late Outcomes of Endovascular and Open Revascularization for Nonatherosclerotic Renal Artery Disease

Ham SW, Kumar SR, Wang BR, et al (Univ of Southern California, Los Angeles, CA)

Arch Surg 145:832-839, 2010

Objective.—To evaluate the long-term outcome of endovascular and open treatment for nonatherosclerotic renal artery disease (NARAD).

Design.—Retrospective review.

Setting.—Academic institution.

Patients.—Fifty-five patients (47 women; mean age, 40 years) with NARAD. Underlying disease included Takayasu arteritis in 31 and fibromuscular dysplasia in 24.

Interventions.—Open revascularization and renal artery percutaneous transluminal angioplasty with or without stenting.

Main Outcome Measures.—Primary, primary assisted, and secondary patency rates; blood pressure; antihypertensive medication requirements; renal function; and mortality.

Results.—Seventy-nine renal interventions were performed, including 59 aortorenal bypass (16 ex vivo), 3 visceral-renal bypass, 12 endovascular (8 percutaneous transluminal angioplasty and 4 stent placements) procedures, and 5 nephrectomies. There were no inhospital deaths. During a mean follow-up of 75 months, 1-, 3-, and 5-year primary patency rates for any intervention were 87%, 75%, and 75%, respectively; primary assisted/secondary patency rates were 92%, 86%, and 86%, respectively. Endovascular interventions at 1, 3, and 5 years had primary patency rates of 73%, 49%, and 49%, respectively, and primary assisted/secondary patency rates of 83%, 83%, and 83%, respectively. For open revascularization, 1-, 3-, and 5-year primary patency rates were 91%, 80%, and 80%, respectively; primary assisted/secondary patency rates were 94%, 87%, and 87%, respectively. For both interventions, blood pressure and the number of antihypertensives used were reduced compared with preintervention values (all $P < .05$). Serum creatinine level and estimated glomerular filtration rate were also improved after revascularization (both $P < .05$). There were 6 deaths. Five- and 10-year actuarial survival rates were 94% and 78%, respectively.

Conclusions.—Endovascular and open management of NARAD confers long-term benefit for blood pressure, renal function, renal artery/graft patency, and survival. Open revascularization results in superior 1- and 5-year outcomes compared with endovascular management and provides the most durable outcome for NARAD.

▶ Of patients with nonatherosclerotic renal artery disease (NARAD) with correctable hypertension, fibromuscular dysplasia and Takayasu arteritis are the most common etiologies. It is generally agreed that open or endovascular revascularization is preferred over medical management alone in patients with severe hypertension associated with NARAD. In addition, percutaneous transluminal angioplasty is generally considered the first-line therapy for fibro-muscular disease, while patients with Takayasu arteritis are felt best treated with open revascularization. Some do argue that endovascular therapy is the preferred initial treatment in patients with Takayasu arteritis as well.[1] The purpose of this article was to evaluate the long-term outcome of endovascular and open treatment of NARAD. The authors have demonstrated that both open and endovascular intervention can be safe and effective in managing renal artery—mediated hypertension and renal dysfunction associated with NARAD. The patients are not randomized, and any conclusion is somewhat weakened by the study design, but in general, the data indicate that primary open revascularization provides superior outcome with respect to patency with equivalent safety compared with endovascular intervention. The authors' conclusion is that open revascularization should be considered selectively as the first-line of therapy for NARAD in the young patient with moderate to complex renal artery disease. This conclusion is clearly suggested, but not confirmed, by the data.

G. L. Moneta, MD

Reference

1. Sharma S, Saxena A, Talwar KK, Kaul U, Mehta SN, Rajani M. Renal artery stenosis caused by nonspecific arteritis (Takayasu disease): results of treatment with percutaneous transluminal angioplasty. *AJR Am J Roentgenol.* 1992;158: 417-422.

Leiomyosarcoma of the Inferior Vena Cava: Clinicopathologic Study of 40 Cases
Laskin WB, Fanburg-Smith JC, Burke AP, et al (Northwestern Memorial Hosp, Chicago, IL; Armed Forces Inst of Pathology, Warsaw, Poland; et al)
Am J Surg Pathol 34:873-881, 2010

This report details the clinicopathologic features and follow-up data on 40 cases of inferior vena cava leiomyosarcoma, a rare sarcoma with a poor prognosis. Study cohort consisted of 31 females and 9 males (mean age, 53 y), whose material was accessioned to the Armed Forces Institute of Pathology between 1976 and 2008. Inferior vena cava leiomyosarcomas ranged in size from 3.5 to 15.0 (median, 8.5) cms, and most involved the middle segment of the vessel and grew extraluminally. Eleven leiomyosarcomas were French Federation Nationale des Centres de Lutte Contre le Cancer (FNCLCC) histologic grade I; 21, grade II; and 5 were grade III. Eleven of 33 patients managed by complete or radical resection had involved surgical margins. Twenty of the 34 patients (59%) with clinical follow-up data (mean, 33.5; median, 51 mo) died of sarcoma-related complications and 9 (26%) of unknown causes. The 5-year and 10-year survival rates after resection without documented residual macroscopic disease were 50% and 22%, respectively. Two patients are alive without disease 9 and 18 years after last surgical intervention. Suprahepatic vena caval and right atrial involvement by tumor, predominant intraluminal tumor growth, and residual postsurgical macroscopic disease were factors that statistically correlate with death within 2 years. By univariate analysis, intraluminal tumor ($P = 0.03$), liver injury or failure (compromised liver) ($P = 0.01$), and moderate to poor tumor differentiation ($P = 0.03$) were associated with increased tumor-related mortality, whereas a compromised liver ($P = 0.01$) was the only factor correlated with mortality by multivariate analysis. Our study concludes that a macroscopic resection

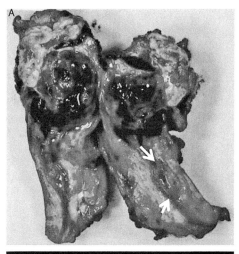

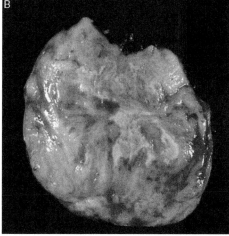

FIGURE 1.—A, Longitudinally opened inferior vena cava reveals a rounded mass protruding into the lumen of the vessel and extending caudally in a cord-like fashion (arrows). This level I-II tumor was predominantly intraluminal [case 36; French Federation Nationale des Centres de Lutte Contre le Cancer (FNCLCC) grade 2]. B, Macroscopic cut surface of an IVCL. Tumor has a focally trabeculated appearance with a yellow, geographic-shaped area of necrosis, and reddish-purple foci of hemorrhage [case 25; French Federation Nationale des Centres de Lutte Contre le Cancer (FNCLCC) grade 2]. For interpretation of the references to color in this figure legend, the reader is referred to web version of this article. (Reprinted from Laskin WB, Fanburg-Smith JC, Burke AP, et al. Leiomyosarcoma of the inferior vena cava: clinicopathologic study of 40 cases. *Am J Surg Pathol.* 2010;34:873-881.)

of localized inferior vena cava leiomyosarcoma provides the best chance for long-term survival, suprahepatic tumors often result in early death, and a compromised liver correlates with overall poor survival, but French Federation Nationale des Centres de Lutte Contre le Cancer grading does not affect prognosis (Fig 1).

▶ Leiomyosarcoma is the most common sarcoma that affects the venous system and nearly 50% arise in the inferior vena cava.[1] However, leiomyosarcoma of the inferior vena cava accounts for only about 0.5% of adult soft tissue sarcomas.[2] Overall prognosis is thought to be poor, with metastatic disease occurring primary to liver and lung and recurrent disease contributing to tumor-related mortality as well. In this report, the authors detailed the clinical pathologic features and follow-up data on 40 cases of inferior vena cava leiomyosarcoma accessioned to the Armed Forces Institute of Pathology between 1976 and 2008. This very large series confirms the poor prognosis associated with these tumors and the seemingly obvious fact that incomplete resection is associated with a poor short-term survival. Nevertheless, it is interesting to note that the growth pattern, extraluminal versus intraluminal (Fig 1), and the status of the patients' overall hepatic function also appear to be important prognostic factors in patients with this rare malignancy.

G. L. Moneta, MD

References

1. Kavorkian J, Cento DP. Leiomyosarcoma of large arteries and veins. *Surgery.* 1973;73:390-400.
2. Hollebeck ST, Grobmyer SR, Kent KC, Brennan MF. Surgical treatment and outcomes of patients with primary inferior vena cava leiomyosarcoma. *J Am Coll Surg.* 2003;197:575-579.

Normal CSF ferritin levels in MS suggest against etiologic role of chronic venous insufficiency
Worthington V, Killestein J, Eikelenboom MJ, et al (UCL Inst of Neurology, London, UK; Free Univ Med Ctr, Amsterdam, the Netherlands)
Neurology 75:1617-1622, 2010

Objectives.—Chronic cerebrospinal venous insufficiency (CCSVI) has been suggested to be a possible cause of multiple sclerosis (MS). If the presumed mechanism of venous stasis—related parenchymal iron deposition and neurodegeneration were true, then upregulation of intrathecal iron transport proteins may be expected.

Methods.—This was a cross-sectional (n = 1,408) and longitudinal (n = 29) study on CSF ferritin levels in patients with MS and a range of neurologic disorders.

Results.—Pathologic (>12 ng/mL) CSF ferritin levels were observed in 4% of the control patients (median 4 ng/mL), 91% of patients with superficial siderosis (75 ng/mL), 73% of patients with a subarachnoid hemorrhage

(59 ng/mL), 10% of patients with relapsing-remitting MS (5 ng/mL), 11% of patients with primary progressive MS (6 ng/mL), 23% of patients with secondary progressive MS (5 ng/mL), and 23% of patients with meningoencephalitis (5 ng/mL). In MS, there was no significant change of CSF ferritin levels over the 3-year follow-up period.

Conclusion.—These data do not support an etiologic role for CCSVI-related parenchymal iron deposition in MS (Figs 1 and 2).

▶ A new and controversial hypothesis suggests that disease progression in multiple sclerosis (MS) may be related to chronic cerebrospinal venous insufficiency (CCSVI) and resulting toxic effects of parenchymal iron deposition in the central nervous system (CNS).[1] When iron is present in the CNS it simulates intrathecal expression of ferritin.[2] An indirect test for deposition of iron in the CNS is therefore quantification of ferritin. The authors postulated that if CSSVI leads to parenchymal iron deposition in MS, there ought to be increased cerebrospinal fluid (CSF) ferritin levels. They quantified CSF ferritin levels from a previously published cohort with clinically definite MS.[3,4] The current study consists of both a cross-sectional and longitudinal component. In the cross-sectional part of the study, CSF ferritin levels in patients with MS were compared with those in patients with subarachnoid hemorrhage and occult bleeding (siderosis). There were no impressive differences of CSF ferritin levels in the patients with MS compared with the controls (Figs 1 and 2). The data therefore do not support the chronic CCSVI hypothesis for MS. The authors, however, point out several shortcomings of their study, including the fact that ferritin is only an indirect marker for CSF iron deposition and that they have no longitudinal data on CSF ferritin levels in the control subjects. This precludes conclusions about variations over time of individual CSF ferritin levels in an assumed normal population. Also, regarding magnetic resonance imaging, they do not have T2 imaging data

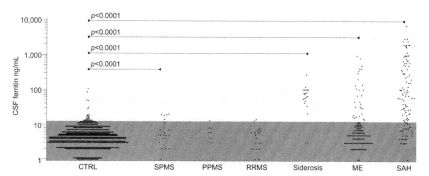

FIGURE 1.—CSF ferritin levels. The normal range (<12 ng/mL) is indicated by the gray shaded area. Elevated CSF ferritin levels were observed in a significant proportion of patients with secondary progressive multiple sclerosis (SPMS) (23%, $p < 0.0001$), siderosis (91%, $p < 0.0001$), meningoencephalitis (23%, $p < 0.0001$), and subarachnoid hemorrhage (SAH) (73%, $p < 0.0001$). The proportion of elevated CSF ferritin levels was statistically comparable between the control group (4%) and patients with primary progressive multiple sclerosis (PPMS) (11%) and relapsing-remitting multiple sclerosis (RRMS) (10%). ME = meningoencephalitis. (Reprinted from Worthington V, Killestein J, Eikelenboom MJ, et al. Normal CSF ferritin levels in MS suggest against etiologic role of chronic venous insufficiency. *Neurology.* 2010;75:1617-1622, with permission from AAN Enterprises, Inc.)

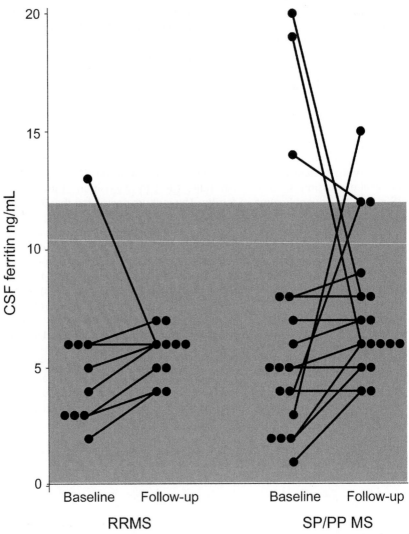

FIGURE 2.—Change of CSF ferritin levels in patients with multiple sclerosis between baseline and follow-up. An increase of CSF ferritin above the upper range of normal was observed in one patient with secondary progressive multiple sclerosis (SPMS) only. In all other patients, CSF ferritin levels either remained or dropped into the normal range (gray shaded area). PPMS = primary progressive multiple sclerosis; RRMS = relapsing-remitting multiple sclerosis. (Reprinted from Worthington V, Killestein J, Eikelenboom MJ, et al. Normal CSF ferritin levels in MS suggest against etiologic role of chronic venous insufficiency. *Neurology*. 2010;75:1617-1622, with permission from AAN Enterprises, Inc.)

potentially permitting correlation of CSF ferritin levels with parenchymal iron deposition or markers of CCSVI.

G. L. Moneta, MD

References

1. Singh AV, Zamboni P. Anomalous venous blood flow and iron deposition in multiple sclerosis. *J Cereb Blood Flow Metab.* 2009;29:1867-1878.
2. Keir G, Tasdemir N, Thompson EJ. Cerebrospinal fluid ferritin in brain necrosis: evidence for local synthesis. *Clin Chim Acta.* 1993;216:153-166.
3. Petzold A, Eikelenboom MJ, Gveric D, et al. Markers for different glial cell responses in multiple sclerosis: clinical and pathological correlations. *Brain.* 2002;125:1462-1473.
4. Polman CH, Reingold SC, Edan G, et al. Diagnostic criteria for multiple sclerosis: 2005 revisions to the "McDonald Criteria". *Ann Neurol.* 2005;58:840-846.

Preoperative Angiography and Transarterial Embolization in the Management of Carotid Body Tumor: A Single-Center, 10-Year Experience
Li J, Wang S, Zee C, et al (The First Affiliated Hosp of Sun Yat-sen Univ, Guangzhou, China; Keck School of Medicine of Univ of Southern California, Los Angeles, CA)
Neurosurgery 67:941-948, 2010

Background.—Sixty percent of paragangliomas are located unilaterally at the carotid bifurcation. These are referred to as carotid body tumors (CBTs).

Objective.—To present our 10-year experience in the management of patients with CBTs, and to evaluate the efficacy of angiography and preoperative embolization technique in this retrospective study.

Methods.—Sixty-two patients with surgically removed CBTs (Shamblin class II and III), were divided into two groups. Group I, the preoperative embolization group, included 33 patients with 11 class II lesions and 25 class III lesions. Group II, the group that had surgery only, without preoperative embolization, included 29 patients with 9 class II lesions and 21 class III lesions. Comparisons were made between the groups in terms of mean intraoperative blood loss, mean operation time, mean postoperative hospital stay, and clinical complications.

Results.—In group I, post-embolization angiography demonstrated complete tumor devascularization in 25 (76%) lesions and partial devascularization in 11 (24%) lesions. All but 1 (2%) lesion were completely excised. Mean intraoperative blood loss, mean operation time, and mean hospital stay were 354.8 ± 334.4 mL, 170.3 ± 75.4 min, 8.0 ± 2.1 days in group I and 656.4 ± 497.4 mL, 224.6 ± 114.0 min, 9.5 ± 3.5 days in group II, respectively. In group II, 27 lesions (91%) were completely removed. The transient ischemic attack (TIA) and cranial nerve injury incidence rates were 10.3% and 13.8% in group II and only 3% for TIA in group I.

Conclusion.—These results suggest angiography is highly valuable for the diagnosis of CBT. Preoperative selective embolization of CBT is an effective and safe adjunct for surgical resection, especially for Shamblin class II and III tumors.

▶ Carotid body tumors (CBTs) are often hypervascular. The blood supply is primarily from the external carotid artery. Larger CBTs (Shamblin class II, those that partially surround the internal and external carotid arteries, and Shamblin class III, those that completely surround the carotid bifurcation and/or internal carotid artery) can be difficult to remove, and excessive blood loss is possible given the hypervascular nature of the tumors (Fig 3 in the original article). Some surgeons therefore advocate preoperative embolization of larger, Shamblin class II and III, CBTs (Fig 1 in the original article). Others feel preoperative embolization is unnecessary and has added risk of neurologic complication. The authors present a series of 62 patients with Shamblin class II or III tumors that were operated over 10 years in their institution. This is the largest published series of CBTs operated with preoperative embolization. Apparently, although not specifically mentioned, there were no significant complications associated with the preoperative embolization, and the procedure was successful a large majority of the time. It is unclear how the patients were allocated to group I or group II, with allocation likely on the basis of surgeon preference. It is also unclear whether inclusion into group I or group II changed over time and that the same proportion was operated by the same surgeons in group I and group II. Therefore, the benefits of preoperative embolization in terms of operative time and blood loss, while potentially ascribed to the procedure, may also be surgeon-specific Nevertheless, it does appear that preoperative embolization of larger CBTs can be done with technical success. It may facilitate removal of the tumor. Other than time and expense, the article does not indicate any potential drawback to preoperative embolization of large CBTs. The combination of an experienced interventionalist and an experienced surgeon is likely to provide the best results for resection of larger CBTs.

G. L. Moneta, MD

Results of Superior Vena Cava Reconstruction With Externally Stented-Polytetrafluoroethylene Vascular Prostheses

Okereke IC, Kesler KA, Rieger KM, et al (Indiana Univ School of Medicine, Indianapolis)
Ann Thorac Surg 90:383-387, 2010

Background.—Resection and reconstruction of the superior vena cava (SVC) is occasionally required in the surgical treatment of intrathoracic neoplasms or symptomatic occlusion secondary to benign causes. We reviewed our institutional experience with SVC reconstruction using externally stented-polytetrafluoroethylene vascular prostheses.

Methods.—From 1991 to 2009, medical records of 38 patients who underwent SVC resection and reconstruction with externally stented-polytetrafluoroethylene vascular prostheses were reviewed. Indications for surgery were malignancy in 34 (89%) patients (germ cell, 13; thymoma, 10; lung cancer, 9; sarcoma, 2) and benign symptomatic occlusion in 4 (11%) patients.

Results.—Eighteen patients (47%) underwent right innominate vein to SVC interposition graft reconstruction, which became the favored approach during the study interval when resection of the innominate confluence was necessary. Eight patients (21%) had left innominate vein to SVC interposition grafts, earlier in the series or when the right innominate vein was unavailable. Nine patients (24%) received graft interposition of the proximal to distal SVC. The remaining 3 patients had a Y reconstruction. There were 2 perioperative mortalities. Follow-up averaged 15 months (range, 1 to 113 months), including 11 (29%) patients who died of disease. All patients demonstrated minimal to no brachiocephalic swelling at last follow-up. Twenty (53%) patients underwent imaging after an average of 24 months (range, 1 to 113 months) with only two grafts demonstrating complete occlusion.

Conclusions.—Although several SVC reconstructive techniques have been described, externally stented-polytetrafluoroethylene vascular prostheses are

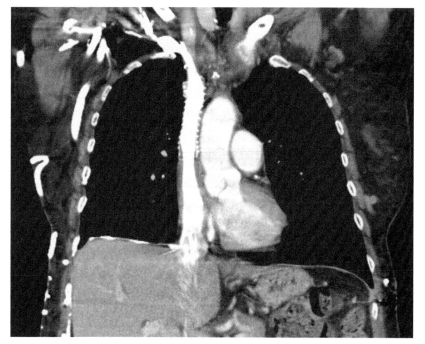

FIGURE 1.—Computed tomography scan displaying patency of externally stented-polytetrafluoroethylene graft from the right innominate vein to superior vena cava with ligation of the left innominate vein. Note slight oversizing of the externally stented-polytetrafluoroethylene graft compared with the right innominate vein. (This article was published in The Annals of Thoracic Surgery, Okereke IC, Kesler KA, Rieger KM, et al. Results of superior vena cava reconstruction with externally stented-polytetrafluoroethylene vascular prostheses. *Ann Thorac Surg.* 2010;90:383-387. Copyright The Society of Thoracic Surgeons 2010.)

readily available for off-the-shelf use. In our experience, patency rates are high, and patients who do demonstrate graft thrombosis have minimal to no symptoms.

▶ Superior vena cava (SVC) obstruction, whether benign or malignant, can result in facial swelling, dyspnea, and stridor. The SVC, depending on individual circumstance, may be reconstructed with autogenous tissue, stents, or grafts. In this article, the authors describe experience with SVC reconstruction using externally supported polytetrafluoroethylene grafts (Fig 1). This is a series of SVC reconstructions primarily for malignant disease. Therefore, even though the study spans 20 years, follow-up averaged only 2 years. There are several technical points that are worth noting. It does not appear that warfarin anticoagulation is required. If graft occlusion occurs, it appears to be well tolerated. In the discussion section of the article, the authors detail methods to avoiding graft kinking, particularly with sternotomy closure. They note that reconstruction of only one innominate vein when SVC innominate confluence was involved provided adequate results. They note that although it is technically more difficult to perform a right innominate vein–to-graft anastomosis than a left innominate vein anastomosis, the right anastomosis results in minimal graft angulation and direct downward blood flow into the right atrium. The authors also note that sternal retractors should be partially closed before creating the second anastomosis in a left innominate–to-SVC reconstruction. Performing both anastomoses with sternal distraction results in graft kinking with sternotomy closure.

G. L. Moneta, MD

Vascular Function and Circulating Progenitor Cells in Thromboangitis Obliterans (Buerger's Disease) and Atherosclerosis Obliterans

Idei N, Nishioka K, Soga J, et al (Hiroshima Univ Graduate School of Biomed Sciences, Japan)
Hypertension 57:70-78, 2011

Thromboangitis obliterans (TAO; Buerger's disease) and atherosclerosis obliterans (ASO) are associated with endothelial dysfunction. The purpose of this study was to evaluate the role of circulating progenitor cells (CPCs) in endothelial function in patients with TAO and ASO. We measured flow-mediated vasodilation (FMD), nitroglycerine-induced vasodilation, and circulating CPCs in 30 patients with TAO and 30 age- and sex-matched healthy subjects and in 40 patients with ASO. FMD was smaller in both the TAO group and ASO group than in the control group (6.6 ± 2.7%, 5.7 ± 3.3% versus 9.5 ± 3.1%, $P<0.0001$, respectively). There was no significant difference in FMD between the TAO group and ASO group. Nitroglycerine-induced vasodilation was similar in the 3 groups. The number of and migration of circulating CPCs were similar in the TAO group and control group, whereas the number of and migration of circulating CPCs were significantly lower in the ASO group than in other groups (ASO 553 ± 297/mL versus TAO 963 ± 543/mL; control 1063 ± 426/mL

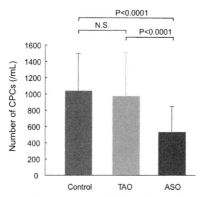

FIGURE 2.—B, Comparisons of the number of CPCs in the normal control subjects, patients with TAO, and patients with ASO. (Reprinted from Idei N, Nishioka K, Soga J, et al. Vascular function and circulating progenitor cells in thromboangitis obliterans (Buerger's disease) and atherosclerosis obliterans. *Hypertension.* 2011;57:70-78, with permission from American Heart Association, Inc.)

and ASO 36 ± 18/hpf versus TAO 62 ± 23/hpf; control 68 ± 18/hpf, $P<0.0001$, respectively). There was a significant relationship between the number of and migration of CPCs and FMD ($r=0.43$ and $r=0.40$, $P<0.0001$, respectively). FMD was impaired in patients with TAO as well as in patients with ASO compared to that in normal control subjects, and the number of and function of circulating CPCs were not decreased in patients with TAO. These findings may partially explain why there are differences in cardiovascular morbidity and mortality rates between patients with TAO and patients with ASO (Fig 2B).

▶ A healthy endothelium mediated mainly by nitric oxide maintains vascular structure and tone by regulating the balance between vasoconstriction and vasodilation, growth promotion and growth inhibition, and antioxidation and pro-oxidation.[1] Both Buerger disease and atherosclerosis are associated with endothelial dysfunction.[2] However, while the mortality rate of patients with atherosclerosis is higher than age-matched controls, the mortality rate of patients with Buerger disease is not.[3] The number of circulating progenitor cells (CPCs) appears to correlate with endothelial function, and the number of CPCs may be a predictor of cardiovascular events.[4] Given the discrepancy between apparent cardiovascular death rates in patients with atherosclerosis versus those with Buerger disease, the authors thought to evaluate the role of CPCs and endothelial function in patients with Buerger disease compared with patients with atherosclerosis. Preservation of CPCs in Buerger disease may allow mitigation of the effects of inflammatory-induced oxidative stress and oxidative dysfunction associated with Buerger disease. The authors found that patients with Buerger disease have a normal number (Fig 2B) and function of CPCs that may contribute to restoration of endothelial function in these patients, resulting in either reduction or inhibition of the adverse cardiovascular outcomes predicted by endothelial dysfunction.

G. L. Moneta, MD

References

1. Vanhoutte P. Endothelium and control of vascular function. State of the Art lecture. *Hypertension.* 1989;13:658-667.
2. Makita S, Nakamura M, Murakami H, Komoda K, Kawazoe K, Hiramori K. Impaired endothelium-dependent vasorelaxation in peripheral vasculature of patients with thromboangiitis obliterans (Buerger's disease). *Circulation.* 1996; 94:II211-II215.
3. Criqui MH, Langer RD, Fronek A, et al. Mortality over a period of 10 years in patients with peripheral arterial disease. *N Engl J Med.* 1992;326:381-386.
4. Werner N, Kosiol S, Schiegl T, et al. Circulating endothelial progenitor cells and cardiovascular outcomes. *N Engl J Med.* 2005;353:999-1007.

17 Venous Thrombosis and Pulmonary Embolism

Factors affecting outcome of open and hybrid reconstructions for nonmalignant obstruction of iliofemoral veins and inferior vena cava
Garg N, Gloviczki P, Karimi KM, et al (Mayo Clinic, Rochester, MN)
J Vasc Surg 53:383-393, 2011

Objectives.—To identify factors affecting long-term outcome after open surgical reconstructions (OSR) and hybrid reconstructions (HR) for chronic venous obstructions.

Methods.—Retrospective review of clinical data of 60 patients with 64 OSR or HR for chronic obstruction of iliofemoral (IF) veins or inferior vena cava (IVC) between January 1985 and September 2009. Primary end points were patency and clinical outcome.

Results.—Sixty patients (26 men, mean age 43 years, range 16-81) underwent 64 procedures. Ninety-four percent had leg swelling, 90% had venous claudication, and 31% had active or healed ulcers (CEAP classes: C3 = 30, C4 = 12, C5 = 8, C6 = 12). Fifty-two OSRs included 29 femorofemoral (Palma vein: 25, polytetrafluoroethylene [PTFE]: 4), 17 femoroiliac-inferior vena cava (IVC) (vein: 3, PTFE: 14) and six complex bypasses. Twelve patients had HR, which included endophlebectomy, patch angioplasty, and stenting. Early graft occlusion occurred after 17% of OSR and 33% HR. Discharge patency was 96% after OSR, 92% after HR. No mortality or pulmonary embolism occurred. Five-year primary and secondary patency was 42% (95% confidence interval [CI] 29%-55%) and 59% (CI 43%-72%), respectively. For Palma vein grafts it was 70% and 78%, for femoroiliac and ilio-infrahepatic IVC bypasses it was 63% and 86%, and for femoro-infrahepatic IVC bypasses it was 31% and 57%, respectively. Complex OSRs and hybrid procedures had 28% and 30% 2-year secondary patency, respectively. The only factor that significantly affected graft patency in multivariate analysis was May-Thurner syndrome with associated chronic venous thrombosis. For HR, stenting into the common femoral vein patch vs iliac stents only significantly increased patency. At last follow-up, 60% of the patients had no venous claudication and no or minimal swelling. All ulcers with patent grafts healed but 50% of these recurred.

Conclusions.—Both OSR and HR are viable options if endovascular procedures fail or are not feasible. Palma vein bypass and femoroiliac or iliocaval PTFE bypasses have excellent outcomes with good symptomatic relief.

▶ With the development of improved endovascular technologies, there has been a renewed interest in the treatment of lower extremity venous outflow. Large self-expanding stents have been used to treat both acute and chronic obstructions of the iliac veins with good results. This therapy works best in non-thrombotic patients but has also been quite successful in thrombotic patients with appropriate anticoagulation.

The increase in investigation of patients with lower extremity venous claudi-cation, severe swelling, and ulceration has led to the identification of several patients whose iliofemoral (IF) venous occlusions cannot be successfully treated with endovascular techniques. As such, today's modern vascular surgeon needs to be facile in open techniques to correct severe lower extremity venous outflow obstruction.

In this report, Dr Garg and colleagues from the Mayo Clinic examined several factors affecting long-term outcomes of open surgical reconstructions and hybrid reconstructions of IF veins and the inferior vena cava over a 25-year period.

In their review, they found a 78% patency rate at 5 years with the cross-femoral venous bypass or Palma procedure. This is consistent with previous reports showing patency rates to be between 70% and 83% at 3 to 5 years. Results were the best in patients with good inflow and no significant infrain-guinal venous obstruction and incompetence. Furthermore, they found that endoscopic vein harvest significantly increased primary failure in comparison to open greater saphenous vein harvest.

Hybrid reconstructions included 9 patients with unilateral common femoral vein (CFV) endophlebectomy and patch angioplasty with proximal stent place-ment and 3 patients with bilateral iliac stent placement (unilateral phlebectomy and patch). Overall, these procedures had worse long-term patency than bypass. In addition, endophlebectomy without CFV stent extension had early failure. In these cases, extension of stent into the CFV patch is important and significantly improves long-term patency. It has been shown that stenting across the inguinal ligament is safe in the venous circulation, and it is more harmful to leave a diseased segment of vein without a stent rather than stent across the ligament.

D. L. Gillespie, MD, RVT

Iliofemoral stenting for venous occlusive disease

Titus JM, Moise MA, Bena J, et al (Cleveland Clinic Foundation, OH)
J Vasc Surg 53:706-712, 2011

Background.—Venous hypertension is a significant cause of patient morbidity and decreased quality of life. Common etiologies of venous hypertension include deep venous thrombosis (DVT) or congenital abnormalities resulting in chronic outflow obstruction. We have implemented an aggressive endovascular approach for the treatment of iliac venous occlusion with angioplasty and stenting. The purpose of this study was to determine the patency rates with this approach at a large tertiary care center.

Materials/Methods.—All patients undergoing iliofemoral venous angioplasty and stenting over a 4-year period were identified from a vascular surgical registry. Charts were reviewed retrospectively for patient demographics, the extent of venous system involvement, the time course of the venous pathology, and any underlying cause. Technical aspects of the procedure including previous angioplasty or stenting attempts and presence of collaterals on completion venogram were then recorded. Patency upon follow-up was determined using primarily ultrasound scans; other imaging methods were used if patency was not clear using an ultrasound scan.

Results.—A total of 36 patients (40 limbs) were stented from January 2005 through December 2008. Of these patients, 27 were women (75%). Both lower extremities were involved in 4 patients. Thrombolysis was performed in 19 patients (52.8%). Thrombosis was considered acute (<30 days) in 13 patients (38%). The majority of patients who had a recognized underlying etiology were diagnosed with May-Thurner syndrome (15 patients; 42%). In 9 patients, an etiology was not determined (25%). The mean follow-up time period in the study population was 10.5 months. One stent in the study occluded acutely and required restenting. Primary patency rates at 6, 12, and 24 months were 88% (75.2-100), 78.3% (61.1-95.4), and 78.3% (61.1-95.4), respectively. Secondary patency rates for the same time frames were 100% (100.0, 100.0), 95% (85.4, 100.0), and 95% (85.4, 100.0). Better outcomes were seen in stenting for May-Thurner syndrome and idiopathic causes, whereas external compression and thrombophilia seemed to portend less favorable outcomes ($P < .001$). Symptomatic improvement was reported in 24 of 29 patients (83%) contacted by telephone follow-up.

Conclusion.—Iliofemoral venous stenting provides a safe and effective option for the treatment of iliac venous occlusive disease. Acceptable patency rates can be expected through short-term follow-up, especially in the case of May-Thurner syndrome. Further experience with this approach and longer-term follow-up is necessary. Thrombophilia workup should be pursued aggressively in this population, and further studies should be undertaken to determine the optimal length of anticoagulation therapy after stent placement.

▶ Iliofemoral venous stenting for venous outflow obstruction of the lower extremity has been shown to be safe and effective. It has been popularized by Drs Raju and Neglen from Mississippi as an effective therapy in both thrombotic and nonthrombotic patients. This article by Titus et al reports on the experience of the Cleveland Clinic with this therapy. Of note, this report combines 19 (51%) patients with acute thrombosis requiring venous thrombolysis. In addition, it included several nonthrombotic iliac vein obstructions as well as chronically occluded patients with history of thrombophilia. This article shows that the principles of venous stenting can be generalized to other institutions outside of Mississippi but is really too small to substantially affect the field overall. As stated by the authors, their primary and secondary patency rates at 2 years of 78% and 95%, respectively, are comparable to those found by previous studies.

To date, the concept of venous stenting has been proven; however, there are numerous questions yet to be answered. The authors point out that little is known about how long patients should remain on anticoagulation after stenting, whether patients with nonthrombotic iliac vein obstructions be treated as aggressively as those with thrombosis, and whether any kind of inferior vena cava filter is needed to protect these patients from symptomatic pulmonary embolism.

D. L. Gillespie, MD, RVT

Fondaparinux for the Treatment of Superficial-Vein Thrombosis in the Legs
Decousus H, for the CALISTO Study Group (Université Jean-Monnet, Saint-Etienne, France; et al)
N Engl J Med 363:1222-1232, 2010

Background.—The efficacy and safety of anticoagulant treatment for patients with acute, symptomatic superficial-vein thrombosis in the legs, but without concomitant deep-vein thrombosis or symptomatic pulmonary embolism at presentation, have not been established.

Methods.—In a randomized, double-blind trial, we assigned 3002 patients to receive either fondaparinux, administered subcutaneously at a dose of 2.5 mg once daily, or placebo for 45 days. The primary efficacy outcome was a composite of death from any cause or symptomatic pulmonary embolism, symptomatic deep-vein thrombosis, or symptomatic extension to the saphenofemoral junction or symptomatic recurrence of superficial-vein thrombosis at day 47. The main safety outcome was major bleeding. The patients were followed until day 77.

Results.—The primary efficacy outcome occurred in 13 of 1502 patients (0.9%) in the fondaparinux group and 88 of 1500 patients (5.9%) in the placebo group (relative risk reduction with fondaparinux, 85%; 95% confidence interval [CI], 74 to 92; P<0.001). The incidence of each component of the primary efficacy outcome was significantly reduced in the fondaparinux group as compared with the placebo group, except for the outcome of death (0.1% in both groups). The rate of pulmonary embolism or deep-vein thrombosis was 85% lower in the fondaparinux group than in the placebo group (0.2% vs. 1.3%; 95% CI, 50 to 95; P<0.001). Similar risk reductions were observed at day 77. A total of 88 patients would need to be treated to prevent one instance of pulmonary embolism or deep-vein thrombosis. Major bleeding occurred in one patient in each group. The incidence of serious adverse events was 0.7% with fondaparinux and 1.1% with placebo.

Conclusions.—Fondaparinux at a dose of 2.5 mg once a day for 45 days was effective in the treatment of patients with acute, symptomatic superficial-vein thrombosis of the legs and did not have serious side effects. (Funded by GlaxoSmithKline; ClinicalTrials.gov number, NCT00443053.)

▶ Patients with isolated supraventricular tachycardia (SVT) may develop more serious manifestations of venous thrombosis with an 8.3% incidence of symptomatic venous thromboembolic (VTE) complications at 3 months and an estimated 3% to 4% risk of deep venous thrombosis or pulmonary embolism (PE).[1] SVT has no agreed-upon treatment strategy with therapy varying from observation to use of anti-inflammatory agents to anticoagulation or surgery. It does not appear that therapeutic or intermediate doses of low-molecular-weight heparin (LMWH) provide substantial benefit over low-dose (prophylactic) LMWH regimes in treatment of SVT. It does appear that treatment for < 30 days is ineffective, as many symptomatic thromboembolic complications of SVT occur after 30 days.[2,3] To help to clarify pharmacologic treatment of SVT, the authors conducted the Comparison of Arixtra and Lower Limb Superficial Vein Thrombosis with Placebo trial evaluating the efficacy of fondaparinux in reducing symptomatic VTE complications or death in patients with acute isolated SVT of the legs. Looking at the results of the trial and focusing on the number needed to treat to prevent 1 episode of PE with fondaparinux in patients with SVT, that number would be 300. This is similar to the number needed to treat with LMWH compared with placebo or no treatment in trials of VTE prophylaxis in acutely ill medical patients.[4] Treatment with fondaparinux also reduced risk of symptomatic recurrence of SVT and extension to the saphenofemoral junction. Since both of these events may result in escalation of therapy, these end points also appear clinically relevant. Overall, the data indicate that with pharmacologic therapy, it is possible to improve the natural history of SVT. Of course, the cost-effectiveness and effects on quality of life of the 45-day treatment regime of fondaparinux for SVT will need to be evaluated in the context of the cost of fondaparinux and diagnostic testing to determine eligibility for treatment.

G. L. Moneta, MD

References

1. Decousus H, Quéré I, Presles E, et al. Superficial venous thrombosis and venous thromboembolism: a large, prospective epidemiologic study. *Ann Intern Med.* 2010;152:218-224.
2. Superficial Thrombophlebitis Treated By Enoxaparin Study Group. A pilot randomized double-blind comparison of a low-molecular-weight heparin, a nonsteroidal anti-inflammatory agent, and placebo in the treatment of superficial vein thrombosis. *Arch Intern Med.* 2003;163:1657-1663.
3. Prandoni P, Tormene D, Pesavento R, et al. High vs. low doses of low-molecular-weight heparin for the treatment of superficial vein thrombosis of the legs: a double-blind, randomized trial. *J Thromb Haemost.* 2005;3:1152-1157.
4. Dentali F, Douketis JD, Gianni M, Lim W, Crowther MA. Meta-analysis: anticoagulant prophylaxis to prevent symptomatic venous thromboembolism in hospitalized medical patients. *Ann Intern Med.* 2007;146:278-288.

Influence of preceding length of anticoagulant treatment and initial presentation of venous thromboembolism on risk of recurrence after stopping treatment: analysis of individual participants' data from seven trials
Boutitie F, Pinede L, Schulman S, et al (Hospices Civils de Lyon, France; Infirmerie Protestante, Lyon, France; Karolinska Hosp, Stockholm, Sweden; et al)
BMJ 342:d3036, 2011

Objective.—To determine how length of anticoagulation and clinical presentation of venous thromboembolism influence the risk of recurrence after anticoagulant treatment is stopped and to identify the shortest length of anticoagulation that reduces the risk of recurrence to its lowest level.

Design.—Pooled analysis of individual participants' data from seven randomised trials.

Setting.—Outpatient anticoagulant clinics in academic centres.

Population.—2925 men or women with a first venous thromboembolism who did not have cancer and received different durations of anticoagulant treatment.

Main Outcome Measure.—First recurrent venous thromboembolism after stopping anticoagulant treatment during up to 24 months of follow-up.

Results.—Recurrence was lower after isolated distal deep vein thrombosis than after proximal deep vein thrombosis (hazard ratio 0.49, 95% confidence interval 0.34 to 0.71), similar after pulmonary embolism and proximal deep vein thrombosis (1.19, 0.87 to 1.63), and lower after thrombosis provoked by a temporary risk factor than after unprovoked thrombosis (0.55, 0.41 to 0.74). Recurrence was higher if anticoagulation was stopped at 1.0 or 1.5 months compared with at 3 months or later (hazard ratio 1.52, 1.14 to 2.02) and similar if treatment was stopped at 3 months compared with at 6 months or later (1.19, 0.86 to 1.65). High rates of recurrence associated with shorter durations of anticoagulation were confined to the first 6 months after stopping treatment.

Conclusion.—Three months of treatment achieves a similar risk of recurrent venous thromboembolism after stopping anticoagulation to a longer course of treatment. Unprovoked proximal deep vein thrombosis and pulmonary embolism have a high risk of recurrence whenever treatment is stopped.

▶ Randomized data indicate that at least 3 months of anticoagulation is preferable to shorter periods to reduce recurrent venous thromboembolic (VTE) events after an initial episode of deep vein thrombosis (DVT) or pulmonary embolism (PE). The studies evaluating optimal length of vitamin K antagonist treatment following VTE have been limited by the fact that such studies have compared 2 lengths of treatment. With only 2 lengths of treatment compared in individual studies, no study could tell if the superior length of treatment from one individual study was actually optimal length of treatment. Perhaps a third treatment duration could result in even better clinical outcomes. The authors of this study pooled their data from a total of 7 individual comparative trials using a spectrum of lengths treatment evaluated for VTE. Their primary goal was to identify the shortest length of treatment that reduces the risk of recurrent VTE to its lowest value after stopping treatment with vitamin K antagonist. They also sought to determine the optimal length of treatment using vitamin K antagonists according to specific subgroups at time of presentation, VTE association (such as proximal or distal DVT or PE), and whether thrombus recurrence was influenced by a temporary risk factor or whether the VTE was unprovoked. The primary implication of this study is that patients with a VTE event who do not have an obvious indication for indefinite anticoagulation treatment can stop vitamin K antagonist treatment after their initial VTE event after 3 months. The analysis also suggested that patients with unprovoked proximal DVT or PE will have higher recurrence if they are treated only for 3 months rather than 6 months. Limitations of this study include the fact that D-dimer levels and vascular laboratory assessment of the status of the venous thrombus at the end of anticoagulation were not included as potential variables influencing duration of anticoagulation. Perhaps patients with unprovoked VTE will in the future be better stratified by additional variables to determine who will benefit from longer durations of anticoagulation and who will have a low risk of recurrence with only 3 months of treatment.

G. L. Moneta, MD

Recurrent Deep Vein Thrombosis: Long-Term Incidence and Natural History
Labropoulos N, Jen J, Jen H, et al (Stony Brook Univ Med Ctr, NY)
Ann Surg 251:749-753, 2010

Objective.—To determine the long-term incidence, risk factors, and associated morbidity and mortality of recurrent deep vein thrombosis (DVT).

TABLE 4.—Incidence of Recurrent DVT According to Risk Factor

No. Recurrences	Spontaneous	BMI >30	Cancer	Surgery	Trauma	Thrombophilia	Disc AC	Shorter AC	Pregnancy	HT	Long Travel	Medical Diseases
1	5	2	3	2	0	5	3	2	2	1	0	2
2	1	1	2	1	0	2	1	0	1	0	0	0
3	1	0	1	0	0	1	0	0	0	0	0	0
4	0	0	0	0	0	1	0	0	0	0	0	0
Total	7/11	3/18	6/9	3/32	0/15	9/24	4/12	2/9	3/8	1/5	0/2	2/8

BMI indicates body-mass index; Disc AC, discontinuation of anticoagulation; AC, anticoagulation; HT, hormone therapy.

Summary Background Data.—Few studies have examined the long-term natural history and impact of recurrent DVT.

Methods.—We conducted a prospective observational study that followed 153 consecutive patients with an acute first episode of DVT. Clinical examination and ultrasound were performed serially for at least 5 years. Location and extent of the initial DVT, recurrence, pulmonary embolism, cause of mortality, signs and symptoms of post thrombotic syndrome (PTS), and the risk factors were recorded.

Results.—The incidence of recurrence at 5 years was 26.1%. Patients with both proximal and distal DVT had a higher recurrence rate than proximal (17/48 35% vs. 12/49, 24%, $P = 0.27$) or calf alone (11/56, 20%, $P = 0.08$). Unprovoked DVT and age >65 years were associated with higher recurrence rates ($P < 0.001$; relative risk [RR]: 2.9, 95% confidence interval [CI]: 1.5–5.7) and ($P = 0.025$; RR: 1.5, 95% CI: 1–2.3), respectively. Thrombophilia was not associated with increased risk of recurrence ($P = 0.21$). Patients with DVT due to surgery or trauma had a lower recurrence ($P < 0.001$). Ipsilateral recurrence was associated with increased severity of PTS ($P < 0.001$; RR: 1.6, 95% CI: 1.4–2.2). PE occurred 47 times, 12 (25%) of which were fatal events.

Conclusions.—Factors associated with a higher rate of recurrence included unprovoked DVT and age >65. Elevated thrombus burden had a trend towards higher risk. Patients with surgery and trauma had low recurrence rates. Ipsilateral recurrence was strongly associated with PTS. PE occurred frequently and was a common cause of death (Table 4).

▶ The reported incidence of recurrent venous thromboembolism (VTE) is up to 40% at 10 years, with most recurrent VTE occurring after anticoagulation has been discontinued. Whereas much is known about recurrent deep vein thrombosis (DVT), there are actually few long-term studies examining factors influencing recurrent DVT and its natural history. This study has severe limitations due to sample size. The number of patients is too small to provide meaningful subgroup analysis (Table 4). The number of patients ultimately dying of pulmonary embolism is a bit shocking, but perhaps what is most interesting in this field is the increasing frequency of articles contradicting the widely held belief that thrombophilia is a risk factor for recurrence of VTE.[1] Clearly, as in this study, many patients with thrombophilia have other risk factors for VTE that make it difficult to independently assess the impact of thrombophilia on VTE recurrence. Despite the results here, until there are larger and better studies examining the impact of thrombophilia on VTE recurrence, it is best to still consider thrombophilia as a risk factor for recurrent VTE.

G. L. Moneta, MD

Reference

1. Prandoni P, Noventa F, Ghirarduzzi A, et al. The risk of recurrent venous thromboembolism after discontinuing anticoagulation in patients with acute proximal deep vein thrombosis or pulmonary embolism. A prospective cohort study in 1,626 patients. *Haematologica.* 2007;92:199-205.

Risk of Recurrent Venous Thrombosis in Homozygous Carriers and Double Heterozygous Carriers of Factor V Leiden and Prothrombin G20210A

Lijfering WM, Middeldorp S, Veeger NJGM, et al (Univ Med Ctr Groningen, the Netherlands; Academic Med Ctr, Amsterdam, the Netherlands; et al)
Circulation 121:1706-1712, 2010

Background.—Homozygous or double heterozygous factor V Leiden and/or prothrombin G20210A is a rare inherited thrombophilic trait. Whether individuals with this genetic background have an increased risk of recurrent venous thrombosis is uncertain.

Methods and Results.—A case-control design within a large cohort of families with thrombophilia was chosen to calculate the risk of recurrent venous thrombosis in individuals with homozygosity or double hetero-zygosity of factor V Leiden and/or prothrombin G20210A. Cases were individuals with recurrent venous thrombosis, and controls were those with only 1 venous thrombosis. The cohort consisted of 788 individuals with venous thrombosis; 357 had factor V Leiden, 137 had prothrombin G20210A, 27 had factor V Leiden and/or prothrombin G20210A homo-zygosity, and 49 had double heterozygosity for both mutations. We iden-tified 325 cases with recurrent venous thrombosis and 463 controls with only 1 venous thrombosis. Compared with noncarriers, crude odds ratio for recurrence was 1.2 (95% confidence interval, 0.9 to 1.6) for hetero-zygous carriers of factor V Leiden, 0.7 (95% confidence interval, 0.4 to 1.2) for prothrombin G20210A, 1.2 (95% confidence interval, 0.5 to 2.6) for homozygous carriers of factor V Leiden and/or prothrombin G20210A, and 1.0 (95% confidence interval, 0.6 to 1.9) for double heterozygotes of both mutations. Adjustments for age, sex, family status, first event type, and concomitance of natural anticoagulant deficiencies did not alter the risk estimates.

Conclusions.—In this study, individuals with homozygous factor V Leiden and/or homozygous prothrombin G20210A or double hetero-zygous carriers of factor V Leiden and prothrombin G20210A did not have a high risk of recurrent venous thrombosis.

▶ Thrombophilia is generally acknowledged as a risk factor for first-time venous thrombosis. Factor V Leiden has prevalence within the Caucasian population of approximately 5%, and the prothrombin G20210A mutation has a prevalence of approximately 2% in the Caucasian population. Double hetero-zygotes for the prothrombin gene mutation and factor V Leiden are infrequent (approximately 0.1%,).[1] Homozygosity for prothrombin G20210A and factor V Leiden is quite rare with a prevalence of 0.014% for homozygosity for prothrombin G20210A and 0.02% for homozygosity for factor V Leiden.[2,3] Risk for initial venous thrombosis is clearly higher in heterozygote and homozy-gote carriers of factor V Leiden and prothrombin G20210A. Heterozygote carriers of factor V Leiden have an approximately 5 times increased risk for initial venous thrombosis, while homozygote carriers have an 18-fold increased risk for initial venous thrombosis. Individuals heterozygous for both factor V Leiden and prothrombin G20210A have approximately 20-fold risk for initial venous thrombosis. Based on increased risk for initial venous thrombosis, it has generally been assumed that patients with thrombophilia on the bases of genetic abnormalities for factor V Leiden and prothrombin G20210A would also have increased risk for recurrent venous thrombosis. The assumption, of course, is that the risk of recurrence is driven by the same factors that prompted the initial venous thrombosis and that the thrombophilia is a much stronger risk factor for recurrent venous thrombosis then the residual of the initial venous thrombosis. There are, however, few data to suggest that thrombophilia secondary to factor V Leiden and prothrombin G20210A actually does increase the risk of recurrent venous thrombosis. Some studies have suggested that thrombophilia secondary to factor V Leiden and prothrombin G20210A mutations actually do not increase the risk of recurrent venous thrombosis and therefore argue against testing for these genetic defects in individuals with an unprovoked first-time venous thrombosis.[4,5] The study found patients with venous thromboses who are homozygous for factor V Leiden and/or prothrombin G20210A or double heterozygous carriers of factor V Leiden and prothrombin G20210A do not have high risk of recurrent venous thrombosis. This has major implications for the evaluation of patients with a first-time unprovoked venous thrombosis. It suggests that evaluation for factor V Leiden and prothrombin G20210A mutations has little clinical implication or benefit for the individual with a first-time venous thrombosis. After all, if recurrence of first-time venous thrombosis is not increased by the presence of these mutations, then there is no need to test for them in the patient with an initial unprovoked venous thrombosis. The information in this study does not apply to individuals with multiple recurrent venous thrombi. It is also important to consider, because these mutations are genetic, whether it is still reasonable to perform thrombophilia testing in the patients with first-time venous thrombosis so that family members can be appropriately counseled.

G. L. Moneta, MD

References

1. Emmerich J, Rosendaal FR, Cattaneo M, et al. Combined effect of factor V Leiden and prothrombin 20210A on the risk of venous thromboembolism—pooled analysis of 8 case-control studies including 2310 cases and 3204 controls. Study Group for Pooled-Analysis in Venous Thromboembolism. *Thromb Haemost.* 2001;86: 809-816.
2. Poort SR, Rosendaal FR, Reitsma PH, Bertina RM. A common genetic variation in the 3'-untranslated region of the prothrombin gene is associated with elevated plasma prothrombin levels and an increase in venous thrombosis. *Blood.* 1996; 88:3698-3703.
3. Rosendaal FR, Koster T, Vandenbroucke JP, Reitsma PH. High risk of thrombosis in patients homozygous for factor V Leiden (activated protein C resistance). *Blood.* 1995;85:1504-1508.
4. Christiansen SC, Cannegieter SC, Koster T, Vandenbroucke JP, Rosendaal FR. Thrombophilia, clinical factors, and recurrent venous thrombotic events. *JAMA.* 2005;293:2352-2361.
5. Baglin T, Luddington R, Brown K, Baglin C. Incidence of recurrent venous thromboembolism in relation to clinical and thrombophilic risk factors: prospective cohort study. *Lancet.* 2003;362:523-526.

Superficial Venous Thrombosis and Venous Thromboembolism: A Large, Prospective Epidemiologic Study

Decousus H, for the POST (Prospective Observational Superficial Thrombophlebitis) Study Group (Univ Hosp, Saint-Étienne, France; et al)
Ann Intern Med 152:218-224, 2010

Background.—Superficial venous thrombosis (SVT) is perceived to have a benign prognosis.

Objective.—To assess the prevalence of venous thromboembolism in patients with SVT and to determine the 3-month incidence of thromboembolic complications.

Design.—National cross-sectional and prospective epidemiologic cohort study (ClinicalTrials.gov registration number: NCT00818688).

Setting.—French office- and hospital-based vascular medicine specialists.

Patients.—844 consecutive patients with symptomatic SVT of the lower limbs that was at least 5 cm on compression ultrasonography.

Measurements.—Incidence of venous thromboembolism and extension or recurrence of SVT in patients with isolated SVT at presentation.

Results.—Among 844 patients with SVT at inclusion (median age, 65 years; 547 women), 210 (24.9%) also had deep venous thrombosis (DVT) or symptomatic pulmonary embolism. Among 600 patients without DVT or pulmonary embolism at inclusion who were eligible for 3-month follow-up, 58 (10.2%) developed thromboembolic complications at 3 months (pulmonary embolism, 3 [0.5%]; DVT, 15 [2.8%]; extension of SVT, 18 [3.3%]; and recurrence of SVT, 10 [1.9%]), despite 540 patients (90.5%) having received anticoagulants. Risk factors for complications at 3 months were male sex, history of DVT or pulmonary embolism, previous cancer, and absence of varicose veins.

Limitation.—The findings are from a specialist referral setting, and the study was terminated before the target patient population was reached because of slow recruitment.

Conclusion.—A substantial number of patients with SVT exhibit venous thromboembolism at presentation, and some that do not can develop this complication in the subsequent 3 months.

▶ While superficial venous thrombosis (SVT) is known to be painful and relatively common, it is thought to have a benign prognosis. However, there is accumulating evidence that SVT often occurs with deep venous thrombosis (DVT) or pulmonary embolism (PE). DVT appears to be present in about 6% to 53% of patients with SVT and PE between 0% and 10% of patients with SVT.[1] The authors performed this large observational study to determine the prevalence of concurrent SVT and venous thromboembolism (VTE), to assess how SVT is treated, and to determine the 3-month incidence of thromboembolic complications in patients with SVT. Risk factors for VTE complications in patients presenting with SVT were also determined. The study indicates that symptomatic SVT is not necessarily benign. About one-quarter of the patients will have symptomatic PE or DVT at presentation. An additional 10% will develop some manifestation of VTE or complication of their SVT at 3 months. Given the percentage of patients who present for evaluation of symptoms consistent with SVT and who actually have DVT at presentation, it would appear prudent to perform a venous ultrasound examination in all patients with symptomatic SVT. This would appear especially so if the physician does not wish to prescribe anticoagulation for treatment of SVT. Patients with identifiable risk factors for development of VTE following SVT should be considered for follow-up duplex ultrasonography if the patient is not going to be treated with anticoagulation.

G. L. Moneta, MD

Reference

1. Leon L, Giannoukas AD, Dodd D, Chan P, Labropoulos N. Clinical significance of superficial vein thrombosis. *Eur J Vasc Endovasc Surg.* 2005;29:10-17.

Vena Cava Filter Occlusion and Venous Thromboembolism Risk in Persistently Anticoagulated Patients: A Prospective, Observational Cohort Study

Hajduk B, Tomkowski WZ, Małek G, et al (The Natl Tuberculosis and Lung Diseases Res Inst, Warsaw, Poland; et al)
Chest 137:877-882, 2010

Background.—Inferior vena cava (IVC) filter placement may be life-saving, but after contraindications to anticoagulation remit, patient management is uncertain.

Methods.—We followed patients who had venous thromboembolism, followed by treatment with permanent IVC filter placement, and were anticoagulated long-term as soon as safety allowed. We conducted annual physical examinations and ultrasound surveillance of the lower extremity deep veins and of the IVC filter site. Clot detected at the filter site was treated with graded intensities of anticoagulation, depending on the clot burden.

Results.—Symptomatic DVT occurred in 24 of 121 patients (20%; 95% CI, 14%-28%); symptomatic pulmonary embolism (one fatal) was diagnosed in six patients (5%; 95% CI, 2%-10%). There were 45 episodes of filter clot in 36 patients (30%; 95% CI, 22%-38%). The rate of major bleeding (6.6%) was similar to that of a concurrent persistently anticoagulated cohort without IVC filters (5.8%).

Conclusions.—If therapeutic anticoagulation can be safely begun in patients with IVC filters inserted after venous thromboembolism, further management with clinical surveillance, including ultrasound examination of the IVC filter and graded degrees of anticoagulation therapy if filter clot is detected, has a favorable prognosis. This approach appears valid for patients with current IVC filter and can serve as a comparison standard in subsequent clinical trials to optimize clinical management of these patients.

▶ Inferior vena cava (IVC) filters are frequently used in patients who fail antico-agulation, who have risk factors that preclude anticoagulation, and, increasingly, for prophylaxis. Despite the availability of removable IVC filters, many are never removed. There are also many patients with IVC filters placed before removable filters became available. It is known that thrombus can form within the filter and propagate, reducing filter patency, reducing lower extremity venous return, and increasing risk of lower extremity DVT.[1] In addition, it appears impaired IVC venous return can lead to collateral venous return with recurrence of pulmonary embolism.[2] Therefore, in patients whose contraindication to anticoagulation remits or who can be anticoagulated with an IVC filter, some physicians will offer indefinite anticoagulation to patients with permanent IVC filters.

The authors hypothesized that in patients with IVC filters, anticoagulation indefinitely would be effective in preventing filter occlusion and venous thrombotic complications. They prospectively evaluated the effect of long-term anti-coagulation on the frequency of symptomatic venous thromboembolism and IVC patency and flow impairment in a cohort of patients with IVC filters and a management protocol for dealing with filter clot. Based on their results, the authors are proposing an ultrasound-based stringent follow-up protocol for patients with permanently implanted IVC filters. Their protocol appeared effective but, of course, the data apply only to those patients who can be anticoagu-lated. Certainly, the data would be more convincing if independent observers had confirmed the status of the IVC filter by ultrasound examination. Nevertheless, the idea of serially following IVC filters and increasing the intensity of anticoagulation or of monitoring of anticoagulation in response to ultrasound-detected filter clot is interesting. Who will provide such monitoring is a question, but logically, those who perform procedures on patients should be vested in the long-term outcome and monitoring of those procedures.

G. L. Moneta, MD

References

1. Tardy B, Mismetti P, Page Y, et al. Symptomatic inferior vena cava filter throm-bosis: clinical study of 30 consecutive cases. *Eur Respir J.* 1996;9:2012-2016.
2. Piccone VA Jr, Vidal E, Yarnoz M, Glass P, LeVeen HH. The late results of caval ligation. *Surgery.* 1970;68:980-998.

Isolated Gastrocnemius and Soleal Vein Thrombosis: Should These Patients Receive Therapeutic Anticoagulation?
Lautz TB, Abbas F, Walsh SJN, et al (Northwestern Univ, Chicago, IL)
Ann Surg 251:735-742, 2009

Objective.—To determine the incidence of isolated gastrocnemius and soleal vein thrombosis (IGSVT) and the effect of anticoagulation on venous thromboembolism (VTE) events in patients with IGSVT.

Summary Background Data.—Although IGSVT is diagnosed with increasing frequency, the clinical significance and optimal management remains unknown.

Methods.—Vascular laboratory studies from April 2002 to April 2007 were retrospectively reviewed to identify patients with IGSVT. Medical records were reviewed for demographic data, risk factors, treatment modalities, and VTE events. Univariate and multivariate analysis were performed.

Results.—Of 38,426 lower extremity venous duplex studies, 406 patients with IGSVT were included in this study. Mean follow-up was 7.5 ± 11 months. The overall incidence of VTE among the entire cohort was 18.7%, which included 3.9% pulmonary embolism and 16.3% deep venous thrombosis, with 1.5% of patients having both pulmonary embolism and deep venous thrombosis. However, the incidence of VTE was 30% (36/119) and 27% (13/48) in patients who received no or prophylactic anticoagulation, respectively, but only 12% in patients treated with therapeutic anticoagulation (23/188; *P* = 0.0003). Multivariate analysis identified lack of therapeutic anticoagulation (*P* = 0.017) and history of VTE (*P* = 0.011) as independent predictors of subsequent VTE development. The rate of IGSVT resolution during follow up was 61.2% with therapeutic anticoagulation, but only 40.0% and 41.0% with prophylactic or no anticoagulation, respectively (*P* = 0.003).

Conclusions.—IGSVT is associated with a clinically significant rate of VTE which is dramatically reduced with therapeutic anticoagulation. These data warrant further investigation, taking into account the risks and benefits of anticoagulation (Fig 4B, C).

▶ Recent studies have demonstrated the significance of calf vein thrombosis but only a few have focused on optimal management of isolated gastrocnemius

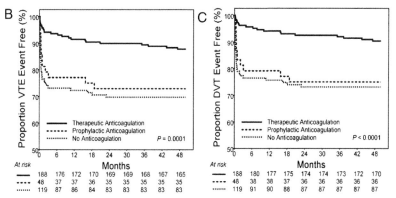

FIGURE 4.—Kaplan-Meier analysis of patients with isolated gastrocnemius and soleal vein thrombosis (IGSVT). Kaplan-Meier curves show (B) the proportion of patients that remain event-free for all VTE events (*P* = 0.0001), (C) DVT (*P* < 0.0001). (Reprinted from Lautz TB, Abbas F, Walsh SJN, et al. Isolated gastrocnemius and soleal vein thrombosis: should these patients receive therapeutic anticoagulation? *Ann Surg.* 2009;251:735-742.)

and soleal vein thrombi (IGSVT). The incidence and prevalence of IGSVT appear to be significant, with IGSVT accounting for 15% to 25% of patients with lower extremity thrombus on venous duplex examinations.[1] There are very few studies quantifying the natural history of IGSVT and the effects of anticoagulation or no anticoagulation on IGSVT propagation or resolution. A combination of the overall awareness of the problem of venous thrombo-embolism, high-resolution modern duplex scanners, and highly skilled vascular technologists has, however, led to increased recognition of the prevalence and incidence of IGSVT. Accumulating data suggest that IGSVT may not be benign and that its natural history may be favorably influenced by anticoagulation. However, there is no randomized study of the efficacy of anticoagulation in patients with IGSVT. In retrospective studies such as this, it may be that high-risk patients with anticoagulation may have therapy withheld, and those same risk factors contribute to the apparent adverse natural history of IGSVT. With increasing numbers of IGSVT cases being recognized, a multicenter randomized trial of the efficacy of anticoagulation in patients with IGSVT will be required to guide therapy of this increasingly recognized condition. Until that happens, data such as these (Figs 4B and 4C) should lead to strong consideration of anticoagulation in patients with IGSVT.

G. L. Moneta, MD

Reference

1. Labropoulos N, Webb KM, Kang SS, et al. Patterns and distribution of isolated calf deep vein thrombosis. *J Vasc Surg.* 1999;30:787-791.

Risk of Symptomatic DVT Associated With Peripherally Inserted Central Catheters
Evans RS, Sharp JH, Linford LH, et al (Intermountain Healthcare, Salt Lake City, UT; Med Ctr, Salt Lake City, UT; et al)
Chest 138:803-810, 2010

Background.—Previous studies undertaken to identify risk factors for peripherally inserted central catheter (PICC)-associated DVT have yielded conflicting results. PICC insertion teams and other health-care providers need to understand the risk factors so that they can develop methods to prevent DVT.

Methods.—A 1-year prospective observational study of PICC insertions was conducted at a 456-bed, level I trauma center and tertiary referral hospital affiliated with a medical school. All patients with one or more PICC insertions were included to identify the incidence and risk factors for symptomatic DVT associated with catheters inserted by a facility-certified PICC team using a consistent and replicated approach for vein selection and insertion.

Results.—A total of 2,014 PICCs were inserted during 1,879 distinct hospitalizations in 1,728 distinct patients for a total of 15,115 days of

PICC placement. Most PICCs were placed in the right arm (76.9%) and basilic vein (74%) and were double-lumen 5F (75.3%). Of the 2,014 PICC insertions, 60 (3.0%) in 57 distinct patients developed DVT in the cannulated or adjacent veins. The best-performing predictive model for DVT (area under the curve, 0.83) was prior DVT (odds ratio [OR], 9.92; *P* < .001), use of double-lumen 5F (OR, 7.54; *P* < .05) or triple-lumen 6F (OR, 19.50; *P* < .01) PICCs, and prior surgery duration of >1 h (OR, 1.66; *P* = .10).

Conclusions.—Prior DVT and surgery lasting >1 h identify patients at increased risk for PICC-associated DVT. More importantly, increasing catheter size also is significantly associated with increased risk. Rates of PICC-associated DVT may be reduced by improved selection of patients and catheter size.

▶ Peripherally inserted central catheters (PICCs) are cost-effective and relatively safe for providing long-term intravenous access for extended total parenteral nutrition, antibiotic therapy, and chemotherapy. PICC lines, however, are also associated with the development of catheter-associated deep venous thrombosis (DVT). The authors sought to identify risk factors for PICC-associated DVT. Assessment for DVT in the patients in this study, however, occurred only in symptomatic patients. Therefore, the actual true incidence of PICC-associated DVT is likely to be much higher than that documented. It is doubtful the clinical correlates associated with PICC-induced DVT (prior DVT and surgery lasting > 1 hour) will have much impact on the selection of patients for PICC placement. Physicians may, however, choose to treat patients with these identified correlates with enhanced prophylaxis following PICC placement. The data would also suggest it is important to minimize the size of the catheter to reduce the development of symptomatic PICC-associated DVT.

G. L. Moneta, MD

Standard Prophylactic Enoxaparin Dosing Leads to Inadequate Anti-Xa Levels and Increased Deep Venous Thrombosis Rates in Critically Ill Trauma and Surgical Patients
Malinoski D, Jafari F, Ewing T, et al (Univ of California, Orange)
J Trauma 68:874-880, 2010

Background.—Deep venous thromboses (DVT) continue to cause significant morbidity in critically ill patients. Standard prophylaxis for high risk patients includes twice-daily dosing with 30 mg enoxaparin. Despite prophylaxis, DVT rates still exceed 10% to 15%. Anti-Xa levels are used to measure the activity of enoxaparin and 12-hour trough levels ≤0.1 IU/mL have been associated with higher rates of DVT in orthopedic patients. We hypothesized that low Anti-Xa levels would be found in critically ill trauma and surgical patients and that low levels would be associated with higher rates of DVT.

Methods.—All patients on the surgical intensive care unit (ICU) service were prospectively followed. In the absence of contraindications, patients were given prophylactic enoxaparin and anti-Xa levels were drawn after the third dose. Trough levels ≤0.1 IU/mL were considered low. Screening duplex exams were obtained within 48 hours of admission and then weekly. Patients were excluded if they did not receive a duplex, if they had a prior DVT, or if they lacked correctly timed anti-Xa levels. DVT rates and demographic data were compared between patients with low and normal anti-Xa levels.

Results.—Data were complete for 54 patients. Eighty-five percent suffered trauma (Injury Severity Score of 25 ± 12) and 74% were male. Overall, 27 patients (50%) had low anti-Xa levels. Patients with low anti-Xa levels had significantly more DVTs than those with normal levels (37% vs. 11%, $p = 0.026$), despite similar age, body mass index, Injury Severity Score, creatinine clearance, high risk injuries, and ICU/ventilator days.

Conclusion.—Standard dosing of enoxaparin leads to low anti-Xa levels in half of surgical ICU patients. Low levels are associated with a significant increase in the risk of DVT. These data support future studies using adjusted-dose enoxaparin.

▶ In prospectively screened intensive care unit patients and up to 70% of severely injured trauma patients, deep venous thrombosis (DVT) rates of those who are untreated range from 13% to 31%. Prophylactic low-molecular-weight heparin (LMWH) is superior to low-dose heparin in preventing venous thromboembolic (VTE) complications when the injury severity score is > 9. Other studies, however, have failed to confirm that LMWH is superior to low-dose heparin or that chemical prophylaxis is more effective than mechanical prophylaxis alone. Standard prophylaxis in higher-risk trauma or surgical patients includes twice daily dosing with 30 mg of enoxaparin but can still result in DVT rates of 10% to 15%. Some patients experience altered pharmacokinetics and pharmacodynamics of LMWH reflected in low trough anti-Xa levels with standard prophylactic dosing of LMWH. The authors hypothesized that low anti-Xa levels would be found in critically ill, trauma, and surgical patients treated with standard prophylactic doses of LMWH and that such patients would have higher rates of DVT. Their hypothesis may be correct in that the data provide at least a partial explanation for the continued high rates of VTE complications in the injured patient despite protocols of chemical and mechanical VTE prophylaxis. It remains to be seen whether prophylactic dosing of LMWH stratified for anti-Xa levels would be both effective and cost-effective in reducing VTE complications in the injured patient or critically ill surgical patient.

G. L. Moneta, MD

Prognostic Significance of Deep Vein Thrombosis in Patients Presenting with Acute Symptomatic Pulmonary Embolism

Jiménez D, the RIETE Investigators (Ramón y Cajal Hosp, Madrid, Spain; et al)
Am J Respir Crit Care Med 181:983-991, 2010

Rationale.—Concomitant deep vein thrombosis (DVT) in patients with acute pulmonary embolism (PE) has an uncertain prognostic significance.

Objectives.—In a cohort of patients with PE, this study compared the risk of death in those with and those without concomitant DVT.

Methods.—We conducted a prospective cohort study of outpatients diagnosed with a first episode of acute symptomatic PE. Patients underwent bilateral lower extremity venous compression ultrasonography to assess for concomitant DVT.

Measurements and Main Results.—The primary study outcome, all-cause mortality, and the secondary outcome of PE-specific mortality were assessed during the 3 months of follow-up after PE diagnosis. Multivariate Cox proportional hazards regression was done to adjust for significant covariates. Of 707 patients diagnosed with PE, 51.2%(362 of 707) had concomitant DVT and 10.9% (77 of 707) died during follow-up. Patients with concomitant DVT had an increased all-cause mortality (adjusted hazard ratio [HR], 2.05; 95% confidence interval [CI], 1.24 to 3.38; $P = 0.005$) and PE-specific mortality (adjusted HR, 4.25; 95% CI, 1.61 to 11.25; $P = 0.04$) compared with those without concomitant DVT. In an external validation cohort of 4,476 patients with acute PE enrolled in the international multicenter RIETE Registry, concomitant DVT remained a significant predictor of all-cause (adjusted HR, 1.66; 95% CI, 1.28 to 2.15; $P < 0.001$) and PE-specific mortality (adjusted HR, 2.01; 95%CI, 1.18 to 3.44; $P = 0.01$).

Conclusions.—In patients with a first episode of acute symptomatic PE, the presence of concomitant DVT is an independent predictor of death in the ensuing 3 months after diagnosis. Assessment of the thrombotic burden should assist with risk stratification of patients with acute PE.

▶ Mortality rates during the first 3 months of treatment following an objectively confirmed diagnosis of acute pulmonary embolism (PE) vary from 1.4% to 17.4%. Variability in mortality likely illustrates differences in the clinical spectrum of patients with PE. In patients with PE, early deaths are secondary to PE-associated complications, whereas underlying medical problems cause most late deaths.[1] Up to 61% of patients with acute PE have concomitant deep vein thrombosis (DVT).[2] The prognostic significance of finding both DVT and PE at the time of presentation of PE is debated. Some studies note that a diagnosis of proximal DVT is an independent predictor of adverse outcome, including death or recurrent PE. Other studies have not confirmed these findings.[3,4] The data provide the strongest evidence to date that a first episode of acute symptomatic PE with a concurrent diagnosis of DVT imparts increased risk of subsequent DVT and PE (Fig 3 in the original article) and all-cause and PE-specific mortality in the first 3 months following diagnosis of PE (Fig 2 in the original article). Although it may be argued that a patient with a diagnosed PE does not need investigation for lower-extremity DVT in that the PE is going to be treated with heparin anyway, the current data suggest that patients with PE should undergo lower-extremity venous ultrasound for prognostic purposes and risk stratification. This may identify patients at high risk of early death who may benefit from more intensive surveillance or aggressive therapy. Alternatively, patients without concurrent DVT and diagnosed with PE may be considered for partial or complete outpatient treatment of the PE.

G. L. Moneta, MD

References

1. Conget F, Otero R, Jiménez D, et al. Short-term clinical outcome after acute symptomatic pulmonary embolism. *Thromb Haemost.* 2008;100:937-942.
2. Bradley MJ, Alexander L. The role of venous colour flow Doppler to aid the non-diagnostic lung scintigram for pulmonary embolism. *Clin Radiol.* 1995;50: 232-234.
3. Wicki J, Perrier A, Perneger TV, Bounameaux H, Junod AF. Predicting adverse outcome in patients with acute pulmonary embolism: a risk score. *Thromb Haemost.* 2000;84:548-552.
4. Girard P, Sanchez O, Leroyer C, et al. Deep venous thrombosis in patients with acute pulmonary embolism: prevalence, risk factors, and clinical significance. *Chest.* 2005;128:1593-1600.

Comparison of the clinical history of symptomatic isolated muscular calf vein thrombosis versus deep calf vein thrombosis
Galanaud J-P, the OPTIMEV SFMV investigators (Montpellier Univ Hosp, France; et al)
J Vasc Surg 52:932-938, 2010

Background.—Half of all lower limb deep vein thromboses (DVT) are distal DVT that are equally distributed between muscular calf vein thromboses (MCVT) and deep calf vein thromboses (DCVT). Despite their high prevalence, MCVT and DCVT have never been compared so far, which prevents possible modulation of distal DVT management according to the kind of distal DVT (MCVT or DCVT).

Methods.—Using data from the French, multicenter, prospective observational OPTimisation de l'Interrogatoire dans l'évaluation du risque throMbo-Embolique Veineux (OPTIMEV) study, we compared the clinical presentation and risk factors of 268 symptomatic isolated DCVT and 457 symptomatic isolated MCVT and the 3-month outcomes of the 222 DCVT and 390 MCVT that were followed-up.

Results.—During the entire follow-up, 86.5% of DCVT patients and 76.7% of MCVT patients were treated with anticoagulant drugs ($P = .003$). MCVT was significantly more associated with localized pain than DCVT (30.4% vs 22.4%, $P = .02$) and less associated with swelling (47.9% vs 62.7%, $P < .001$). MCVT and DCVT patients exhibited the same risk factors profile, except that recent surgery was slightly more associated with DCVT (odds ratio, 1.70%; confidence interval, 1.06-2.75), and had equivalent comorbidities as evaluated by the Charlson index. At 3 months, no statistically significant difference was noted between MCVT and DCVT in death (3.8% vs 4.1%), venous thromboembolism recurrence (1.5% vs 1.4%), and major bleeding (0% vs 0.5%).

Conclusion.—Isolated symptomatic MCVT and DCVT exhibit different clinical symptoms at presentation but affect the same patient population. Under anticoagulant treatment and in the short-term, isolated distal DVT constitutes a homogeneous entity. Therapeutic trials are needed to determine a consensual mode of care of MCVT and DCVT.

▶ Using data from the prospective, multicenter, observational OPTimisation de l'Interrogatoire dans l'évaluation du risque throMbo-Embolique Veineux (OPTIMEV) study,[1] this subset analysis shows that isolated muscular and distal calf vein thrombosis might have different clinical symptoms on presentation but have the same patient risk profile and same early outcomes (recurrent venous thromboembolism, major bleeding, or death) at 3 months, suggesting that both forms of isolated distal calf vein thrombosis may represent a homogenous entity. While most patients in this study received anticoagulation, some did not, and limitations include the usual post hoc analysis study design flaws. While risk profiles and outcomes for both muscular and distal calf vein thrombosis may have been equivalent, with most patients receiving anticoagulation, any additional conclusions are skewed. The more important question remains unanswered about whether patients with isolated distal calf vein thrombosis either in the muscular or deep vein levels need to be anticoagulated at all compared with more proximal deep vein thrombosis, or whether there is a difference between these entities when anticoagulation is not used.

M. A. Passman, MD

Reference

1. Galanaud JP, Sevestre-Pietri MA, Bosson JL, et al. Comparative study on risk factors and early outcome of symptomatic distal versus proximal deep vein thrombosis: results from the OPTIMEV study. *Thromb Haemost.* 2009;102:493-500.

Cost-effectiveness of guidelines for insertion of inferior vena cava filters in high-risk trauma patients
Spangler EL, Dillavou ED, Smith KJ (Univ of Pittsburgh School of Medicine, PA; Univ of Pittsburgh Med Ctr, PA)
J Vasc Surg 52:1537-1545, 2010

Background.—Inferior vena cava filters (IVCFs) can prevent pulmonary embolism (PE); however, indications for use vary. The Eastern Association for the Surgery of Trauma (EAST) 2002 guidelines suggest prophylactic IVCF use in high-risk patients, but the American College of Chest Physicians

(ACCP) 2008 guidelines do not. This analysis compares cost-effectiveness of prophylactic vs therapeutic retrievable IVCF placement in high-risk trauma patients.

Methods.—Markov modeling was used to determine incremental cost-effectiveness of these guidelines in dollars per quality-adjusted life-years (QALYs) during hospitalization and long-term follow-up. Our population was 46-year-old trauma patients at high risk for venous thromboembolism (VTE) by EAST criteria to whom either the EAST (prophylactic IVCF) or ACCP (no prophylactic IVCF) guidelines were applied. The analysis assumed the societal perspective over a lifetime. For base case and sensitivity analyses, probabilities and utilities were obtained from published literature and costs calculated from Centers for Medicare & Medicaid Services fee schedules, the Healthcare Cost &Utilization Project database, and *Red Book* wholesale drug prices for 2007. For data unavailable from the literature, similarities to other populations were used to make assumptions.

Results.—In base case analysis, prophylactic IVCFs were more costly ($37,700 vs $37,300) and less effective (by 0.139 QALYs) than therapeutic IVCFs. In sensitivity analysis, the EAST strategy of prophylactic filter placement would become the preferred strategy in individuals never having a filter, with either an annual probability of VTE of ≥9.6% (base case, 5.9%), or a very high annual probability of anticoagulation complications of ≥24.3% (base case, 2.5%). The EAST strategy would also be favored if the annual probability of venous insufficiency was <7.69% (base case, 13.9%) after filter removal or <1.90% with a retained filter (base case, 14.1%). In initial hospitalization only, EAST guidelines were more costly by $2988 and slightly more effective by .0008 QALY, resulting in an incremental cost-effectiveness ratio of $383,638/QALY.

Conclusions.—Analysis suggests prophylactic IVC filters are not cost-effective in high-risk trauma patients. The magnitude of this result is primarily dependent on probabilities of long-term sequelae (venous thromboembolism, bleeding complications). Even in the initial hospitalization, however, prophylactic IVCF costs for the additional quality-adjusted life years gained did not justify use.

▶ With growing concern over increased use of inferior vena cava filters, especially for venous thromboembolism prophylaxis in trauma patients, this study uses Markov modeling to compare hypothetical pathways based on prophylactic placement in high-risk trauma patients as recommended by the Eastern Association for the Surgery of Trauma 2002 guidelines and against placement as per the American College of Chest Physicians 2008 guidelines. Based on probability assignments of long-term sequelae, with adjustment made for possible filter retrieval, the analysis here suggests that filters are not cost effective for prophylactic use in high-risk trauma patients. Unfortunately, this study is limited by the several layers of assumptions used, so at best this conclusion should be tempered by the Markov study design and subsequent analysis. In reality, there are too many interdependent variables based on weak clinical evidence to draw any solid direction. Real-world data are still desperately needed to support the wide scope of filter use in current clinical practice. Until then, filter usage should be limited and, if used as a bridge for prophylaxis, should be proactively removed as soon as possible once risk of thromboembolism has subsided or until pharmacologic thromboprophylaxis can be initiated.

M. A. Passman, MD

18 Chronic Venous and Lymphatic Disease

Randomized clinical trial of different bandage regimens after foam sclerotherapy for varicose veins
O'Hare JL, Stephens J, Parkin D, et al (Gloucestershire Royal Hosp, Gloucester, UK)
Br J Surg 97:650-656, 2010

Background.—This trial compared outcomes after foam sclerotherapy in patients wearing compression bandaging for 24 h or 5 days after treatment.

Methods.—Consecutive patients with primary uncomplicated varicose veins were randomized after foam sclerotherapy treatment. The primary endpoint was 6-week Aberdeen Varicose Vein Severity Score (AVVSS) and Burford pain score.

Results.—Some 124 legs were randomized, 61 to 24 h and 63 to 5 days of bandaging. Target vein occlusion rates at 6-week duplex imaging were 90 and 89 per cent respectively ($P = 0·842$). There was no significant difference in phlebitis after 2 weeks ($P = 0·445$) or skin discoloration after 6 weeks (46 *versus* 40 per cent; $P = 0·546$). There was no significant difference in the change in AVVSS from baseline to 2 weeks ($-0·29$ *versus* $-0·80$; $P = 0·717$) or to 6 weeks ($-5·89$ *versus* $-5·14$; 95 per cent confidence interval (c.i.) for the difference $-3·29$ to $1·80$; $P = 0·563$), or in change in Burford pain score from baseline to 2 weeks ($-9·04$ *versus* $-2·80$; $P = 0·248$) or to 6 weeks ($-17·32$ *versus* $-8·46$; 95 per cent c.i. for the difference $-19·06$ to $1·33$; $P = 0·088$), or in change in Short Form 36 score from baseline to 6 weeks ($2·02$ *versus* $1·74$; $P = 0·903$).

Conclusion.—There was no advantage to compression bandaging for more than 24 h when thromboembolus deterrent stockings were worn for the remainder of 14 days. Registration number: NCT00991497 (http://www.clinicaltrials.gov).

► In Great Britain, 80% of the members of the Vascular Society of Great Britain and Ireland who responded to a questionnaire and who also treated patients with sclerotherapy indicated that they used compression bandages, and 90% subsequently used compression stockings following compression bandaging. Duration of treatment ranged from 1 to 7 days for initial bandages with compression stockings used for 7 to 14 days, with some surgeons recommending compression stockings for up to 3 months. The authors sought to determine whether duration of bandaging could be reduced following foam sclerotherapy for truncal varices. Foam sclerotherapy is, in fact, replacing liquid sclerotherapy as the preferred method of sclerotherapy for patients with truncal varicosities. Compression following treatment is essential to optimal results. However, as the authors point out with respect to foam sclerotherapy, the optimal duration of compression following treatment has not been adequately studied. This study is good news for patients. Compression bandages are not comfortable, and the results indicate that 24 hours of compressive bandaging followed by a thromboembolus deterrent (TED) stocking for a total of 2 weeks is just as efficacious as 5 days of compressive bandaging followed by a TED stocking for a total of 2 weeks. The study provides practical guidance for posttherapy bandaging of patients undergoing foam sclerotherapy.

G. L. Moneta, MD

Randomized clinical trial of VNUS® ClosureFAST™ radiofrequency ablation *versus* laser for varicose veins
Shepherd AC, Gohel MS, Brown LC, et al (Charing Cross Hosp, London, UK)
Br J Surg 97:810-818, 2010

Background.—Endovenous laser ablation (EVLA) and radiofrequency ablation (RFA) are both associated with excellent technical, clinical and patient-reported outcomes for the treatment of varicose veins. The aim of this study was to compare the techniques in a randomized clinical trial.

Methods.—Consecutive patients with primary great saphenous vein reflux were randomized to EVLA (980 nm) or RFA (VNUS® Closure-FAST™) at a single centre. The primary outcome measure was post-procedural pain after 3 days. Secondary outcome measures were quality of life at 6 weeks, determined by the Aberdeen Varicose Vein Questionnaire (AVVQ) and Short Form 12 (SF-12®), and clinical improvement assessed by the Venous Clinical Severity Score (VCSS). Analyses were performed on the basis of intention to treat using multivariable linear regression.

Results.—Some 131 patients were randomized to EVLA (64 patients) or RFA (67). Mean(s.d.) pain scores over 3 days were $26 \cdot 4(22 \cdot 1)$ mm for RFA and $36 \cdot 8(22 \cdot 5)$ mm for EVLA ($P = 0 \cdot 010$). Over 10 days, mean(s.d.) pain scores were $22 \cdot 0(19 \cdot 8)$ mm *versus* $34 \cdot 3(21 \cdot 1)$ mm for RFA and EVLA respectively ($P = 0 \cdot 001$). The mean(s.d.) number of analgesic tablets used was lower for RFA than for EVLA over 3 days ($8 \cdot 8(9 \cdot 5)$ *versus* $14 \cdot 2(10 \cdot 7)$; $P = 0 \cdot 003$) and 10 days ($20 \cdot 4(22 \cdot 6)$ *versus* $35 \cdot 9(29 \cdot 4)$ respectively; $P = 0 \cdot 001$). Changes in AVVQ, SF-12® and VCSS scores at 6 weeks were similar in the two groups: AVVQ ($P = 0 \cdot 887$), VCSS ($P = 0 \cdot 993$), SF-12® physical component score ($P = 0 \cdot 276$) and mental component score ($P = 0 \cdot 449$).

Conclusion.—RFA using VNUS® ClosureFAST™ was associated with less postprocedural pain than EVLA. However, clinical and quality-of-life improvements were similar after 6 weeks for the two treatments. Registration number: ISRCTN66818013 (http://www.controlled-trials.com).

▶ Endovenous ablative procedures have largely replaced standard saphenous stripping for treatment of saphenous reflux in patients with primary varicose veins. Advantages include fewer complications, decreased postprocedural pain, faster recovery, and faster return to work. An additional theoretical advantage of endovenous procedures is reduced neovascularization in the groin, potentially leading to lower recurrence rates and late follow-up.[1] At the time of publication of this article, only 1 small randomized trial has compared VNUS ClosureFAST and endovenous laser ablation (EVLA).[2] This study compares the most-used technique for EVLA in Great Britain (980-nm wavelength and bare fiber) versus the most popular radiofrequency ablation (RFA) system, VNUS ClosureFAST in Great Britain.

The study demonstrated that VNUS ClosureFAST results in significantly less pain than 980-nm EVLA for ablation of the greater saphenous veins in treatment of patients with varicose veins (Fig 3 in the original article). The study supports previous publications that demonstrate less postprocedural pain after RFA but failed to show differences in outcomes after 1 month.[3] It is important to note that patients in this study were treated under general anesthesia, so the adequacy of tumescence used during the procedure was not possible to assess. However, EVLA is continuing to be refined. There are newer fibers with longer wavelengths and jacketed laser fibers that appear to be associated with lower postintervention pain scores.[4] Data comparing these new devices to the VNUS closure system will be required.

G. L. Moneta, MD

References

1. Theivacumar NS, Darwood R, Gough MJ. Neovascularisation and recurrence 2 years after varicose vein treatment for sapheno-femoral and great saphenous vein reflux: a comparison of surgery and endovenous laser ablation. *Eur J Vasc Endovasc Surg.* 2009;38:203-207.
2. Almeida JI, Kaufman J, Göckeritz O, et al. Radiofrequency endovenous Closure-FAST versus laser ablation for the treatment of great saphenous reflux: a multicenter, single-blinded, randomized study (RECOVERY study). *J Vasc Interv Radiol.* 2009; 20:752-759.
3. Morrisson N. Saphenous ablation: what are the choices, laser or RF energy. *Semin Vasc Surg.* 2005;18:15-18.
4. Almeida J, Mackay E, Javier J, Mauriello J, Raines J. Saphenous laser ablation at 1470 nm targets the vein wall, not blood. *Vasc Endovascular Surg.* 2009;43: 467-472.

Desmuslin gene knockdown causes altered expression of phenotype markers and differentiation of saphenous vein smooth muscle cells

Xiao Y, Huang Z, Yin H, et al (First Affiliated Hosp of Sun Yat-sen Univ, Guangzhou, People's Republic of China; Memorial Hosp of Sun Yat-sen Univ, Guangzhou, People's Republic of China)
J Vasc Surg 52:684-690, 2010

Objective.—Phenotypic alterations of vascular smooth muscle cells (VSMCs) appear critical to the development of primary varicose veins. Previous study indicated desmuslin, an intermediate filament protein, was differentially expressed in smooth muscle cells (SMCs) isolated from varicose veins; thus, it was naturally hypothesized that altered desmuslin expression might in turn affect the functioning of VSMCs, leading to the phenotypic alterations and varicose vein development.

Methods.—In this study, expression of desmuslin in normal human saphenous vein SMCs was knocked down using small interfering RNA (siRNA), and control cells were treated with a scrambled siRNA sequence. The levels of several phenotypic markers including smooth muscle (SM) α-actin and smooth muscle myosin heavy chain (SM-MHC) were assessed. Collagen formation, matrix metalloproteinase expression (MMP-2), and cytoskeletal and morphological changes were also examined.

Results.—SMCs treated with desmuslin siRNA exhibited significantly increased levels of collagen synthesis and MMP-2 expression and decreased expression levels of SM α-actin, SM-MHC, and smoothelin and exhibited disassembly of actin stress fibers when compared with the control cells. Changes in cell morphology and actin fiber networks in VSMCs treated with desmuslin siRNA were consistent with a lower degree of differentiation.

Conclusions.—These results indicated desmuslin expression is required for the maintenance of VSMC phenotype. Decreased desmuslin expression may affect differentiation of VSMCs and ultimately contribute to the development of varicose veins.

▶ The pathophysiology of varicose vein formation, a disease which affects millions of individuals, is not known. In this elegant study, the authors studied the effects on smooth muscle (SM) cell differentiation and function by silencing an important regulatory protein called desmuslin. Desmuslin is a type VI intermediate fiber (IF) protein and a component of the extensive cytoskeletal network. IF cytoskeleton is a dynamic signaling platform involved in cell growth, differentiation, and other fundamental biological activities. The same authors demonstrated that desmuslin was significantly downregulated in SM cells isolated from varicose veins. In this study, the authors postulated that inhibition of desmuslin expression in human saphenous vein SM cells may deleteriously affect the functioning of venous wall causing phenotypic alterations that may contribute to the development of varicose veins. By using small interfering RNA on desmuslin gene knockdown, the study found that SM cells decreased the expression of SM-actin, SM—myosin heavy chain, and smoothelin and exhibited disassembly of actin stress fibers when compared with the control cells. In addition there was increased expression of collagen and MMP-2. The importance of the study's findings is that desmuslin is indeed required for proper SM cell phenotype and function, at least in vitro, and dysregulation of desmuslin in SM cells may lead to alterations in the vein wall and eventual varicose vein formation. However, the study was an in vitro analysis of SM cells, and future research will need to assess, especially in animal models, how the inhibition of desmuslin affects intact vein tissue function.

J. D. Raffetto, MD

Ultrasound-guided foam sclerotherapy is a safe and clinically effective treatment for superficial venous reflux
Bradbury AW, Bate G, Pang K, et al (Birmingham Univ, UK)
J Vasc Surg 52:939-945, 2010

Objective.—To test the hypothesis that ultrasound-guided foam sclerotherapy (UGFS) is a safe and durable treatment for superficial venous reflux (SVR) associated with CEAP clinical grade 2-6 disease.

Methods.—This was an interrogation of a prospectively gathered computerized database.

Results.—Between March 23, 2004 and December 31, 2009, 977 patients (1252 legs) underwent UGFS for unilateral (702 legs) or bilateral (550 legs) SVR in association with CEAP clinical grade 2-3 (n = 868), 4 (n = 232), or 5/6 (n = 152) disease. The following reflux in 1417 venous segments was treated: primary great saphenous vein (GSV) (n = 745); recurrent GSV (n = 286), primary small saphenous vein (SSV) (n = 189), recurrent SSV (n = 50); primary anterior accessory saphenous vein (AASV) (n = 93); recurrent AASV (n = 46); vein of the popliteal fossa (VOPF) (n = 5), and Giacomini vein (GV) (n = 3). Three hundred forty-eight legs (27.8%) had undergone previous surgery. Three patients suffered post-UGFS deep vein thrombosis (DVT) and one a pulmonary embolus (PE), all within the first month (0.4% venous thrombo-embolic complication rate). Five patients (0.5%) had transient visual disturbance at the time of, or shortly after, treatment. No other neurologic or serious complications were reported. During a mean (range) follow-up of 28 (<1 to 68) months, 161 (12.9%) legs underwent a further session of UGFS for truncal VV at a mean (range) of 17 (<1 to 63) months following the first treatment. In 52 legs, retreatment was due to the development of new SVR and in 109 legs was for true recurrence (8.7% complete or partial recanalization rate leading to treatment). There was no significant difference in retreatment rates between UGFS for GSV and SSV reflux or between UGFS for primary or recurrent disease.

Conclusion.—UGFS for CEAP 2-6 SVR is associated with a low complication and retreatment rate. However, as patients are at risk of developing

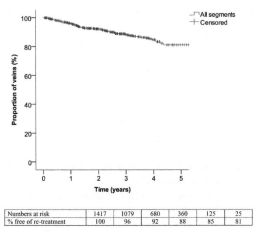

| Numbers at risk | 1417 | 1079 | 680 | 360 | 125 | 25 |
| % free of re-treatment | 100 | 96 | 92 | 88 | 85 | 81 |

FIGURE 2.—Kaplan-Meier plot showing freedom for any reintervention of all 1417 treated venous segments. (Reprinted from Bradbury AW, Bate G, Pang K, et al. Ultrasound-guided foam sclerotherapy is a safe and clinically effective treatment for superficial venous reflux. *J Vasc Surg.* 2010;52:939-945. Copyright 2010, with permission from The Society for Vascular Surgery.)

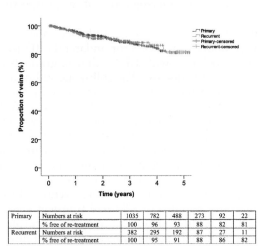

Primary	Numbers at risk	1035	782	488	273	92	22
	% free of re-treatment	100	96	93	88	82	81
Recurrent	Numbers at risk	382	295	192	87	27	11
	% free of re-treatment	100	95	91	88	86	82

FIGURE 4.—Kaplan-Meier plot comparing freedom from any reintervention in patients undergoing ultrasound-guided foam sclerotherapy (UGFS) for primary (n = 1035) and recurrent disease (n = 382) (P =.884 log-rank test; 95% CI 4.97-5.27). (Reprinted from Bradbury AW, Bate G, Pang K, et al. Ultrasound-guided foam sclerotherapy is a safe and clinically effective treatment for superficial venous reflux. *J Vasc Surg.* 2010;52:939-945. Copyright 2010, with permission from The Society for Vascular Surgery.)

recurrent and new SVR they should be kept under review. Further UGFS for new or recurrent disease is simple, safe, and effective (Figs 2 and 4).

▶ The treatment for superficial venous reflux has largely been supplanted by endovenous treatments. Patients with symptomatic superficial venous reflux can easily be treated with endovenous ablations on an ambulatory basis with excellent clinical outcomes and early return to activity and work. Although widely used in Europe and Latin America, foam sclerotherapy for superficial venous insufficiency is not widely used as the primary treatment modality in the United States. Interestingly, in the United States, although not Food and Drug Administration approved, foam sclerotherapy is used to treat recurrences in recanalized venous segments that have failed other endovenous treatment ablations of the superficial axial venous system as well as trunk varices. Major concerns relate to possible microfoam bubble air emboli through patent foramen ovale and with possible neurologic sequelae. This study is a large non-randomized prospective series from a single center evaluating 977 patients in 1252 legs treating primary and recurrent superficial venous insufficiency by ultrasound-guided foam sclerotherapy (UGFS). In the entire cohort, 0.4% suffered a venous thromboembolism, all occurring within the first month of treatment and none fatal; 0.5% of patients reported transient visual disturbances and no other neurologic events occurred; and at a mean of 17 months there were 8.7% recurrences following the first treatment of foam sclerotherapy. Freedom from any reintervention at 5 years for all 1417 treated truncal segments was well above 80% (Fig 2). There was no significant difference in overall (recurrent and new reflux combined) retreatment rates following first UGFS for primary or recurrent disease (Fig 4). From this study, it would appear that UGFS is a good first-line treatment for both primary and recurrent superficial venous disease, with excellent outcomes and low complication rates. Further randomized clinical trials are necessary to evaluate different treatment modalities with longer follow-up and also with quality-of-life and cost analysis.

J. D. Raffetto, MD

19 Technical Notes

Final Results of the Protected Superficial Femoral Artery Trial Using the FilterWire EZ System

Müller-Hülsbeck S, Hümme TH, Schäfer JP, et al (Academic Teaching Hosps Flensburg, Germany; Univ Hosps Schleswig-Holstein—Campus Kiel, Germany; et al)
Cardiovasc Intervent Radiol 33:1120-1127, 2010

The purpose of this study was to evaluate the safety and efficacy of debris-capture for distal protection using the FilterWire EZ Embolic Protection System (Boston Scientific, Mountain View, CA) with the additional aim to further define the incidence of distal embolization during superficial femoral artery (SFA) interventions. A prospective, single-centre registry was designed to evaluate the performance of the FilterWire EZ in capturing debris during standard SFA percutaneous intervention. The PRO-RATA study included 30 patients suitable for PTA (Fontaine IIb to III or Rutherford I to II classification). The primary end points were occurrence of distal embolization or decreased runoff, improvement in ankle—brachial index (ABI) after the procedure, and number of filters containing emboli. Secondary end points included major adverse events (i.e., procedure- or device-related death and/or clinical target lesion revascularisation), device delivery, deployment success, and incidence of embolic recovery (patients with device success exhibiting embolic protection in the filter). Procedural success was determined as ≤30% residual stenosis with no worsening of distal runoff as determined on angiography. A total of 29 patients (age 66.2 ± 12 years; total no. of limbs = 30; total no. of lesions = 30) suitable for PTA were enrolled in the study between February 2007 and March 2008. There were 26 patients with claudication (Fontaine IIB) and 3 patients with stage IV peripheral vascular disease. In one patient, lesions in both legs were treated. No procedural or device-related complications occured. The average degree of stenosis was 86 ± 7%. Stenosis length ranged from 8 to 88 mm. The average degree of residual stenosis was 10 ± 10%. ABI improved from 0.56 ± 0.16 to 0.92 ± 0.19 ($P < 0.05$). No restenosis or dissection was seen at 1-month ultrasound follow-up. Macroscopic debris was found in 27 of 30 filters of all distal protection devices used in all 29 patients. Debris particle size ranged from 90 to 2000 μm (1200 ± 640). Histological debris analysis showed platelets, erythrocytes, inflammatory cells, extracellular matrix, and cholesterol as being the major components of emboli. Additional immunochemistry showed no correlation between lesion morphology and debris components.

313

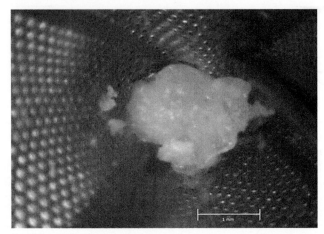

FIGURE 2.—Photograph showing visible debris within the filter tip after PTA of a short-distant SFA stenosis using an EPD (FilterWire EZ) for treatment of claudication. Bar = 1 mm. (With kind permission from Springer Science+Business Media: Müller-Hülsbeck S, Hümme TH, Schäfer JP, et al. Final results of the protected superficial femoral artery trial using the FilterWire EZ system. *Cardiovasc Intervent Radiol.* 2010;33:1120-1127, with permission from Springer Science+Business Media, LLC and the Cardiovascular and Interventional Radiological Society of Europe (CIRSE).)

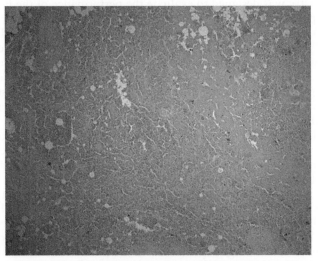

FIGURE 3.—Hematoxylin-and-eosin staining of filter debris showing debris and blood components consisting of platelets, erythrocytes, inflammatory cells, extracellular matrix, and cholesterol. (With kind permission from Springer Science+Business Media: Müller-Hülsbeck S, Hümme TH, Schäfer JP, et al. Final results of the protected superficial femoral artery trial using the FilterWire EZ system. *Cardiovasc Intervent Radiol.* 2010;33:1120-1127, with permission from Springer Science+Business Media, LLC and the Cardiovascular and Interventional Radiological Society of Europe (CIRSE).)

The FilterWire EZ is easy and safe to handle. The system caused no complications. In all cases, macroscopic debris was captured. Using a distal protection device during femoropopliteal interventions has the potential to prevent migration of debris, which may be important for high-risk patients with limited distal runoff (Figs 2 and 3).

▶ This is a small, single-center, nonrandomized, commercially sponsored study with the first author having a consulting arrangement with the study sponsor. The study is obviously good marketing material for the manufacturer of the FilterWire EZ System. However, assuming the author's observations are accurate, the study should bring some measure of concern to all who perform catheter-based superficial femoral artery interventions, as these interventions seem to be nearly uniformly associated with distal embolization. Long-term clinical implications of these distal emboli remain to be defined. But as someone once said, "They may not be bad, but they can't be good." The true clinical utility of embolic protection devices in all vascular beds remains an intriguing and certainly potentially profitable avenue of research.

G. L. Moneta, MD

20 Miscellaneous

Cognitive Functioning, Retirement Status, and Age: Results from the Cognitive Changes and Retirement among Senior Surgeons Study
Drag LL, Bieliauskas LA, Langenecker SA, et al (Univ of Michigan Health System, Ann Arbor)
J Am Coll Surg 211:303-307, 2010

Background.—Accurate assessment of cognitive functioning is an important step in understanding how to better evaluate both clinical and cognitive competence in practicing surgeons. As part of the Cognitive Changes and Retirement among Senior Surgeons study, we examined the objective cognitive functioning of senior surgeons in relation to retirement status and age.

Study Design.—Computerized cognitive tasks measuring visual sustained attention, reaction time, and visual learning and memory were administered to both practicing and retired surgeons at annual meetings of the American College of Surgeons. Data from 168 senior surgeons aged 60 and older were compared with data from 126 younger surgeons aged 45 to 59, with performance below 1.5 standard deviations or more indicating a significant difference between the groups.

Results.—Sixty-one percent of practicing senior surgeons performed within the range of the younger surgeons on all cognitive tasks. Seventy-eight percent of practicing senior surgeons aged 60 to 64 performed within the range of the younger surgeons on all tasks compared with 38% of practicing senior surgeons aged 70 and older. Forty-five percent of retired senior surgeons performed within the range of the younger surgeons on all tasks. No senior surgeon performed below the younger surgeons on all 3 tasks.

Conclusions.—The majority of practicing senior surgeons performed at or near the level of their younger peers on all cognitive tasks, as did almost half of the retired senior surgeons. This suggests that older age does not inevitably preclude cognitive proficiency. The variability in cognitive performance across age groups and retirement status suggests the need for formal measures of objective cognitive functioning to help surgeons detect changes in cognitive performance and aid in their decisions to retire.

▶ Nearly 20% of practicing physicians are older than 65 years. However, more than 20% of adults older than age 70 years have some form of cognitive impairment.[1] Therefore, there is interest in detection of cognitive deficits to reduce the prevalence of aging physicians with cognitive impairment. The authors have previously shown that measures of cognitive skill, including attention, reaction time, visual learning, and memory, decline with age among surgeons but that subjective evaluation of cognitive decline does not reflect objective measures of cognitive status. In this study, as part of the Cognitive Changes in Retirement Among Senior Surgeon Study, the authors examined objective cognitive function of senior surgeons with respect to retirement status and age. The data indicate that most senior surgeons perform at or near the level of younger surgeons in measures of memory, visual learning, reaction time, and attention. This was so even among retired surgeons and among almost 75% senior surgeons planning to retire within 5 years. Perceived cognitive decline is among many factors entering into a decision to retire. The data suggest objective measures of cognitive function may be useful in aiding senior surgeons in their decision to retire. Given the anticipated shortfall of practicing surgeons in the work force, retention of senior surgeons with intact cognitive function may be one of many factors important in providing adequate health care services to the population in the near and intermediate future.

G. L. Moneta, MD

Reference

1. Plassman BL, Langa KM, Fisher GG, et al. Prevalence of cognitive impairment without dementia in the United States. *Ann Intern Med.* 2008;148:427-434.

Venous and Cerebrospinal Fluid Flow in Multiple Sclerosis: A Case-Control Study
Sundström P, Wåhlin A, Ambarki K, et al (Umeå Univ, Sweden)
Ann Neurol 68:255-259, 2010

The prevailing view on multiple sclerosis etiopathogenesis has been challenged by the suggested new entity chronic cerebrospinal venous insufficiency. To test this hypothesis, we studied 21 relapsing-remitting multiple sclerosis cases and 20 healthy controls with phase-contrast magnetic resonance imaging. In addition, in multiple sclerosis cases we performed contrast-enhanced magnetic resonance angiography. We found no differences regarding internal jugular venous outflow, aqueductal cerebrospinal fluid flow, or the presence of internal jugular blood reflux. Three of 21 cases had internal jugular vein stenoses. In conclusion, we found no evidence confirming the suggested vascular multiple sclerosis hypothesis.

▶ The multiple sclerosis (MS) chronic cerebral spinal venous insufficiency hypothesis suggests that MS may develop secondary to impaired venous outflow from the central nervous system. This new hypothesis concerning the etiology of MS has rapidly gained attention among the media, patients with MS, and the scientific community. The implication is that stenosis of the internal jugular and/or azygos veins may be potentially treated by angioplasty and/or stenting and lead to relief of symptoms in patients with MS.

This article is in sharp contrast with the findings of Zamboni et al[1] in that the authors here are unable to demonstrate differences between cerebral spinal venous drainage between the MS cases and controls. While the study did not address azygos vein blood flow, the data here make it seem likely that any association between chronic cerebral spinal venous insufficiency and MS will be weaker than that previously reported. The study certainly does not provide any support for endovascular treatment in patients with MS. The MS community, neurologists, and vascular interventionalists need to develop a rational and deliberate approach to assessment of this new hypothesis. At this point, it seems irresponsible and perhaps unethical for physicians to encourage expensive (and likely uncovered by insurance) endovascular treatment of the highly vulnerable MS population.

G. L. Moneta, MD

Reference

1. Zamboni P, Galeotti R, Menegatti E, et al. A prospective open-label study of endovascular treatment of chronic cerebrospinal venous insufficiency. *J Vasc Surg.* 2009;50:1348-1358.

Anatomical variations of the femoral vein

Uhl J-F, Gillot C, Chahim M (Univ Paris Descartes, Neuilly-sur-Seine, France; Corentin Celton Hosp, Issy les Moulineaux, France)
J Vasc Surg 52:714-719, 2010

Background.—The venous anatomy is highly variable. This is due to possible venous malformations (minor truncular forms) occurring during the late development of the embryo that produce several anatomical variations in the number and caliber of the main venous femoral trunks at the thigh level. Our aim was to study the prevalence of the different anatomical variations of the femoral vein at the thigh level.

Methods.—This study used 336 limbs of 118 fresh, nonembalmed cadavers. The technique included washing of the whole venous system, latex injection, anatomical dissection, and then painting of the veins.

Results.—The modal anatomy of the femoral vein was found in 308 of 336 limbs (88%). Truncular malformations were found in 28 of 336 limbs (12%); unitruncular configurations in 3% (axo femoral trunk [1%] and deep femoral trunk [2%]). Bitruncular configurations were found in 9% (bifidity of the femoral vein [2%], femoral vein with axio-femoral trunk [5%], and femoral vein with deep femoral trunk [2%]).

Conclusion.—Truncular venous malformations of the femoral vein are not rare (12%). Their knowledge is important for the investigation of the venous network, particularly the venous mapping of patients with cardiovascular disease. It is also important to recognize a bitruncular configuration to avoid potential errors for the diagnosis of deep venous thrombosis of the femoral vein, in the case of an occluded duplicated trunk.

▶ In this study, there is an excellent review of the embryogenesis of the venous system of the lower extremity. The importance is that the venous anatomy is defined by the arrangement of the neuronal network, and the vessel arrangement parallels the nerves. This is possible by the secretion of a vascular endothelial growth factor from the axons and Schwann cells that coat the nerves. There are 3 main nerves determining the venous development: (1) the greater sciatic nerve, (2) the femoral nerve (preaxial nerve), and (3) the postaxial nerve. In most cases (modal anatomy), the femoral vein is the main vessel, but it could be replaced by the axial vein or the deep femoral vein, or it could be separated into 2 main trunks. This study examined the prevalence of the venous anatomy in specially prepared cadavers. The modal anatomy was present in 88% of cadavers, and in 12% there were truncular malformations (replaced axial vein, deep femoral vein, or 2 main trunks). Unitruncular venous systems had venous malformations in 3% of specimens examined with axiofemoral trunk (1%) and deep femoral trunk (2%). Bitruncular venous systems occurred in 9% of extremities evaluated. The importance of this study is that vascular practitioners need to be aware of the variable anatomy and venous malformations. They also need to know that duplicated femoral veins systems are not unusual and can occur bilaterally and have an increased risk for venous thrombosis compared with normal femoral vein anatomy. A limitation of this study is that all of the cadavers were Caucasian; therefore, one has to interpret the data carefully since it may not be entirely applicable to practices with diverse population groups.

J. D. Raffetto, MD

Upper extremity ischemia treated with tissue repair cells from adult bone marrow
Comerota AJ, Link A, Douville J, et al (Toledo Hosp, OH; Univ of Witten-Herdecke, Germany)
J Vasc Surg 52:723-729, 2010

Background.—Unreconstructable critical ischemia with gangrene of the upper extremity is rarely due to atherosclerosis alone, and few treatment options exist. We describe a patient with gangrene of both hands as a result of unreconstructable atherosclerotic disease of both upper extremities who was successfully treated with tissue repair cells (TRCs) produced from the patient's bone marrow.

Methods.—A patient with type 1 diabetes was referred with bilateral upper extremity digital gangrene due to unreconstructable forearm and hand atherosclerosis. He was evaluated for therapeutic angiogenesis using TRCs.

Results.—Following the intramuscular injection of TRCs produced from autologous bone marrow stem cells, the patient demonstrated improved arterial perfusion and a durable clinical response with healing of all amputation sites and cessation of pain.

Conclusions.—The production of TRCs results in the expansion of stem and early progenitor cells, including CD90+ mesenchymal cells and endothelial progenitor cells. This is the first reported case of end-stage upper extremity ischemia treated with TRCs harvested from adult bone marrow.

▶ Unreconstructable peripheral arterial occlusive disease can result in significant limb loss. The majority of these patients have exhausted all surgical and endovascular treatments and are at high risk for major limb amputation. Even rarer are patients who present with upper extremity nonreconstructable arterial occlusive disease, as presented in this case report. This report focuses on the use of tissue repair cells harvested from the patient's bone marrow, which are then processed and cultured to yield the CD90 cell subpopulation shown to contain stem and progenitor cells, including CD90 mesenchymal cells and endothelial progenitor cells. The importance is that the CD90 tissue repair cells contain endothelial progenitor cells that have been shown to possess endothelial tube formation capacity in vivo, providing a scaffold for angiogenesis. The mesenchymal cells are the only progenitor cells that can differentiate into vascular smooth muscle cells, which are extremely important during angiogenesis, secreting a myriad of growth factors, tissue signaling factors, and proangiogenic cytokines. Although the treatment with tissue repair progenitor cells appears appealing, and one should not deny the success of this particular case, it should also be noted that this patient also received 14 hyperbaric oxygen treatments to help heal his hand wounds. As stated in the discussion of this very interesting report, randomized controlled studies are underway and are required to fully assess the potentially promising therapy of stem and progenitor tissue repair cells for advanced vascular ischemia of the limbs. Certain questions that need to be defined: (1) Where is the best location for injecting tissue repair cells; is it directly intramuscularly near the ischemic tissue or at distance, or should it be intra-arterially in the limb in question or combined modalities? (2) What objective measures should be used to assess outcomes? Should all patients receive repeat angiography to demonstrate new vessel growth in the ischemic tissue or is laser Doppler and digit plethysmography adequate as a less invasive means? (3) Should alternative modalities of therapy be combined simultaneously with tissue repair cell injections as done in this case, or should one assess purely the effectiveness of the tissue repair cells' potential and have other arms of the study using more conventional therapies? Finally, cost-effectiveness, quality of life, and long-term outcomes should all be assessed.

J. D. Raffetto, MD

Inelastic bandages maintain their hemodynamic effectiveness over time despite significant pressure loss

Mosti G, Partsch H (M.D. Barbantini Hosp, Lucca, Italy; Private Practice, Wien, Austria)
J Vasc Surg 52:925-931, 2010

Background.—It is widely believed that the loss of compression pressure of inelastic bandages is associated with a loss of efficacy in contrast to elastic material, which maintains its pressure and performance. This study compared the effect exerted by inelastic bandages vs elastic compression stockings on the venous pumping function in patients with severe superficial venous insufficiency immediately after application and 1 week later.

Methods.—Ejection fraction (EF) of the calf pump was measured in 18 patients presenting with bilateral reflux in the great saphenous vein (CEAP C_3-C_5) without any compression and immediately after application of an inelastic bandage on one leg and an elastic compression stocking on the other leg. Measurements were repeated 1 week later, before compression removal. EF was measured using a plethysmographic technique. The changes of interface pressure of the applied compression products were recorded simultaneously with EF measurements.

Results.—After application, bandages and stockings achieved a significant improvement of EF ($P < .001$) that was much more pronounced in the bandaged legs. The median resting pressure was 45 mm Hg (interquartile range, 41-48.5 mm Hg) under the stockings and 64.5 mm Hg (interquartile range, 51-80 mm Hg) under the bandages. After 1 week, EF was still significantly improved in the bandaged leg ($P < .001$), but not under the stockings. At this time, the pressure under the stockings was only slightly reduced (5.9% supine, 3.6% standing), but the mean pressure loss under the bandages was much higher (54.3% supine, 35.4% standing).

Conclusion.—The findings supporting inelastic compression are important in explaining the benefits of its use in chronic venous insufficiency. Inelastic bandages maintain their superior efficacy on the venous pumping function after a wearing time of 1 week, despite a significant loss of pressure.

▶ Contrary to the widely held belief that loss of compression pressure of inelastic bandages over time is associated with loss of efficacy, this study shows that inelastic compression bandages actually maintain superior efficacy on venous physiologic parameters when compared with elastic stockings despite greater loss of pressure than elastic stockings at 1 week. Although a validated model for measuring venous pump function is used in this study, there still may be some confounding variables related to the way plethysmographic measurements are made between the compression layer and the leg that may affect this observation. Regardless, this would be a confounding variable for both groups, so the observed superiority of inelastic bandages on venous physiology on the surface is likely real. While there may be different physiologic explanations for this paradoxical effect, this study does reinforce the physiologic role of inelastic bandages, especially for more severe venous disease, reserving elastic compression modalities for less severe or more ambulatory situations once severe clinical venous disease is under better physiologic control.

M. A. Passman, MD

Article Index

Chapter 1: Basic Considerations

Chapter 2: Coronary Disease

Chapter 3: Epidemiology

Chapter 4: Vascular Laboratory and Imaging

Chapter 5: Perioperative Considerations

Chapter 6: Grafts and Graft Complications

Chapter 7: Aortic Aneurysm

Chapter 8: Abdominal Aortic Endografting

Chapter 9: Visceral and Renal Artery Disease

Chapter 10: Thoracic Aorta

Chapter 11: Leg Ischemia

Chapter 12: Leg Ischemia and Aortoiliac Disease

Chapter 13: Upper Extremity and Dialysis Access

Chapter 14: Carotid and Cerebrovascular Disease

Chapter 18: Chronic Venous and Lymphatic Disease

Chapter 19: Technical Notes

Chapter 20: Miscellaneous

Author Index

Printed and bound by CPI Group (UK) Ltd, Croydon, CR0 4YY

08/05/2025

01864678-0008